CIMETIDINE IN THE 80s

CIMETIDINE IN THE 80s

Edited by

J. H. Baron FRCP

Royal Postgraduate Medical School
Hammersmith Hospital, London, UK

CHURCHILL LIVINGSTONE
EDINBURGH LONDON MELBOURNE AND NEW YORK 1981

CHURCHILL LIVINGSTONE
Medical Division of Longman Group Limited

Distributed in the United States of America by Churchill
Livingstone Inc., 19 West 44th Street, New York, N.Y.
10036, and by associated companies, branches and
representatives throughout the world.

© Longman Group Limited 1981

First published 1981

ISBN 0 443 02540 1

Printed in Great Britain at The Pitman Press, Bath

Preface

Cimetidine has been used in clinical practice for exactly five years. During this time it has radically altered the treatment of patients with duodenal ulcer disease and has also contributed to the management of gastric ulcer and oesophageal reflux disease.

The purpose of the Symposium held on 25–26 March 1981 at the Royal College of Physicians, London, entitled 'Cimetidine in the 80s', was to review our current knowledge on the actions and applications of cimetidine and to answer some of the following questions:

How does cimetidine compare with other drugs?

What are the long-term beneficial and adverse effects of cimetidine?

How does the use of cimetidine in the medical treatment of duodenal ulcer compare with surgical treatment?

What is the optimum dose of cimetidine for healing duodenal ulcers?

What role does cimetidine have in the treatment of haemorrhage and pancreatitis and prior to an anaesthetic?

How does research on cimetidine in other physiological systems contribute to its clinical profile?

I am most grateful to the contributors for their excellent talks and for their cooperation in preparing manuscripts for these Proceedings. Thanks are also due to Professor Clark, Dr Bennett, Mr Alexander-Williams, and Professor Breckenridge for chairing various sessions. I would also like to acknowledge the help and support of the staff at Smith Kline & French who have made both the Symposium and the Proceedings possible.

J. H. Baron

Contributors and Chairmen

J. Alexander-Williams MD FRCS
The General Hospital, Birmingham, UK

K. D. Bardhan DPhil(Oxon) MBBS(Madras) FRCP
Rotherham District General Hospital, Rotherham, UK

J. H. Baron FRCP
Royal Postgraduate Medical School, Hammersmith Hospital, London, UK

J. R. Bennett FRCP
Hull Royal Infirmary, Hull, UK

A. Bernstein MBBCh FRCP
Hope Hospital, Salford, UK

G. Bianchi Porro MD
Ospedale L. Sacco, Milan, Italy

G. Bodemar MD
Linkoping University Hospital, Sweden

G. Bommelaer MD
Hôpital Rangueil, Toulouse, France

M. J. Boyce BSc MRCP
Research Institute, Smith Kline & French Laboratories Limited, Welwyn Garden City, UK

A. M. Breckenridge FRCP
University of Liverpool, Liverpool, UK

R. W. Brimblecombe DSc FRCPath
Research Institute, Smith Kline & French Laboratories Limited,
Welwyn Garden City, UK

C. G. Clark FRCS
University College Hospital Medical School, London, UK

D. G. Colin-Jones MD FRCP
Queen Alexandra Hospital, Cosham, UK

R. J. Crossley BMBCh MPhil BSc
Smith Kline Corporation, Philadelphia, Pennsylvania, USA

V. Eckhardt
University of Mainz, Mainz, West Germany

M. W. L. Gear DM MCh FRCS
Gloucestershire Royal Hospital, Gloucester, UK

R. Gugler
University of Bonn, Bonn, West Germany

R. C. Heading MD FRCP(Ed)
Royal Infirmary, Edinburgh, UK

R. H. Hunt MB MRCP
The Royal Naval Hospital, Gosport, UK

G. D. Kerr FRCP FRACP
Royal Shrewsbury Hospital, Shrewsbury, UK

M. J. S. Langman MD FRCP
City Hospital, Nottingham, UK

R. J. Machell MA MB MRCP
The West Cornwall Hospital, Penzance, UK

J. J. Misiewicz MB BSc FRCP
Central Middlesex Hospital, London, UK

J. Moore MD PhD FFARCS
The Queen's University of Belfast, Belfast, Northern Ireland

T. C. Northfield FRCP
St George's Hospital, London, UK

R. E. Pounder MA MD MRCP
Royal Free Hospital, London, UK

H. G. Rohner
St Barbara-Hospital, Gladbeck, West Germany

D. Rowley-Jones MRCP
*Medical Department, Smith Kline & French Laboratories Limited,
Welwyn Garden City, UK*

V. Speranza MD FACS
University of Rome, Rome, Italy

J. G. Stage MD
Rigshospitalet and Herlev University Hospital, Copenhagen, Denmark

G. N. J. Tytgat
University of Amsterdam, Amsterdam, The Netherlands

C. W. Venables MS FRCS
Newcastle General Hospital, Newcastle upon Tyne, UK

M. R. Vickers PhD
*Research Institute, Smith Kline & French Laboratories Limited,
Welwyn Garden City, UK*

K. G. Wormsley DSc FRCP
Department of Therapeutics, University of Dundee, Dundee, UK

Contents

SESSION 6

SAFETY OF CIMETIDINE IN TREATMENT

Section 1
DUODENAL ULCER

1. Short-term treatment of duodenal ulceration

K. G. Wormsley
Department of Therapeutics, University of Dundee

We do not, at present, know the rate at which duodenal ulcers heal spontaneously. That problem underlies all discussion on the effects of drugs on the rate of healing of ulcers, and thus, for example, we do not actually know whether drugs increase or slow the rate of healing of duodenal ulcers.

The only information which has any bearing on 'spontaneous' healing rates is provided by Bardhan's studies of asymptomatic recurrences discovered during follow-up of ulcers healed after a course of cimetidine. Bardhan found that about two-thirds of the patients developed symptoms after an average of 5 months; about 30 per cent remained asymptomatic and retained their ulcers for 1 to 19 months; and only 1 of 48 patients healed the ulcer. If we can assume that the ulcers remained unhealed during the whole of the time until symptomatic relapse, or re-endoscopy, then clearly the 'spontaneous' rate of healing of duodenal ulcers is very, very slow indeed.

Under these circumstances, the rate of healing observed during treatment with 'placebos' is obviously much increased. In general, the mean overall placebo-associated healing rate is about 15 per cent in the first 14 days, increasing to 24 per cent after 3 weeks of 'treatment' with placebo (Table 1.1). When placebos

Table 1.1 Rate of healing of ulcers

Days treated	Cimetidine		Placebo	
	% healed	Median	% healed	Median
7	20-23	21.5	8-15	11.5
14	33-57	48	8-43	15
21	54-77	67	13-53	24
28	27-93	73	0-79	42
Carbenoxolone				
21		30		25
28		58		50

have been used to 'control' treatment with an 'active' drug for 4 weeks, an average rate of healing of 42 per cent of placebo-treated patients has been observed worldwide, with a range of 0 to 79 per cent (Table 1.2). As has been

3

Table 1.2 Healing of ulcers

	% healing in first month
Spontaneous	?
Placebo	42 (0-79)
Cimetidine	73 (27-93)

noted previously, there appear to be marked regional differences in placebo-associated rates of healing, ranging from averages of 27 per cent during 4 weeks in the UK and 24 per cent in 6 weeks in South Africa, to values of 60 per cent in 4 weeks in the Federal Republic of Germany and countries in Eastern Europe (Czechoslovakia and Hungary). The highest average placebo-associated healing rates have been recorded in Poland, with one reported value of 53 per cent in two weeks (Table 1.3).

Table 1.3 Placebo healing rates

Country	N	Weeks	%
UK	143 (10-37)	4	29 (10-41)
UK	27	12	33
Italy	758 (13-181)	4	32 (0-63)
Eire	35	4	40
Belgium and Holland	73	4	40
France	87	4	56
F.R. Germany	123 (22-40)	4	60 (40-79)
Switzerland	164 (19-58)	4	57 (55-63)
Norway	72 (20-28)	4	50 (46-60)
Czechoslovakia	55	4	60
Hungary	20	4	60
Poland	36	2	53
Poland	26	3	58
Hong Kong	24	4	17
USA	340 (12-142)	4	49 (39-79)
Canada	60	6	48
Mexico	18	6	50
Australia	102 (17-42)	6	37 (20-59)
S. Africa	117 (18-31)	6	24 (16-42)

There has been a lot of speculation about the causes of the differences in healing rates during administration of placebo. Specifically, we do not know whether the differences are attributable to the direct effects of different sorts of placebo (for example, lactose — often used as excipient — has been noted to heal experimental ulcers, while the use of 'emergency' antacids has converted many, or most, studies or parts of studies into 'pseudo-placebo' trials); to the unequal effects of 'placebo-treatment' on different population groups; or to quantitatively variable interference (either augmenting or retarding) with a placebo-induced healing effect by uncontrolled, unrecognised or 'unimportant' extraneous factors (such as perhaps smoking or dietary habits).

In all recorded studies, the rate of healing of duodenal ulcers during treatment with cimetidine has been greater than placebo (Table 1.4). However, the rates of healing during treatment with cimetidine and with placebo have been reported to

Table 1.4 Ulcer healing with cimetidine

	N	Weeks	Cimetidine % healed	N	Placebo % healed	P
UK	441 (11-75)	4	73 (44-85)	151	31	S
UK	118 (11-38)	6	69 (62-96)	33	21	S
Italy	395	4	77	166	36	S
Sweden	54	6	87	38	34	S
Norway	20	4	85	20	60	NS
France	109	4	69	99	55	S
Switzerland	101	4	81	106	58	NS
F.R. Germany	99	4	76	101	62	NS
S. Africa	55	6	75	38	42	S
Australia	43	6	84	42	38	S
USA	264	4	58	195	41	NS

be not significantly different in individual and collected studies from Norway and continental Europe (Federal Republic of Germany, Switzerland) principally because the rates of healing during treatment with placebo have been high, so that the numbers of patients in the individual studies have not been sufficiently large to convert a 'trend' into 'statistical significance'. In the USA, the differences between the rates of healing during treatment with cimetidine and placebo are not statistically significantly different for a different reason — because the proportion of patients healing during treatment with cimetidine is considerably less than in Europe, so that the difference from placebo is also 'too small', relative to the number of treated patients, to permit dignifying the beneficial 'trend' during treatment with cimetidine with statistical significance. These statistical 'errors' (especially of the 'type 2' sort) and woes have been over-emphasised in my opinion. That is to say, it seems to me reasonable to combine trends in a series of studies, especially if many are 'undoubtedly' significant. Since **all** studies have shown that ulcers heal faster during treatment with cimetidine than placebo, it seems to me that the beneficial healing effects of cimetidine are proven, even in countries with apparent individually insignificant differences. There is one corollary. In the latter countries (e.g. USA, FRG) it is not permissible to infer, from trials in which some other drug has been compared with cimetidine, that the drug is 'better than' placebo, unless a significant number of trials show better healing rates with the test drug than with cimetidine.

Unlike the situation during healing with placebo, where the increase in the rate of healing is exponential with time (Table 1.1), the majority of studies of cimetidine show that the highest rates of healing occur during the first week of treatment, following which there is a gradual and then rapid decrease in the rate at which residual ulcers heal. In this connection, there has been a certain amount of fairly sterile argument about whether or not there is a population with ulcers which cannot be healed. In a number of studies in which 'completeness' of healing has been recorded (Table 1.5), 91 to 100 per cent of duodenal ulcers have

Table 1.5 Completeness of healing with cimetidine

N	Weeks	Healed	%
11	12	11	100
96	12	94	98
113	12	111	98
33	6	30	91
18	8	17	94
23	6	22	96

been found to heal in 6 to 12 weeks of treatment with cimetidine. We do not yet know why some ulcers take longer to heal than others (other than that the initial size of the ulcer is obviously one of the determinants of the rate of healing) but it does seem that in many countries the majority of ulcers do heal during treatment with cimetidine.

A large number (over 20) of drugs or groups of drugs have now been shown to 'heal' ulcers more rapidly than placebo. (The most important details are summarised in Table 1.6). A few points require emphasis. I have not found a single study in which comparison of some other drug with cimetidine has shown a 'significant' difference in the rate of healing between the two compounds. Yet analyses of the ranks of the differences between the proportions of the ulcers healing with cimetidine and the trial drugs show that most of the latter drugs heal ulcers uniformly less well than cimetidine. The only 'discordant' result is

Table 1.6 Four to six-week healing rates

Drug	No. of patients	No. of trials (with cimetidine)	% healed	
Placebo	1893		42	*
Cimetidine	1739	46	73	
Ranitidine	241	8(3)	80	NA
Pirenzepine	505	20(5)	56	*
Anticholinergics	83	5(2)	72	*
Antacids	172	7(5)	66	*
DeNol	266	12(5)	78	0
Caved S	53	2(2)	62	*
Carbenoxolone	258	13(4)	64	*
Trithiozine	324	7(2)	53	*
Trimipramine	109	3(2)	70	*
Sucralfate	297	9(4)	75	NA
Gliptide	54	2(1)	63	*

Rank compared with cimetidine:
* Less
0 More
NA Not available

provided by DeNol, for which three of five studies (from Australia) show results identical with cimetidine, while one trial each from Belgium and the UK reported greater proportions of ulcers healing with DeNol than cimetidine. Since in both of these latter studies the cimetidine-associated healing rates were low (57 per cent) compared with 'national' average rates of healing (76 and 73 per cent, respectively), I cannot interpret these results. The more usual situation is that cimetidine has a uniform advantage of 10 to 20 per cent over the other trial drug (Table 1.7). I conclude that cimetidine is better able to heal duodenal ulcers than

Table 1.7 Percentage healed with cimetidine compared with another drug

Cimetidine	Comparison drug
	Carbenoxolone
72	58
68	53
72	61
70	50
	Trithiozine
80	74
90	80
	Pirenzepine
77	55
75	50
75	79
82	71
90	76

most, if not all, of the other drugs, being used in the treatment of duodenal ulcer at present (except perhaps ranitidine, about which insufficient information is available). It is necessary to add that all the drugs mentioned in Table 1.6 heal duodenal ulcers better than placebo, using as criterion of 'better' an almost uniformly higher proportion of ulcers healed during trials with the test drug, compared with placebo (even if the differences in individual trials have been regarded as statistically 'not significant').

And yet, after all, the prize must go to acetazolamide, since this drug has been reported to heal 92 per cent of 1211 Roumanian patients with duodenal ulcer in two weeks, compared with 36 per cent of 568 patients treated with placebo. We are never going to see better results than those, I imagine. However, for those wishing to dabble in modern therapeutics, there clearly remains a wide choice of 'remedies' for duodenal ulcer. We do not have enough satisfactory information about any drug other than cimetidine to be able to predict that, as with cimetidine, the proportion of ulcers healable with the drug is nearly 100 per cent. We need this information, because drugs which cannot heal more than 90 per cent of ulcers should not be used in ulcer therapy. The choice between those drugs which are shown to be potentially uniformly efficacious can, and must, be made on the basis of adverse reactions encountered during short- and long-term treatment with the drugs. On that basis it seems that only the H_2 receptor antagonists should be used at present for the treatment of duodenal ulcers (and that ranitidine has, perhaps, theoretical advantages over cimetidine).

Finally, what are the implications of the fact that 20 or more drugs heal duodenal ulcers better than placebo? Since many of the drugs have no physiological or pharmacological actions in common (as far as is known at present), these drugs must either be influencing different aspects of the process of healing or the processes (if any) interfering with mucosal repair. In view of our ignorance both of the pharmacological actions of the drugs and the processes involved in ulcer formation and healing, it seems probable that we are going to have to treat duodenal ulcers empirically, rather than rationally, for a while longer.

ACKNOWLEDGEMENTS

A research grant from the Scottish Hospital Endowments Research Trust is gratefully acknowledged.

FURTHER READING

All the data for this paper are presented in detail in:
Wormsley K 1979 Duodenal ulcer, Vol 2. Eden Press, Montreal
Wormsley K 1981 Duodenal ulcer, Vol 3. Eden Press, Montreal

2. Cimetidine: twice daily administration in duodenal ulcer — results of a UK and Ireland multicentre study

G. D. Kerr*

Royal Shrewsbury Hospital, Shrewsbury, Salop

Cimetidine at the accepted dosage of 200 mg three times daily (t.d.s.) with meals and 400 mg on retiring heals the majority of duodenal ulcers (e.g. Bardhan, 1978). A pharmacological study in healthy volunteers (Burland et al, 1980), however, indicated no significant difference in the reduction of gastric acidity over 24 hours between this dose of cimetidine and a twice daily (b.d.) regime of 400 mg given with breakfast and 400 mg at bedtime.

These results implied that twice daily cimetidine could heal as high a proportion of duodenal ulcers as the present dosage.

The aim of this study was therefore a comparison of the efficacy of cimetidine 400 mg b.d. with that of 200 mg t.d.s. and 400 mg at night in the healing and symptomatic relief of duodenal ulcer.

METHOD

A total of nine centres in the UK and Ireland participated in the trial with the permission of each hospital ethical committee. The study was conducted according to the Declarations of Helsinki and Tokyo.

Patients (minimum age 14 years) with a diagnosis of duodenal ulceration confirmed endoscopically within the previous four days were randomly allocated to receive cimetidine 200 mg t.d.s and 400 mg nocte (Group A) or 400 mg b.d. (Group B). Antacids (as 'Rennies'; Nicholas) were supplied to be taken for symptoms not relieved by cimetidine. The end-point of the trial was ulcer healing defined as complete re-epithelialization of the duodenal ulcer crater, confirmed by endoscopy after four weeks and, in those not healed by this time, after eight weeks. Endoscopic examination was performed by observers who were unaware, in the large majority of cases, of the treatment allocation. Clinical assessment was carried out at weeks one, two and four and, if necessary, at weeks six and eight.

* Dr Kerr presented the results of this study. The following contributed to the study: P. Brown, Royal Shrewsbury Hospital; J. Lennon, J. Crowe, Mater Misericordiae Hospital, Dublin; R. J. McFarland, A. Vargese, Belfast City Hospital; T. C. Northfield, D. Fine, St George's Hospital, London; J. M. Findlay, B. Selby, Bradford Royal Infirmary; J. Temple, H. Bradby, Queen Elizabeth Hospital, Birmingham; C. Gilbertson, Nevill Hall Hospital, Abergavenny; D. L. Carr-Locke, Leicester Royal Infirmary; M.B. McIllmurray, Royal Lancaster Infirmary.

At these times adverse events, whether or not drug-related, were recorded, as were details of ulcer pain and antacid consumption, this information having been previously recorded by patients on a diary card. Compliance was also assessed by returned tablet counts. A full blood count and platelet count together with biochemical tests of renal and liver function were performed before treatment only, unless clinically indicated.

Statistical methods applied to the resulting data comprised the Chi-square test for simple comparisons of the two dosage groups. A log linear approach to multidimensional contingency tables (Bishop et al, 1975) was used to assess the influence of age and/or sex on healing and ulcer pain, whilst the trend in the latter was also considered using a weighted least squares regression analysis. Demographic data were compared using Chi-square, Student's t-, and Mann–Whitney U tests. Differences were regarded as significant when $P < 0.05$.

RESULTS

Of the 198 patients who entered the study, 171 completed the first four weeks of the trial and were eligible for statistical analysis. Of the withdrawals four could have been the result of drug-related adverse effects: one patient developed headaches, another suffered dizziness and two patients developed rashes. All four were in Group B. Reasons for withdrawal of the other 23 patients included concomitant illness, non-compliance with the protocol and social factors. Of those eligible for analysis, 93 patients were allocated to Group A and 78 to Group B. Both groups were comparable with the exception of the median duration of ulcer disease being significantly longer ($P < 0.05$) in Group A (Table 2.1). There were no statistically significant differences between the incidence of healing or symptomatic relief between participating centres.

Table 2.1 Demographic data of the trial population

Dosage regime	1 g/day	400 mg b.i.d.
Number of patients	93	78
Male/female	66/27	47/31
Mean age (years)	46.5	43.9
Ulcer disease duration (years)		
range	0-40	0-48
median	5*	2
Ulcer symptoms duration (months)		
mean	2.8	2.1

*P<0.05

Ulcer healing
Data on ulcer healing were available for 170 patients. With this sample size, the probabilities of failing to detect a true difference between healing rates of 20 per cent at the 5 per cent level of significance (one-tailed) are between 0.1 and 0.2 after four weeks treatment and 0.05 and 0.1 after eight weeks.

Sixty-three of 92 (69 per cent) patients in Group A had healed ulcers after four weeks compared with 51 of 78 (66 per cent) patients in Group B. By eight weeks a cumulative total of 81 of 90 (90 per cent) patients in Group A had healed ulcers compared with 67 of 76 (88 per cent) patients in Group B. There were no statistically significant differences in healing rates between the two groups. Two patients from each group who had unhealed ulcers did not return for further assessment after week 4.

An interesting finding was that patients aged 60 years or over did not respond as well as those under 60. Twenty-five of 32 (78 per cent) patients in the older age group healed their ulcers compared·with 123 of 134 (92 per cent) younger patients ($P < 0.05$). This result was independent of dosage group.

Ulcer pain
Daytime pain and night time pain were considered separately and there was a substantial reduction in the symptoms of patients in both groups during the course of the study (Figures 2.1 and 2.2).

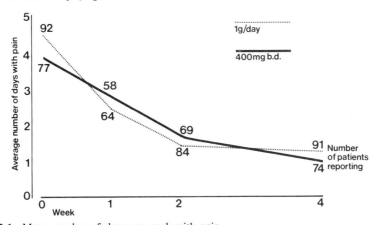

Figure 2.1 Mean number of days per week with pain.

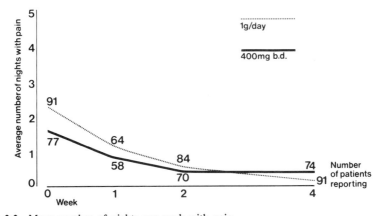

Figure 2.2 Mean number of nights per week with pain.

There was a significantly greater fall in the mean number of days per week with pain in patients in Group A compared with Group B during the first two weeks ($P = 0.03$ week 1; $P = 0.04$ week 2). Patients in Group A, however, had a higher frequency of pain at the start of the trial than those in Group B.

After week 2, pain reduction in both groups was comparable, although the numbers between weeks 4 and 8 were too small for any reliable statistical comparison to be made.

The proportion of patients with daytime pain during the week preceding the start of treatment was higher in Group A (77/90 patients; 86 per cent) than Group B (57/77 patients; 74 per cent). These proportions decreased over the following four weeks, and no statistically significant difference between the groups was detectable at any stage.

No statistically significant differences between the two groups were seen with respect to night pain, although prior to treatment those in Group A suffered more pain, as judged by the average number of nights with pain (Figure 2.2), than those in Group B.

It is apparent that the largest decrease in day and night pain took place during the first two weeks of treatment in both groups.

Antacid consumption
The proportion of patients known to have taken antacids during the first week of therapy amounted to 70 per cent in each group.

The actual numbers of antacid tablets consumed per week were not reliably recorded and varied considerably in both groups (range 0–32 for those in Group A and 0–34 for those in Group B). The mean total consumption for each group for weeks 1–4 was very similar. Median consumption was greater in Group B during week 1 of the trial: 5 vs. 3 in Group A.

Adverse events
In addition to the four patients withdrawn from the trial, adverse events, defined as any symptom occurring during treatment and not present before the trial, occurred in 35 patients in Group A and 28 in Group B. In total 54 events were reported by patients in Group A, of which 31 were gastro-intestinal in nature and were largely related to ulcer symptomatology. The corresponding figure for Group B was 50 events, of which 24 were classed as gastrointestinal. The adverse events experienced by the patients who remained in the trial were largely of a minor nature and did not necessitate any change in treatment. Of note, however, was a 27-year-old male patient in Group A who developed alopecia areata confined to the beard within a week of commencing treatment with cimetidine. Hair growth slowly returned to normal on discontinuation of the drug after ulcer healing.

No further haematological or biochemical tests were considered necessary in any patient.

DISCUSSION

The healing rate of 69 per cent following four weeks treatment with cimetidine 1 g/day is consistent with the results from trials of similar methodology as reviewed by Bardhan (1978). The 66 per cent healing rate on cimetidine 400 mg b.d. is comparable. As expected, the incidence of healing increased with the longer duration of treatment to cumulative proportions of 90 per cent and 88 per cent respectively at eight weeks. Age appeared to be a factor influencing overall healing but numbers are too small in the subgroup of 60 years and over to allow any conclusion from this observation.

There was rapid, effective and comparable reduction of pain in both groups. The lower median antacid consumption in the group on 1 g/day could indicate that more frequent administration of cimetidine provided more even relief of pain. Patients in the group receiving twice daily cimetidine may have required extra antacid during the day as the effect of the morning dose wore off. However, as symptoms were reduced to a similar level in both groups by the end of the first week, this observation could also imply that the two extra administrations of cimetidine were having a 'placebo' effect on pain.

Twice daily dosing is likely to improve patient compliance, decreases the total amount of ingested drug and is cheaper. We feel therefore that as there is no significant clinical difference between the two doses there may be an advantage in using cimetidine 400 mg b.d. to heal duodenal ulcers.

REFERENCES

Bardhan K D 1978 Cimetidine in duodenal ulceration. In: Wastell C, Lance P (eds) Cimetidine: Proceedings of the Westminster Hospital Symposium. Churchill Livingstone, Edinburgh, p 31-56

Bishop Y M N, Sienberg S E, Holland P W 1975 Discrete multivariate analysis. MIT Press, Cambridge, Massachusetts, USA

Burland W L B, Brunet P L, Hunt R H, Melvin M A, Mills J G, Vincent D, Milton-Thompson G J 1980 Comparison of the effects on intragastric acidity of SK&F 92994 and two dose regimens of cimetidine. Hepatogastroenterology Suppl (XI International Congress of Gastroenterology) 259

3. Cimetidine: twice daily administration in duodenal ulcer — results of a European multicentre study

V. Eckardt

Department of Medicine, University of Mainz, West Germany

The effectiveness of cimetidine in healing duodenal ulcers has been demonstrated in many controlled trials (Bank et al, 1976; Bardhan et al, 1979; Binder et al, 1978; Blackwood et al, 1976; Bodemar et al, 1977; Gillespie et al, 1977; Gillies et al, 1978; Gray et al, 1977; Hetzel et al, 1978; Northfield and Blackwood, 1977; Peter et al, 1978; Ubilluz, 1979). Although the daily dosage of cimetidine varied between 800 and 2000 mg, healing rates in the majority of these studies were remarkably similar.

The standard daily dosage of 1.0 g cimetidine divided in four doses is based on the results of pharmacological studies which show that 200 mg cimetidine with meals inhibits the mean intragastric hydrogen ion activity by 57 per cent (Pounder et al, 1977) and that inhibition of nocturnal acid secretion is most marked with a bedtime dose of 400 mg (Blackwood and Northfield, 1977).

However, it has recently been demonstrated that daytime acid secretion could similarly be reduced by a single morning dose of 400 mg (Burland et al, 1980). Furthermore, it has not been proved that the degree of acid inhibition is an accurate predictor of the magnitude of the therapeutic response. In fact, previous studies in a small number of subjects comparing 800 mg cimetidine with either 1.2 or 1.6 g cimetidine daily did not reveal any significant difference in duodenal ulcer healing (Blackwood et al, 1976; Bodemar et al, 1977).

METHOD

The study was performed in 43 centres in nine European countries using a common protocol. A total of 633 outpatients with active duodenal ulcer disease confirmed by fibre-optic endoscopy entered the trial within four days of the initial endoscopy. Pregnant and lactating women were excluded from the study.

All patients gave informed consent to the study and the trial was carried out according to the Declaration of Helsinki.

Patients were randomly allocated to either the standard dose of 1 g cimetidine divided in four doses (200 mg three times a day with meals and 400 mg at bedtime) or 400 mg cimetidine twice daily at breakfast and bedtime. No other treatment was allowed except antacids which could be taken as frequently as

14

required for the relief of ulcer pain which was not controlled by the trial medication.

The patients were provided with diary cards and kept a daily record of the number and severity of attacks of ulcer pain and the number of antacid tablets taken.

They were interviewed and examined at fortnightly intervals. After four weeks of treatment endoscopy was repeated and the trial ended if the ulcer had healed. Patients whose ulcers had not healed at that time continued treatment for another four weeks at which time a third endoscopy was performed. Ulcer healing was defined as complete disappearance of all ulcers and erosions.

The trial design was single blind in that the endoscopist was unaware of the treatment allocation.

For statistical analysis the G^2 test (log linear model, four-way contingency tables), the x^2 test and Fisher's exact test were used.

RESULTS

Of the 633 patients who initially entered the trial 50 defaulted and had to be excluded from the data analysis. Of the remaining 583 patients 302 received the q.i.d. dosage and 281 were allocated to the b.d. regimen.

The treatment groups were comparable in terms of sex, age, smoking habits and ulcer size (Table 3.1) and no difference was observed between the two groups from country to country.

Table 3.1 Pre-trial population

	q.i.d.	b.d.
Sex		
Females	76	81
Males	226	200
Age (years)		
Mean	45.5	46.6
Smoking habits		
Smoking	193	173
Not smoking	102	100
Not known	8	7
Ulcer size (mm²)		
Small (0-50)	127	120
Medium (50-200)	93	74
Large (200)	24	26

Ulcer healing
After four weeks 77 per cent of patients on the q.i.d. regimen and 73 per cent on the b.d. dosage had healed ulcers (Table 3.2). A small group of subjects was reinvestigated after six weeks instead of four weeks. Their healing rates did not differ significantly from the healing rates in patients endoscoped after four

Table 3.2 Healing rates at four weeks

Country	q.i.d.		b.d.		Total patients
	H/T*	%	H/T*	%	
Belgium	21/24	88	20/23	87	47
France	30/39	77	28/37	76	76
Germany	55/63	87	47/59	80	122
Holland	3/3	100	2/2	100	5
Portugal	12/13	92	16/19	84	32
Spain	27/48	56	23/45	51	93
Scandinavia	2/2	100	2/2	100	4
UK	38/53	72	30/42	71	95
Overall	188/245	77	168/229	73	474

*Number of patients healed/treated.

weeks. Patients not healed after four weeks of treatment were re-endoscoped at eight weeks. At this time the cumulative healing rate for all patients was again similar in patients randomized to the q.i.d. regimen (95 per cent) and patients allocated to the b.d. regimen (93 per cent) (Table 3.3).

Table 3.3 Overall healing rates

	q.i.d.		b.d.	
	H/T*	%	H/T*	%
4 weeks	188/245	77	168/229	73
6 weeks	47/57	82	41/52	79
8 weeks**	229/241	95	208/224	93
Total 583	302		281	

* Number of patients healed/treated.
** Cumulative with 4 weeks.

Though healing rates varied greatly between different countries, no difference was observed at four weeks between the two treatment groups in the various countries. At eight weeks, only in the UK was a significant difference observed between the two treatment groups ($P < 0.05$): 98 per cent of the UK patients had healed ulcers with the q.i.d. regimen as opposed to 88 per cent with the b.d. regimen.

Pain relief

The mean number of days and nights with pain steadily decreased in both treatment groups (Figures 3.1 and 3.2) and there was no significant difference between the groups at any time during the observation period. In addition, if patients who did not have healed ulcers after four weeks of treatment were analyzed separately, no significant difference was observed between the two treatment groups. With the exception of a small subgroup of non-smokers in Italy who experienced less pain with the q.i.d. dosage (100 per cent versus 63 per cent; $P < 0.05$), pain relief was similar with both regimens when the data were analyzed for each country separately.

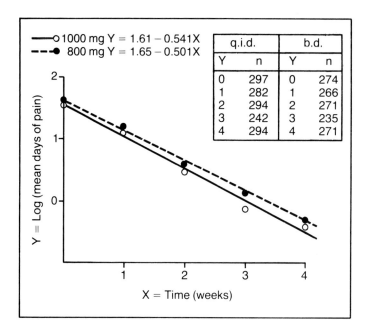

Figure 3.1   Mean number of days with pain, on log scale.

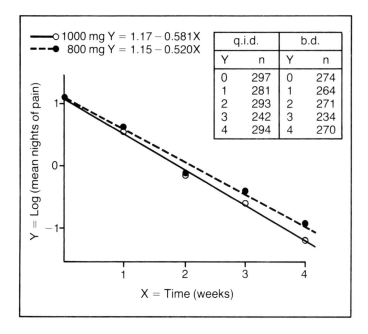

Figure 3.2   Mean number of nights with pain, on log scale.

Antacid consumption

Detailed analysis of total doses of antacids consumed during the study was not possible as the antacids used varied greatly within and between countries. However, when the data were analyzed according to the number of patients taking or not taking antacids no differences were observed between the two treatment groups (Figure 3.3).

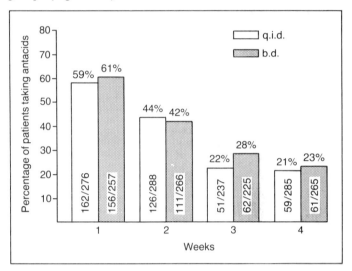

Figure 3.3 Overall antacid consumption in the q.i.d. and b.d. treatment groups.

Antacid consumption was similar for both treatment groups in each country at one, two and three weeks. Only in Germany was the number of patients taking antacids during the fourth week greater in the b.d. regimen.

Adverse events

A total of 81 adverse events were reported by 57 patients with similar frequency in both treatment groups (Table 3.4). In only two cases did these reactions

Table 3.4 Adverse events

Type of adverse event	q.i.d.	b.d.
Rash–pruritus	7	5
Musculo-skeletal (lumbago)	1	—
Vertigo–headache–dizziness	8	11
Confusion–depression/irritability	6	3
Nausea/diarrhoea	10	5
Weight increase	—	1
Phlebitis	—	3
Dyspnoea/tonsillitis	1	1
Urinary disorder	2	—
Gynaecomastia	—	2
Amenorrhoea	—	2
Tiredness/pain	8	5
Total 81	43	38

necessitate withdrawal of treatment: one elderly patient developed mental confusion which subsided when the drug was withdrawn and recurred upon rechallenge; the other patient complained of headache and refused further treatment.

CONCLUSIONS

The results of this single-blind randomized multicentre trial show that the administration of 400 mg cimetidine twice daily is as effective in the treatment of active duodenal ulcer disease as the currently used q.i.d. regimen with 1 g cimetidine per day. Both treatment regimens result in similar healing rates and similar decreases in ulcer pain and antacid consumption. Whether analyzed overall or by country, no significant differences were found between the two dosage regimens with the exception of a few small subgroups. Since the b.d. regimen improves the cost benefit ratio and may result in better patient compliance, 400 mg cimetidine twice daily should be the preferred dosage in the treatment of active duodenal ulcer disease.

SUMMARY

Cimetidine 800 mg/day (as 400 mg twice daily) and 1 g/day (spread over four doses) was compared in a single-blind randomized multicentre trial of duodenal ulcer healing.

After 4 weeks the ulcers of 188 of the 245 patients (77 per cent) treated with the q.i.d. regimen had healed compared with 168 of the 229 patients (73 per cent) receiving the b.d. dosage.

Symptomatic improvement and antacid consumption were similar in both treatment groups throughout the observation period. With the exception of a few small subgroups similar results were observed when the data were analyzed for each country separately.

It is concluded that 400 mg cimetidine twice daily is as effective as the currently used q.i.d. regimen with 1 g cimetidine per day and should be the preferred dosage in the treatment of duodenal ulcer disease.

REFERENCES

Bank S, Barbezat G O, Novis B H, Ou Tim L, Odes H S, Helman C, Narunsky L, Duys P J, Marks I N 1976 Histamine H_2-receptor antagonists in the treatment of duodenal ulcers. South African Medical Journal 50:1781-1785

Bardhan K D et al 1979 Comparison of two doses of cimetidine and placebo in the treatment of duodenal ulcer: a multicentre trial. Gut 20:68-74

Binder H J, Cocco A, Crossley R J, Finkelstein W, Font R, Friedman G, Groarke J, Hughes W, Johnson A F, McGuigan J E, Summers R, Vlahevic R, Wilson E C, Winship D H 1978 Cimetidine in the treatment of duodenal ulcer. A multicenter double blind study. Gastroenterology 74:380-388

Blackwood W S, Maugdal D P, Pickard R G, Lawrence D, Northfield T C 1976 Cimetidine in duodenal ulcer. Controlled trial. Lancet 2:174-176

Blackwood W S, Northfield T C 1977 Nocturnal gastric acid secretion: effect of cimetidine and interaction with anti-cholinergics. In: Burland W L, Simkins M A (eds) Cimetidine: Proceedings of the Second International Symposium on histamine H_2-receptor antagonists. Excerpta Medica, Amsterdam, Oxford, p 124-130

Bodemar G, Norlander B, Walan A 1977 Cimetidine in the treatment of active peptic ulcer disease. In Burland W L, Simkins M A (eds) Cimetidine: Proceedings of the Second International Symposium on histamine H_2-receptor antagonists. Excerpta Medica, Amsterdam, Oxford, p 224-239

Burland W L, Brunet P L, Hunt R H, Melvin M A, Mills G J, Vincent D, Milton-Thompson G J 1980 Comparison of the effect on 24-hour intragastric acidity of SKF 92994 and two dose regimens of cimetidine. Hepatogastroenterology Suppl (International Congress of Gastroenterology), p 259

Gillespie G, Gray G R, Smith I S, Mackenzie I, Crean G P 1977 Short-term and maintenance cimetidine treatment in severe duodenal ulceration. In: Burland W L, Simkins M A (eds) Cimetidine: Proceedings of the Second International Symposium on histamine H_2-receptor antagonists. Excerpta Medica, Amsterdam, Oxford, p 240-247

Gillies R R, Archambault A, Kinnear D G, Lacerte M 1978 Controlled comparison of two dosage regimens of cimetidine in duodenal ulcer. Gastroenterology 74:396

Gray G R, McKenzie I, Smith I S, Crean G P, Gillespie G 1977 Oral cimetidine in severe duodenal ulceration. A double-blind controlled trial. Lancet 1:4-7

Hetzel D J, Hansky J, Shearman D J, Konman M G, Hecker R, Taggart G J, Jackson R, Gabb B W 1978 Cimetidine treatment of duodenal ulceration. Gastroenterology 74:389-392

Northfield T C, Blackwood W S 1977 Short communication: controlled clinical trial of cimetidine for duodenal ulcer. In: Burland W L, Simkins M A (eds) Cimetidine: Proceedings of the Second International Symposium on histamine H_2-receptor antagonists. Excerpta Medica, Amsterdam, Oxford, p 224-247

Peter P, Kiene K, Gonvers J J, Pelloni S, Weber K, Sonnenberg A, Schmitz H, Richter O, Hofstetter J R, Blum A L, Strohmeyer G 1978 Cimetidin in der Behandlung des Ulcus duodeni. Deutsche Medizinische Wochenschrift 103:1163-1166

Pounder R E, Williams J G, Hunt R H, Vincent S H, Milton-Thompson G J, Misiewicz J J 1977 The effects of oral cimetidine on food-stimulated gastric acid secretion and 24-hour intragastric acidity. In: Burland W L, Simkins M A (eds) Cimetidine: Proceedings of the Second International Symposium on histamine H_2-receptor antagonists. Excerpta Medica, Amsterdam, Oxford, p 189-204

Ubilluz R 1979 Cimetidine in the treatment of active duodenal ulcer: a double blind study. Current Therapeutic Research 25:243-250

4. Healing of duodenal ulcer with twice daily oxmetidine, part 1

H.-G. Rohner*, G. Brandstätter, P. Kratochvil, J. Kollmeier and R. Gugler
*St. Barbara-Hospital, Gladbeck, West Germany

Oxmetidine is a new histamine H_2-receptor antagonist which differs from cimetidine in that it contains an isocytosine ring as a side-chain instead of a cyanoguanidine group. Studies in healthy volunteers and in duodenal ulcer patients have indicated that oxmetidine is more potent than cimetidine on a molar basis, but has a similar duration of effect (Brunet et al, 1980).

In this randomised controlled double-blind trial the effect of oxmetidine on the healing of duodenal ulcers was compared with that of cimetidine.

METHOD

The study was conducted in two centres: Gladbeck, West Germany, and Graz, Austria. The protocol stated that a total number of 100 patients (50 patients per centre) were to be included in the study. Of these 100 patients 99 completed the study; one patient was withdrawn when he developed a rash, possibly due to oxmetidine. This patient still shows the symptoms of urticaria factitia seven months after the trial.

Cimetidine was given in the standard daily dose of 1 g, as three 200 mg doses with meals and 400 mg at night. Oxmetidine was administered 400 mg twice daily. Tablets were packed into blisters of two tablets each for the morning and the night dose, and one tablet to be taken at lunch and with the evening meal. Patients on cimetidine received one placebo tablet (morning); patients on oxmetidine received two placebo tablets (lunch, evening) in their blisters. Tablets of a mild antacid (Gelusil) were permitted if ulcer pain was severe.

The study lasted eight weeks. Patients were asked to visit once a fortnight. Endoscopy was performed at the beginning of the study, after four weeks of treatment, and again after eight weeks if the ulcer had not healed at four weeks. The endpoint of the study was complete healing of the ulcer. At the initial endoscopy the maximum diameter of the ulcer was recorded. At follow-up endoscopies, the size of unhealed ulcers was also determined. The shape of the ulcer and its location in the duodenal bulb were also noted. The presence or absence of ulcer pain was recorded, separately for day and night, on diary cards.

RESULTS

Clinical data for all patients who completed the study are listed in Table 4.1. The mean age of the patients was 45 years, and was not different in the cimetidine and in the oxmetidine groups. Twenty-two per cent of all patients were female with a

Table 4.1 Clinical data

	Cimetidine	Oxmetidine
N	50	49
Age (yr)	44.5 ± 14.3	45.2 ± 13.8
Male/female	42 / 8	35 / 14
No. of smokers	34	35
No. of alcohol drinkers	24	27
Mean duration of ulcer disease (yr)	9.7	9.4
Ulcer size (mm)	7.6 ± 4.1	7.6 ± 4.0
Form (linear/round)	4 / 46	9 / 41

small but not significant difference between the two treatment groups. The smokers and the regular alcohol drinkers were both equally distributed between the cimetidine and the oxmetidine groups.

A large interindividual variation was noted in the duration of the duodenal ulcer disease — from 0 to 40 years. Four patients presented with duodenal ulcer for the first time.

The mean ulcer size was 7.6 mm in the cimetidine as well as in the oxmetidine treated group. In agreement with the protocol, no ulcer was smaller than 3 mm. Ulcers seen in Gladbeck were generally larger than those seen in Graz (Table 4.2). Since some endoscopists feel that the ulcer form is of importance in assessing the treatment response, the ratio of linear (longitudinal) to round ulcers was determined, but was equal in the two treatment groups.

Very few patients needed to use antacid tablets and no difference in antacid consumption existed between the two groups.

Cimetidine compared with oxmetidine
After four weeks of treatment, the ulcers had healed in 37 out of 50 patients treated with cimetidine, and in 38 out of 49 patients treated with oxmetidine (Figure 4.1). Healing rates (74 and 78 per cent respectively) are consistent with healing rates reported in the literature for cimetidine (Wastell, 1978). The difference between the two groups was obviously not significant. After eight weeks treatment, 45 of the cimetidine-treated and 46 of the oxmetidine-treated patients showed healing of their ulcers, representing 90 and 94 per cent healing rates, respectively. Again, this difference was not significant.

Graz compared with Gladbeck
A comparison of the healing rates after 4 weeks in the two centres shows surprising differences. In Gladbeck 88 per cent of the cimetidine-treated ulcers

healed, but only 63 per cent of the oxmetidine-treated ulcers healed (Figure 4.1). This difference was clearly in favour of cimetidine, but did not reach significance.

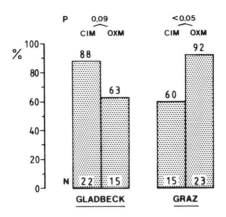

Figure 4.1   Ulcer healing at four weeks: Graz and Gladbeck compared.

In contrast, only 60 per cent of the cimetidine-treated ulcers healed in Graz, while 92 per cent of the oxmetidine-treated ulcers healed (Figure 4.1). This difference was significant at the 5 per cent level, but here oxmetidine was superior. These contradictory results cannot easily be explained. Statistical analysis revealed that the chance of obtaining such conflicting results from two centres is less than one per cent.

At first it seemed that an error in the distribution of tablets might have happened, so that in one centre patients who were allocated to the cimetidine group were actually receiving oxmetidine and vice versa. This possibility was ruled out, however, by two investigations. First, oxmetidine and cimetidine tablets were packed into blisters on two different days that were marked on the blisters at a secret place. From the unused blisters that were sent back to Smith Kline, Dauelsberg, the dates on these blisters were compared with the actual randomisation plan and were found to correspond to the original list. Second, from a large number of blisters returned, tablets were taken for analysis of their cimetidine or oxmetidine content in the clinical pharmacology laboratory in Bonn, and these results also confirmed the randomisation plan.

Table 4.2 shows the clinical data analysed separately for the two centres. Patients in Graz were as a group somewhat older than those in Gladbeck. Sex distribution was only slightly different. Alcohol use and the duration of disease were similar in the two centres and in the respective treatment groups. The ulcer size was consistently larger in the Gladbeck patients than in those from Graz. This might be due to subjective differences in the judgement of ulcer size. Also the ratio of linear to round ulcers was the same in the two centres and in the treatment groups of each centre. As far as the discrepancy in results was concerned, no differences could be found between the two treatment groups in each centre to account for this.

Table 4.2 Clinical data : comparison of two centres

	Gladbeck		Graz	
	Cimetidine	Oxmetidine	Cimetidine	Oxmetidine
N	25	24	25	25
Age (yr)*	42.8 ± 16.0	42.1 ± 12.3	46.2 ± 12.6	48.1 ± 14.8
Male/female	23/2	19/5	19/6	16/9
No. of smokers	15	23	19	12
No. of alcohol drinkers	12	13	12	14
Mean duration of ulcer disease (yr)	8.1	7.4	10.1	10.1
Ulcer				
size (mm)*	10.8 ± 3.4	11.0 ± 3.3	4.3 ± 1.4	4.7 ± 1.7
Form (linear/round)	2/23	4/20	2/23	5/20

*mean ± s.d.

An interesting observation is the difference in smoking habits between the two centres and its effect on the healing of duodenal ulcers in the present study, for a strong difference was observed: 68 per cent of all cimetidine-treated patients and 71 per cent of the oxmetidine-treated patients were smokers (Figure 4.2). Of all patients who did not respond to treatment 92 per cent were smokers, and thus smoking seems to be an important factor in accounting for treatment failures with H_2-receptor antagonists.

In Gladbeck as well as in Graz there were significantly more smokers in the treatment group with the poorer result: 96 per cent in the oxmetidine vs. 48 per cent in the cimetidine group in Gladbeck; 76 per cent in the cimetidine vs. 48 per cent in the oxmetidine group in Graz. These figures correspond to 63 vs. 88 per cent (oxmetidine vs. cimetidine) healing in Gladbeck and 60 vs. 92 per cent (cimetidine vs. oxmetidine) healing in Graz. Smoking therefore is inversely correlated with the healing response of duodenal ulcers. Thus, smoking does explain at least in part the difference in treatment response to cimetidine and oxmetidine between Gladbeck and Graz.

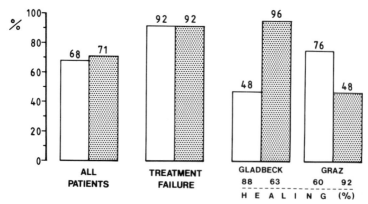

Figure 4.2 Smoking and duodenal ulcer healing: Graz and Gladbeck compared. Open columns = patients treated with cimetidine; hatched columns = patients treated with oxmetidine.

Cimetidine and oxmetidine were equally effective in reducing day pain and night pain in week 2 and week 4 of treatment (Figures 4.3, 4.4). No difference in pain relief existed between the two centres.

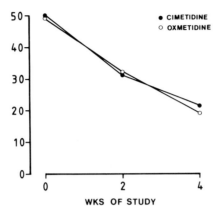

Figure 4.3   Number of patients with day pain at the beginning of the study and at 2 weeks and 4 weeks.

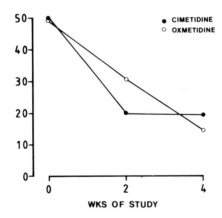

Figure 4.4   Number of patients with night pain at the beginning of the study and at 2 weeks and 4 weeks.

CONCLUSION

1. In a two-centre controlled clinical trial 50 patients were treated with cimetidine and 49 patients with oxmetidine for active duodenal ulcer. Of these 74 per cent healed on cimetidine and 78 per cent healed on oxmetidine after four weeks treatment.

2. Analysis of data from each centre revealed that in Gladbeck cimetidine was superior to oxmetidine, while in Graz oxmetidine was significantly better than cimetidine.

3. Evaluation of the clinical data showed that smoking accounts for most of the difference in treatment response. Smoking appears to be a decisive factor in poor responders to H_2-receptor antagonists in duodenal ulcer.

4. Comparable symptomatic improvement was achieved by cimetidine and oxmetidine, irrespective of the centre.

REFERENCES

Brunet P L, Hunt R H, Melvin M A, Mills J G, Sharpe P, Milton-Thompson G J, Burland W L 1980 Comparison of the effects of SK&F 92994 and cimetidine on food stimulated gastric acid secretion. Hepatogastroenterology Suppl (XI International Congress of Gastroenterology) 260
Wastell C 1978 The problem of duodenal ulcer disease and its treatment with cimetidine. In: Wastell C, Lance P (eds) Cimetidine. The Westminster Hospital Symposium. Churchill Livingstone, Edinburgh, p 3-12

5. Healing of duodenal ulcer with twice daily oxmetidine, part 2

Gabriele Bianchi Porro, Maddalena Petrillo, Marco Lazzaroni and Susanna Leto Di Priolo

Gastrointestinal Unit, Ospedale L. Sacco, Milan

The medical treatment of duodenal ulcer has been dominated by cimetidine for the last few years. The efficacy of this drug in inducing ulcer healing in the short-term is beyond any doubt (Bardhan, 1980). Recently the interest of gastroenterologists has been caught by other drugs of which the mechanism of action is also antisecretory — such as pirenzepine — (Bianchi Porro et al, 1981) or through which the gastric mucosal resistance is enhanced — such as colloidal bismuth subcitrate (Vantrappen et al, 1980).

The most important development, however, is the appearance of the newest H_2-receptor antagonists, the most promising of which is without doubt ranitidine. It has already been demonstrated that this new drug exerts similar ulcer-healing potency in the short-term treatment of peptic ulcer to cimetidine with the advantage of twice daily administration (Misiewicz and Sewing, 1981).

Recently in the Smith Kline & French Research Institute a new histamine H_2 receptor antagonist, oxmetidine dihydrochloride (SKF 92994), has been discovered which is more lipophilic than cimetidine and contains a 5-substituted isocytosine moiety in place of the cyanoguanidine group while retaining the imidazole ring.

A number of studies have now been carried out to investigate the potency and duration of action of oxmetidine as an antisecretory agent in man (Brunet et al, 1980; Burland et al, 1980; Mills et al, 1980). Following intravenous infusion the drug appears on a mg for mg basis to be up to four times as potent as cimetidine but no difference has been observed following oral administration. Recently the effects of four multiple regimens on 24-hour hydrogen ion activity (placebo, oxmetidine 400 mg b.d., cimetidine 400 mg b.d. and cimetidine 1 g daily) have been compared in a group of six ambulant patients (Burland et al, 1980). All treatments reduced intragastric acidity throughout the study period, a more marked response being seen at night. No difference was observed between the duration of action of oxmetidine and cimetidine, and in doses of 400 mg b.d. both produced a marked reduction in the 24-hour gastric acidity.

On the basis of these results further studies to determine the efficacy of oxmetidine in the healing of peptic ulceration seem justified. The aim of the present double-blind trial is to compare the effect of oxmetidine and cimetidine on healing of duodenal ulcer and on ulcer pain and antacid consumption in patients with active ulceration. The preliminary results of this study are presented here.

PATIENTS AND METHODS

Sixty adult patients with endoscopically proven duodenal ulcer were included in the study. Within five days of endoscopic confirmation of ulcer they were randomly allocated in a double-blind manner to oxmetidine 400 mg twice daily or cimetidine 1 g daily. Each patient was also provided with a known supply of antacid tablets (Maalox) to be taken as required for relief of pain. All other therapy for peptic ulcer was withdrawn for the four weeks of the trial. Each patient was provided with diary cards and kept a daily record of the number and severity of pain attacks occurring by day and night, the number of antacid tablets taken and any trial medication not taken. The patients were seen after each week of treatment while laboratory tests were performed before and at the end of the 4 weeks within 48 hours of stopping treatment. The response to treatment was assessed by endoscopy, by symptoms and by antacid consumption. Ulcer healing was defined as complete disappearance of all ulcers and erosions and replacement with either a scar or healthy normal mucosa. An erosion at the site of the original ulcer or in its immediate vicinity was taken as an indication of incomplete healing.

Blindness was assured by giving daily to the patients 6 identical-looking tablets in a blister and asking them to take two tablets after breakfast, one after lunch, one after dinner and two at bedtime. As can be seen from Figure 5.1 two of the

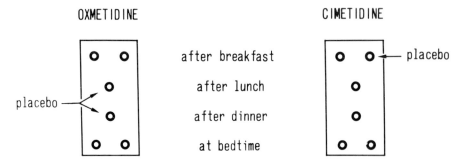

Figure 5.1 The manner in which blindness was maintained in this study.

tablets in the oxmetidine blister were placebo in comparison with only one of the six tablets in the cimetidine blister. So far, 52 of the 60 patients admitted to the study have completed the trial; the interim results presented here have been analysed by a researcher not taking part in the study, so that blindness is maintained.

The data were analysed using either Student's t test, the exact Fisher test, the U Mann–Whitney test or the Wilcoxon's matched-pairs signed-ranks test. P values less than 0.05 were considered significant.

RESULTS

The clinical details of the 52 patients who have completed the trial so far are shown in Table 5.1. The randomisation procedure successfully prevented significant differences between the two groups; in fact they have similar mean

Table 5.1 Clinical details of cimetidine and oxmetidine groups

	Cimetidine	Oxmetidine
Number	26	26
Mean age (years, range)	41.9 (21-68)	45.0 (23-66)
Sex (M/F)	23/3	23/3
Mean duration of disease (years, range)	6.9 (1-20)	11 (1-40)
Mean duration of current relapse (months, range)	1.35 (0-2)	1.57 (0-5)
Smoking history (number)	20	20
Alcohol consumption (number)	19	18
Ulcer type single	26	22
multiple	0	4

age, sex distribution, mean duration of current relapse, smoking history and alcohol consumption. The only difference, although not statistically significant, has been found in mean duration of the disease which appeared greater in the oxmetidine group.

The percentages of patients in each of the two treatment groups who showed complete healing of their ulcers are shown in Table 5.2. Complete healing was observed in 20 (77 per cent) of 26 patients on cimetidine and in 19 (73 per cent) of the 26 treated with oxmetidine. The difference between the two regimens was not significant.

Table 5.2 Endoscopic assessment of ulcer healing after four weeks in oxmetidine and cimetidine groups

Treatment	Total n	Healed $n(\%)$	Not healed $n (\%)$
Cimetidine	26	20 (77)	6 (23)
Oxmetidine	26	19 (73)	7 (27)

Symptomatic response was assessed by calculating the number of days and nights with pain and by quantity of antacid consumption. Mean number of days with pain per week sharply decreased during the first week of treatment especially in the cimetidine group, but there were still patients at the end of the trial with pain. The difference between the two groups was not statistically significant although the decrease between values prior to treatment and those found after 4 weeks appeared highly significant in both treatment groups ($P < 0.01$) (Figure 5.2).

A similar pattern was observed with mean number of nights with pain (Figure 5.2): an important decrease was seen during the first week of treatment but the difference between cimetidine and oxmetidine was not significant. However, in

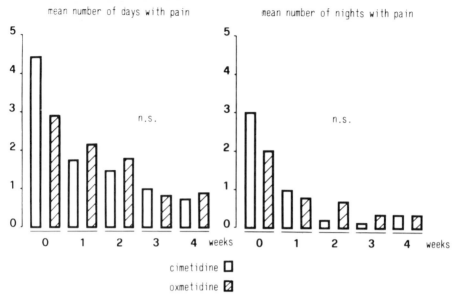

Figure 5.2   Mean number of days and nights with pain during the double-blind trial.

the two regimens the difference between values prior to treatment and those after completion of treatment appeared highly significant ($P < 0.01$).

As far as antacid consumption is concerned the mean consumption per week markedly decreased at the end of the trial in the cimetidine group ($P < 0.01$) but remained practically unchanged in the oxmetidine group; no statistically significant difference, however, was found between the two groups (Figure 5.3).

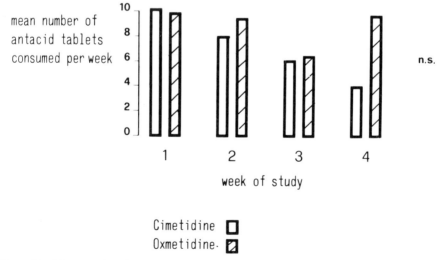

Figure 5.3   Mean number of antacid tablets consumed per week during the oxmetidine vs. cimetidine trial.

Figure 5.4 illustrates the patients' own assessment of their well-being (calculated by the score: 0 very good; 1 good; 2 fair; 3 bad).

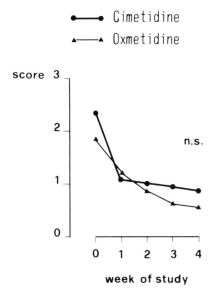

Figure 5.4   Assessment of well-being recorded by 52 patients.

A significant difference between the beginning and the end of treatment occurred with both cimetidine and oxmetidine ($P < 0.01$) but overall the two treatment groups did not differ.

Table 5.3 shows the relationship between ulcer healing and relief of pain. Pain was absent at the end of the trial in 14 out of the 20 patients healed on cimetidine and in 13 of the 19 who healed on oxmetidine. However, there were six patients in each group complaining of pain at the end of trial in spite of endoscopic confirmation of ulcer healing. Moreover there were three and two asymptomatic ulcers respectively in each of the two groups at the end of trial, showing again that factors other than ulcer healing are important for the relief of pain.

Table 5.3 Relationship between relief of pain and healing of ulcer. C = cimetidine, Ox = oxmetidine

		Ulcer			
		healed		not healed	
		No.	%	No.	%
Pain absent	C	14/20	70	3/6	50
	Ox	13/19	69	2/7	71
Pain present	C	6/20	30	3/6	50
	Ox	6/19	31	5/7	71

Eleven patients complained of mild side-effects (five on cimetidine and six on oxmetidine) ranging from headaches and insomnia to constipation, nausea, vomiting and weakness. However, all effects were temporary and did not prevent any patient continuing with treatment.

Biochemical and haematological profiles showed minimal rises in creatinine (three on cimetidine, four on oxmetidine), transaminases (six on cimetidine, one on oxmetidine), alkaline phosphatase (one on cimetidine, three on oxmetidine) and serum urea (one on cimetidine, two on oxmetidine). Moreover in the oxmetidine group one patient (not healed at the final endoscopy) was found to have high values of both transaminases, bilirubin and alkaline phosphatase at the end of the trial. The development of hepatitis was suspected and a liver biopsy performed. He was found to have chronic aggressive hepatitis without any sign of drug-related toxicity. He has been followed since then for nine months; his transaminases are still remarkably abnormal and Hb_cAg still positive, supporting the hypothesis that there is no association between treatment and development of hepatitis.

Serum gastrin and prolactin levels were compared before and after completing the trial (Table 5.4) and no consistent change with either treatment was noted.

Table 5.4 Serum gastrin and prolactin levels before and after four weeks of treatment

	Mean ± SD		
	Pre-treatment	Four weeks	
Serum prolactin (ng/ml): normal range <10 ng/ml			
Cimetidine	8.5 ± 3.4	9.4 ± 3.3	
			n.s.
Oxmetidine	8.5 ± 4.4	8.6 ± 4.6	
Serum gastrin (pg/ml): normal range <150 pg/ml			
Cimetidine	96.1 ± 43.2	98.3 ± 30.9	
			n.s.
Oxmetidine	75.7 ± 18.7	93.5 ± 38.1	

CONCLUSION

This study indicates that oxmetidine 400 mg b.d. and cimetidine 1 g daily in the short-term treatment of duodenal ulcer have similar efficacy with regard to ulcer healing, symptomatic pain relief and antacid consumption. After four weeks treatment changes in laboratory values, when present, were minimal and appeared to be clinically insignificant. In any case these changes are unlikely to limit the clinical application of oxmetidine. If the results of the present trial are confirmed by further studies, oxmetidine 400 mg b.d. might become a good candidate for the treatment of duodenal ulcer and an easier alternative to cimetidine. Such a simplified and more convenient regimen would probably lead to a gain in compliance, inducing the patient to take the drug more regularly.

In conclusion, the results of this trial show that oxmetidine, like ranitidine, is as effective as cimetidine clinically in the short-term management of duodenal ulcer. However, our experience with these newly developed H_2 blockers is too limited to allow any definite conclusion. As recently pointed out by Domschke and Domschke (1980) 'it remains to be seen whether in the long run they are actually more effective, easier to use, safer and, perhaps, less expensive than cimetidine'.

ACKNOWLEDGEMENT

This paper is dedicated to the memory of M. A. Melvin, whose friendship and co-operation made the work possible.

REFERENCES

Bardhan K D 1980 The short and medium term treatment of duodenal ulcer with cimetidine. In: Proceedings of an International Symposium on Recent Advances in Peptic Ulcer, Milan, 10-11 October 1980. Cortina Publications, Verona, in press

Bianchi Porro G, Dal Monte P R, Petrillo M, Giuliani Piccari G, D'Imperio N, Daniotti S 1981 Pirenzepine vs. cimetidine in duodenal ulcer. A double-blind placebo-controlled short-term clinical trial. Digestion, in press

Brunet P L, Hunt R H, Melvin M A, Mills J G, Sharpe P C, Milton-Thompson G J, Burland W L 1980 Comparison of the effects of SK&F 92994 and cimetidine on food stimulated gastric acid secretion. Hepatogastroenterology Suppl (XI Int. Congress of Gastroenterology), E.32.10

Burland W L, Brunet P L, Hunt R H, Melvin M A, Mills J G, Vincent D, Milton-Thompson G J 1980 Comparison of the effects on 24 h intragastric acidity of SK&F 92994 and 20 dose regimens of cimetidine. Hepatogastroenterology Suppl (XI Int. Congress of Gastroenterology) E.32.10

Domschke S, Domschke W 1980 New histamine H_2-receptor antagonists. Hepatogastroenterology 27: 163-168

Mills J G, Hunt R H, Burland W L, Milton-Thompson G J 1980 Impromidine as a gastric secretagogue in comparative studies with a new H_2-receptor antagonist (SK&F 92994). Hepatogastroenterology Suppl (XI Int. Congress of Gastroenterology) E.32.15

Misiewicz J J, Sewing K F R (eds) 1981 Proceedings of the first International Symposium on ranitidine, Hamburg 14 June 1980. Scandinavian Journal of Gastroenterology, suppl. 16, in press

Vantrappen G, Rutgeerts P, Broeckaert L, Janssens J 1980 Randomized open controlled trial of colloidal bismuth subcitrate tablets and cimetidine in the treatment of duodenal ulcer. Gut 21: 329, 333

6. Non-responders to cimetidine treatment, part 1

Richard H. Hunt

Royal Naval Hospital, Haslar, Gosport, Hants

Treatment with cimetidine 1 g/day for four to six weeks will heal 57 to 87 per cent of duodenal ulcers (Burland et al, 1979) while 25 to 40 per cent remain unhealed. In most cases of unhealed ulcer continued treatment with cimetidine ultimately results in healing but the pattern of relapse following cessation of treatment is predictable (Bardhan, 1980; Venables et al, 1978). The failure of ulcers to heal on cimetidine may be due to poor patient compliance, to an endoscopic underestimate of ulcer healing or to the fact that duodenal ulcer is a heterogeneous disease.

Failure to heal, early recurrence after treatment and frequent relapse are of great interest and clearly require further study. During 24-hour studies of intragastric acidity in duodenal ulcer patients treated with cimetidine 1 g/day two distinctive patterns of response have been observed during the overnight period.

METHOD

In the present study we have evaluated a variety of treatments for duodenal ulcer by measuring 24-hour intragastric acidity as described by Pounder et al (1976, 1977). 36 patients with endoscopically proven duodenal ulcers have been studied while in remission receiving either placebo or cimetidine 1 g/day randomly allocated and studied at least one week apart. The patients were unaware of the sequence of treatment. On both study days patients were fully ambulant with a 14Fr Salem sump nasogastric tube left in place, they ate identical meals, consumed the same volume of identical fluids, including beer, and smoked the same number of cigarettes on each study day. Each hour, 3 ml aliquots of gastric contents were aspirated and the hydrogen ion activity determined using a pH meter (Radiometer, Copenhagen). Continuous aspiration was performed by suction pump during the night between 0100 and 0700 and the total acid output for each individual hour calculated.

Six of the patients were studied again under identical conditions at least six months after undergoing proximal gastric vagotomy (PGV), to compare the results of medical treatment with those of surgery in the same individual.

RESULTS

In the 36 duodenal ulcer patients studied, cimetidine in the standard dosage of 1 g/day significantly reduced mean hydrogen ion activity from 38.48 to 18.96 mmol/l (51 per cent) over the whole 24-hour period, while overnight the reduction was from a mean of 49.24 mmol/l to 19.05 mmol/l (61.3 per cent) (Figure 6.1).

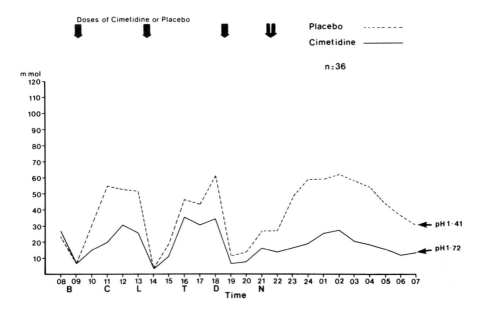

Figure 6.1   The pattern of 24-hour intragastric hydrogen ion activity in 36 patients with duodenal ulcer while taking placebo or cimetidine 200 mg tds and 400 mg nocte. The timing of breakfast, coffee, lunch, tea, dinner and the nightcap are shown. The mean pH is shown on the right.

When these data are looked at for each individual there appear to be two patterns of response, with patients falling clearly into one group or the other. These differences, however, are only apparent overnight and represent either a dramatic response to cimetidine, the patient becoming anacidic (Figure 6.2) or in contrast almost no reduction in acidity (Figure 6.3).

Computer analysis (Hewlett Packard 9845A) confirms this clear separation into two groups during the night-time period. We have chosen to determine an arbitrary separation at 0300 when patients with an intragastric acidity below 5 mmol/l have been declared 'responders' and those above 5 mmol/l 'non-responders', because a natural separation occurs when using this criterion (Table 6.1).

Out of the 36 duodenal ulcer patients there were 19 'responders', 17 of whom had an intragastric hydrogen ion activity of 0 mmol/l at 0300, one of 0.1 mmol/l and one of 4 mmol/l. In contrast the 'non-responders' were all above 11.5

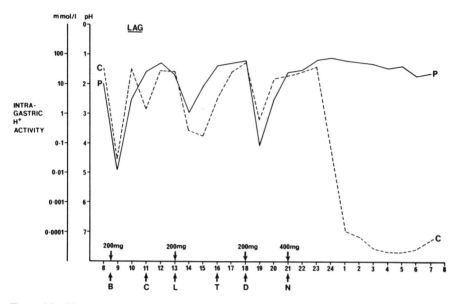

Figure 6.2   The pattern of 24-hour intragastric hydrogen ion activity in a patient who shows a dramatic overnight response to cimetidine treatment. C = cimetidine; P = placebo.

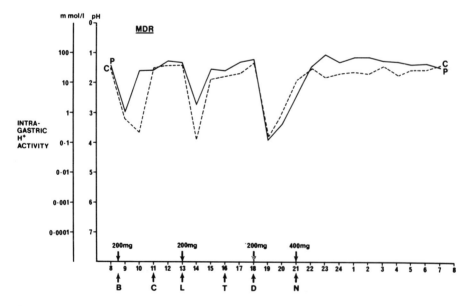

Figure 6.3   The pattern of 24-hour intragastric hydrogen ion activity in a patient who shows almost no response to cimetidine treatment. C = cimetidine; P = placebo.

mmol/l at 0300 (range 11.5–147.0) (Table 6.1). The difference between these two groups was highly significant overnight ($P < 0.001$) (Mann Whitney U test) but not during the daytime.

Table 6.1 Intragastric hydrogen ion activity at 0300 in 36 duodenal ulcer patients treated with cimetidine.

Values below 5 mmol/l ('responders')			Values above 5 mmol/l ('non-responders')		
No.	Name	Value	No.	Name	Value
101	L.A.G.	0	116	M.B.	49
102	M.J.T.	4	117	H.J.D.	43.7
103	B.W.S.	0	118	J.H.	39.8
104	B.C.	0	119	K.R.	35.5
105	H.M.	0.1	120	L.L.M.	55
106	M.H.	0	121	J.D.B.	66.1
107	M.G.	0	122	R.T.	15.1
108	F.T.	0	123	W.T.	50.1
109	F.C.B.	0	124	J.F.	50.12
110	C.D.	0	125	R.M.	17
111	J.A.	0	126	M.R.	11.5
112	K.T.	0	127	B.S.	33.1
113	R.H.	0	132	T.G.	20.9
114	R.F.	0	133	M.L.	26.9
115	G.C.	0	134	M.P.	43.7
128	A.P.C.	0	135	A.G.	50.1
129	G.G.	0	136	R.R.	120.23
130	S.N.	0	137	T.M.	141.25
131	C.E.F.	0	138	B.B.	109.65
			139	J.S.W.	45.71
			140	R.C.	27.54

Analysis of the placebo intragastric hydrogen ion activity for these two groups showed no significant difference during the day but the difference overnight was statistically significant ($P < 0.05$) (Mann Whitney U test) (Figure 6.4).

Six of the patients studied were subsequently operated on for chronic duodenal ulcer and all had a proximal gastric vagotomy. The study was repeated on these six patients not less than six months postoperatively using an identical protocol and diet to the previous study.

In this subgroup of six patients cimetidine reduced mean 24-hour intragastric acidity from 30.75 to 14.11 mmol/l (54.1 per cent) ($P < 0.001$) and nocturnal acidity from 40.6 to 17.3 mmol/l (57.4 per cent) ($P < 0.001$). After PGV all patients were classified as Visick grades I or II and the operation reduced mean 24-hour acidity to 6.25 mmol/l (79.7 per cent).

Three of the six patients operated on had, in the preoperative study, fulfilled our criteria for 'responders' (cimetidine reduced mean nocturnal acidity by 84 per cent) and three were classified as 'non-responders' (with a mean reduction of 46 per cent). Postoperatively there was no significant difference between these two groups in terms of overnight acid output (Figure 6.5).

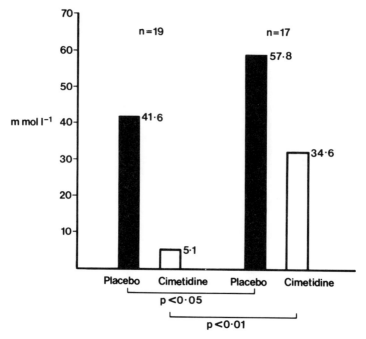

Figure 6.4 The mean nocturnal hydrogen ion activity between 0100 and 0700 showing the two patterns of response.

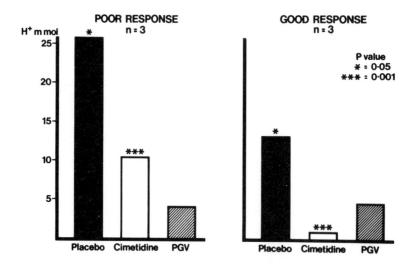

Figure 6.5 The mean nocturnal acid output (0100-0700) in the six patients who underwent PGV showing their response to cimetidine and operation. The results are plotted to show the 'responder' and 'non-responder' groups.

DISCUSSION

The observed variation in response to cimetidine treatment is not easy to explain. Although the patterns of response may represent extremes of the normal spectrum this seems unlikely from the marked separation into two groups which we have observed.

A review of the patient age and sex, medical history, family history, duration of disease, smoking and drinking habits and endoscopic findings showed no differences between the two groups.

The possibility that absorption of cimetidine was either delayed or reduced might account for the lack of inhibition in the 'non-responder' group. An earlier study with metiamide (Milton Thompson et al, 1974) showed that in three patients in whom 59 mg or more metiamide ($<$ 15 per cent of the ingested dose) was recovered from the stomach one hour after administration of a 400 mg dose the pH remained below 7.0 throughout the test, and in one of these patients there was no response to the drug. The remaining eight patients in this study all had residual metiamide of less than 13.5 mg ($<$ 3.4 per cent of the ingested dose) and all became anacidic. These earlier data seemed to suggest that blood levels of cimetidine might be lower in the 'non-responders'. However, preliminary data on overnight cimetidine blood levels in five of seven 'non-responders' whom we are studying prospectively (see below) show that the mean plasma levels for the group as a whole and each individual separately follow the normal absorption pattern after a 400 mg dose of cimetidine (Bodemar et al, 1979).

Although patients with duodenal ulcer tend to have accelerated gastric emptying, prolonged recurrent ulceration of the duodenum may lead to scarring, distortion and stenosis with subsequent delay in gastric emptying. This might explain the findings of Milton-Thompson et al (1974) but does not appear to explain our own findings where blood levels of cimetidine were normal and there were no differences in the length of history, severity of the disease, endoscopic findings, etc.

Two interesting observations which relate to the response of duodenal ulcer patients to cimetidine have been made recently. Venables et al (1978) using the combined pentagastrin/insulin (PG/I) test observed a significant difference in the PG/I maximal acid output ratio between those patients who heal their duodenal ulcer on cimetidine and those who do not. This led them to suggest that the higher pentagastrin response might represent a greater parietal cell mass in those patients with poor healing but they concluded that their observations required further study. Maybury and Carr-Locke (1980) performed an insulin test in 21 duodenal ulcer patients two weeks after starting cimetidine treatment at the standard dosage of 1 g/day. In 13 patients secretion fell within the range established in previously untreated duodenal ulcer and these were predicted to have a high risk of relapse. Those whose secretion was below this range were predicted to have a low risk of relapse. Endoscopic follow-up between 20 and 23 months showed that the probability of predicting relapse using the insulin test in this way was significant ($P < 0.0225$).

In an attempt to apply these observations to our own results we have instituted a prospective study in duodenal ulcer patients using the following clinical criteria for non-response to cimetidine:

1. Failure to respond to treatment with cimetidine 1 g/day.
2. Early relapse after treatment with cimetidine 1 g/day.
3. More than three active duodenal ulcer episodes per year.

Investigations include a history and physical assessment, 24-hour intragastric acidity studies and overnight secretion, overnight cimetidine blood levels, pentagastrin and insulin tests and combined gastric emptying and integrated gastrin response.

To date (March 1981) seven duodenal ulcer patients who have fulfilled the criteria have been studied. All fit clearly into the group designated 'non-responders' using our criteria and have a mean overnight intragastric hydrogen ion activity of 51.9 mmol/l while taking placebo and 49.2 mmol/l while taking cimetidine 1 g/day. The preliminary results of overnight plasma cimetidine levels have already been discussed, but other results are not yet available.

SUMMARY

The pattern of response to standard cimetidine treatment, in terms of reduction of intragastric acidity for patients with duodenal ulcer, seems to separate into two distinct groups during the overnight period. This difference is apparently abolished by proximal gastric vagotomy, and from preliminary studies appears to be related to clinical failure to respond to cimetidine. Blood levels of the drug in the 'non-responders' appear to lie within the normal range and do not explain the observation.

ACKNOWLEDGEMENTS

I am grateful to the Departments of Medical Illustration and Clinical Photography, RNH Haslar, for supplying the illustrations and Miss J. Thompson for typing the manuscript.

REFERENCES

Bardhan K D 1980 Intermittent treatment of duodenal ulcer with cimetidine. British Medical Journal 11: 20-22
Bodemar G, Norlander B, Transson L, Walen A 1979 The absorption of cimetidine before and during maintenance treatment with cimetidine and the influence of a meal on the absorption of cimetidine — studies in patients with peptic ulcer disease. British Journal of Clinical Pharmacology 7: 23-31
Burland W L, Hunt R H, Mills J G, Milton-Thompson G J 1979 Drugs of the decade 1970-79: cimetidine. British Journal of Pharmacotherapy 2: 24-40
Maybury N K, Carr-Locke D L 1980 The value of the new interpretation of the insulin test in predicting duodenal ulcer relapse after treatment with cimetidine. British Journal of Surgery 67: 315-317

Milton-Thompson G J, Williams J G, Jenkins D J A, Misiewicz J J 1974 Inhibition of nocturnal acid secretion in duodenal ulcer by one oral dose of metiamide. Lancet i: 693-694

Pounder R E, Williams J G, Milton-Thompson G J, Misiewicz J J 1976 Effect of cimetidine on 24 hour intragastric acidity in normal subjects. Gut 17: 133-138

Pounder R E, Williams J G, Hunt R H, Vincent S H, Milton-Thompson G J, Misiewicz J J 1977 The effects of oral cimetidine in food stimulated gastric acid secretion and 24 hour intragastric acidity. In: Burland W L, Simkins M A (eds) Cimetidine: Proceedings of the Second International Symposium on histamine H_2 receptor antagonists. Excerpta Medica, Amsterdam, p 189-204.

Venables C W, Stephen J G, Blaire E L, Reed J D, Saunders J D 1978 Cimetidine in the treatment of duodenal ulceration and the relationship of this therapy to surgical management. In: Wastell C, Lance P (eds) Cimetidine: The Westminster Hospital Symposium. Churchill Livingstone, Edinburgh, p 13-27.

7. Non-responders to cimetidine treatment, part 2

K. D. Bardhan

Rotherham District General Hospital, Rotherham

Cimetidine markedly increases duodenal ulcer healing. Pooling the results of 32 double-blind placebo-controlled trials, in a four to six-week period on average 76 per cent of patients on cimetidine healed (693 of 913 patients) compared with only 38 per cent of those on placebo (313 of 830 patients) (for references see Bardhan, 1981). But why do some patients take longer than others to heal? Why do some patients not heal at all? The purpose of this report is to summarise evidence from the literature on this topic and to provide some personal views.

HEALING ON CIMETIDINE AND ON OTHER DRUGS

The majority of duodenal ulcers are thought to heal spontaneously if given enough time. Therefore the principal effect of cimetidine, apart from rapidly relieving symptoms, is to accelerate the healing process. To determine the value of the drug, assessment needs to be made at a time when the difference in healing produced by the drug when compared with placebo is maximal; this time is influenced by the natural history of the disease in the population studied. Thus in Switzerland, where spontaneous healing is rapid, cimetidine does not produce a significantly greater healing than placebo at four weeks (Peter et al, 1978). In the USA spontaneous healing is also rapid; the difference in healing produced by cimetidine when compared with placebo is significant only at two weeks but not at 4 weeks and at 6 weeks (Binder et al, 1978; Collen et al, 1980) (Figure 7.1). In contrast, in other populations where spontaneous healing is slower, the difference in healing produced by cimetidine and by placebo is significant at 4, 6 and 8 weeks and also at 12 weeks (see Bardhan, 1978). Little information is available on healing assessed over longer periods because in most studies those who did not heal after some time on placebo were treated with active drug for ethical reasons. Therefore, it follows that when assessment of healing is made after a short course of treatment, a proportion of patients will be found not to have healed. This is true whether the treatment is with cimetidine or with any of the several agents now shown to be effective in healing duodenal ulcer (for references see Bardhan, 1981; Lenghel et al, 1980; Moshal et al, 1980).

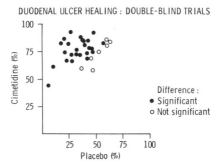

Figure 7.1   Ulcer healing in 32 double-blind short-term trials comparing cimetidine against placebo. Reproduced with the permission of the Editor of *Tropical Gastroenterology*. The original figure was based on 31 studies (for references see Bardhan, 1981). The present figure includes data from an additional study (Collen et al, 1980).

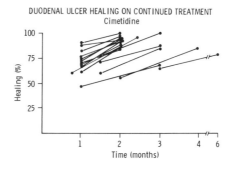

Figure 7.2   The outcome of continuing cimetidine treatment when the ulcer has not healed after a short course. The results of each study are indicated by a pair of closed circles connected by a line. The first circle indicates the time of initial assessment — generally at 1 month or 6 weeks. The second circle indicates the time of final assessment — generally at 2 or 3 months. In every instance healing increased with continued treatment. Reproduced with the permission of the Editor of *Tropical Gastroenterology* (for references see Bardhan, 1981). Data from three further studies are included in this figure (Becker et al, 1980; Martin et al, 1980; Martin et al, 1981).

However, when treatment was continued, the proportion of patients healed also increased; this is a feature not just of cimetidine but of other anti-ulcer drugs (Figures 7.3, 7.4). Once the right conditions are established, healing proceeds at a certain rate, the majority of patients healing quickly but a minority taking a longer time. This is true irrespective of the method by which ulcer healing is produced — whether through reduction of acid by the H_2 receptor antagonists or with antacids, or by providing a 'mucosal seal' with colloidal bismuth or with sucralfate, or by increasing 'mucosal defence' with carbenoxolone. In other words, this is a phenomenon of the healing process and is not specific for any drug.

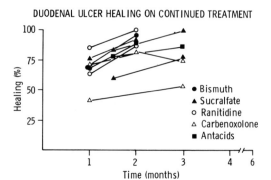

DUODENAL ULCER HEALING ON CONTINUED TREATMENT

Figure 7.3. The outcome of continuing treatment when the ulcer has not healed after a short course. The different symbols represent the various drugs used. The results of each study are indicated by a pair of symbols connected by a line. The first of each pair shows the time of initial assessment of ulcer healing: generally 1 month or 6 weeks. The second of each pair shows the time of final assessment: generally at 2 or 3 months. In every instance, irrespective of the drug used, healing increased with continued treatment. Reproduced with the permission of the Editor of *Tropical Gastroenterology*. Data from two other studies have now been added (Martin et al, 1980; Martin et al, 1981).

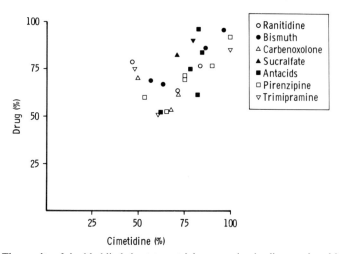

DUODENAL ULCER HEALING : DOUBLE-BLIND TRIALS

Figure 7.4 The results of double-blind short-term trials comparing healing produced by cimetidine with that produced by other drugs. With the permission of the Editor of *Tropical Gastroenterology*. Data from another study have now been included (Martin et al, 1981).

To study this matter further, the rate of healing needs to be measured. This has been done at endoscopy using a special probe which is passed down the biopsy channel. The last 2 cm or so is graduated and is at a right angle to the remainder of the probe. However, being very flexible it can be passed down the biopsy channel and when it protrudes at the distal end, it can be held against the ulcer and measurements taken. In one study, the spontaneous rate of healing in 30 patients with gastric ulcer and 15 patients with duodenal ulcer was examined

(Scheurer et al, 1977). Healing was found to be exponential; by logarithmic transformation, the curve could be converted into a straight line from which the ulcer half-life could be determined. The investigator suggested that measuring this index could become important in therapeutic trials as it did not rely on the precise time taken for an ulcer to heal completely. Furthermore, as it occurred early, presumably the effect of a drug could be assessed at an early stage. These investigators also showed that the rate of healing of duodenal and gastric ulcers was similar (half-life 1.9 weeks and 1.7 weeks respectively); that gastric ulcers took longer to heal because they were generally larger to start with; and that small duodenal ulcers took less time to heal than larger lesions. This method has been applied in a double-blind study on the effect of cimetidine on duodenal ulcer healing. The average half-life for healing on placebo in 6 patients was 20 days, whereas on cimetidine, in another 6 patients, it was only 6 days (Domschke et al, 1977).

However, I have some reservations about the method and these conclusions. First, accurate endoscopic measurement of ulcer size is not easy; it is common experience that the full extent of the ulcer may not be seen or it may be difficult to view the lesion face-on to allow such measurements to be made. When conditions are ideal, quite accurate measurements of the diameter of round ulcers can be made; it is more difficult in ulcers which have an irregular outline. To study only those lesions that can be measured accurately and to exclude the others might introduce a bias. The depth of the ulcer has not been measured and it is possible that this might have some influence on the rate of healing. Despite these problems, the inter-observer variation was remarkably low — only ± 13 per cent (Scheurer et al, 1977). The difficulties in measurement have been highlighted by another study from Switzerland (Sonnenberg et al, 1979). New technical developments have been made by a group in West Germany which will allow more accurate measurements to be made (Dancygier et al, 1980).

Second, do all ulcers heal exponentially? If so, even on cimetidine, ulcers would take a long time to heal and the initial size would be the principal determinant of the healing time. Yet it is common clinical experience that large ulcers may heal more rapidly than tiny ones; this cannot be explained by healing following an exponential course. Further experimental studies in pigs made by the original Swiss group have shown that surgical defects in the stomach did not heal quite in an exponential fashion and that hyperacidity produced by histamine slowed healing. Though these lesions are not the same as peptic ulcers, they do yield some information on re-epithelialisation rates (Halter et al, 1980).

WHY DO SOME ULCERS FAIL TO HEAL RAPIDLY?

In fact the majority of those patients whose ulcers do not heal within four to six weeks will do so when treatment is extended for three or four months. There are several reasons why healing may be 'delayed'.

1. *Semantics.* In most studies on ulcer healing, because of the difficulty in determining the rate of ulcer healing, the end point chosen is complete disappearance of all ulcers and erosions. In the majority of patients with apparent 'delayed healing', the healing process has started and may be nearly complete — most patients are asymptomatic. However, if a tiny ulcer remnant or erosion persists, it is classed as 'not-healed'.

2. *Non-compliance.* As the majority are asymptomatic well before the ulcer heals, the urge to take treatment regularly lessens. This is a well recognised problem and is widespread but there is no ready means to determine its extent and the part it plays in delayed healing. Measuring blood levels of cimetidine gives only a rough guide and unless done as a 'spot-check' does not have much value for it is quite possible that the patient may have taken his tablets regularly just for a day or two before attending the clinic on an appointed day. The usual method is to count the number of tablets returned but again there are potential sources of error here.

3. *'Slow healers'.* Some patients are 'slow-healers'. I have observed that on each occasion they are treated, they take two to three months to heal.

Rare causes of 'resistance to cimetidine'
Patients with the Zollinger–Ellison syndrome are not uncommonly resistant to standard doses of cimetidine. In 1978, the outcome of treatment of 61 patients in the USA was reported. They had all been on cimetidine for a minimum of seven months; over half had been treated for 18 months or longer; nine patients had originally been treated with metiamide and then changed to cimetidine, the total duration of treatment with H_2 antagonists being about three years. Forty of the patients were adequately controlled with cimetidine at a standard dose of 1.2 g daily (in the USA the cimetidine tablets are of 300 mg strength and the standard dose is 1.2 g daily, whereas in the UK the tablets are of 200 mg strength and the standard dose is 1 g daily). Other patients required higher daily doses: 1.5 g in four; 1.8 g in six; 2.2 g in four; and 2.4 g in two. Five patients needed a combination of cimetidine 1.5 g daily as well as an anticholinergic (McCarthy, 1978; McCarthy et al, 1978).

The Danish experience is similar. Fifteen patients were treated for a mean of 10.7 months. Thirteen had been started on cimetidine 1 g daily and two on 1.2 g daily. In one patient the dose had to be increased to 1.2 g; in three patients to 1.4 g; in two patients to 1.6 g and in one patient to 3 g (Stadil and Stage, 1978).

In the UK, Smith Kline and French hold a registry for patients with Zollinger–Ellison syndrome. At the time of writing, 34 patients have been registered of whom three have died. Five patients have no treatment and one is on a combination of an anticholinergic and carbenoxolone; the remainder are on H_2 antagonists. Fifteen patients are on a fixed dose of cimetidine: eight patients on 1 g daily; two patients on 1.6 g daily; three patients on 2 g daily; one patient on 3 g and another patient on 4.8 g daily. A further 11 patients have been on variable doses of cimetidine ranging from 0.4 g to 3 g daily. Details of one patient have not been printed.

Similar observations were made in France. In one study, the combination of cimetidine and the anti-muscarinic agent pirenzipine controlled the acid hypersecretion while cimetidine on its own failed (Mignon et al, 1980a). In another study, cimetidine 2.4 g did not control the hypersecretion but the new H_2 receptor antagonist ranitidine at a dose of 600 mg daily (which is twice the dose required to heal duodenal ulcers) was very effective (Mignon et al, 1980b).

In the USA the combination of vagotomy and cimetidine has been found to be helpful: the operation reduces acid secretion and then standard doses of cimetidine reduce it still further (Richardson et al, 1979). This is in marked contrast to the practice in the days before cimetidine was available: total gastrectomy was the treatment of choice; any less drastic operation was unsuccessful and resulted eventually in increased mortality (Bonfils et al, 1979; Fairclough, 1980; McCarthy, 1980; Marshall and Settles, 1980).

My own experience of Zollinger–Ellison syndrome is limited to only three patients; all were refractory to standard doses of cimetidine. (These are included in the Zollinger–Ellison registry mentioned above.) One patient died of tumour metastases 18 months after the diagnosis had been made. Shortly before he died, he was on cimetidine 3 g daily. The other two patients have been on treatment for almost five years and are well; however, they each need cimetidine 3 g and 250 ml of a potent antacid daily to keep their ulcers healed.

There has been one report so far of a patient with hyperparathyroidism and associated duodenal ulcer whose gastric secretion was resistant to cimetidine (McCarthy et al, 1979). Since then there have been reports that cimetidine can actually reverse hyperparathyroidism (Sherwood et al, 1980 a and b) or reduce parathormone levels or calcium levels in uraemic patients on dialysis (Jacob et al, 1980; Lanier et al, 1980).

However, there are several other reports which show that cimetidine has no effect in hyperparathyroidism (Awoke and Lawrence, 1980; Graziani et al, 1980; Heath, 1980; Ljunghall et al, 1980; Pettengell and Grayson, 1980; Robinson et al, 1980; Vanherweghem et al, 1980).

WHY DOES THE ULCER HEALING RATE VARY?

Virtually nothing is known about this. It has been suggested that the variability of inhibition of acid secretion might play a part. Acid secretion does vary markedly from patient to patient and it is therefore possible that the degree of inhibition will also vary (Baron et al, 1980). This is supported by the finding from Denmark of marked individual variation in the sensitivity to cimetidine. Following a standard dose of cimetidine, plasma levels were found to vary considerably; furthermore, these levels were not accurately reflected by the degree of acid inhibition which also varied markedly. Healing also appeared to occur more slowly in those with high acid secretion but with a low sensitivity to cimetidine (Rune et al, 1979).

In a study from the USA on critically ill patients, cimetidine was given to prevent stress ulceration. A poor correlation was observed between blood levels of the drug and acid inhibition achieved (Cohen et al, 1980). However, circumstances here are rather different from those seen when dealing with the usual ulcer patient and may have had some bearing on these observations.

These findings are in marked contrast to those made by other investigators. Earlier, in the UK, it had been shown that the dose of cimetidine given bore a close relation to the blood levels achieved and that this in turn was closely related to the degree of acid inhibition produced (Pounder et al, 1977). The study from Sweden has shown that the mean blood concentration of cimetidine required to halve pentagastrin-stimulated acid secretion (IC_{50}) was $1.0\,\mu g/ml$ and that on a standard dose of cimetidine of 200 mg 3 times daily and 400 mg at bedtime, this level is maintained for one-third of the day and through the night. There was no development of tolerance to cimetidine: over a year, the blood levels remained constant and continued to inhibit acid effectively. The plasma concentration curves after single doses of cimetidine were also examined. The mean area-under-the-curve following a single 800 mg dose was 2.14 times greater than that after a 400 mg dose and this in turn was 2.05 times greater than that achieved after a 200 mg dose (Bodemar et al, 1979). Similar findings were observed in a study from Holland (Festen et al, 1980). In a study from Scotland, which was unusual in that after three months on cimetidine only 65 per cent of the patients healed and at six months the healing was still only 79 per cent, simultaneous pharmacological studies showed that differences in clinical and endoscopic response to cimetidine could not be explained by differences in the pharmacokinetics between patients (Webster et al, 1980).

Other evidence, albeit indirect, seems to me to argue against differences in acid inhibition being the principal cause of variations in healing rates. First, in my experience, with the exception of those patients who are 'slow-healers' the rate of healing often varies in the same individual at different times. Second, cimetidine in daily doses between 0.8 and 2.0 g produces similar healing rates, i.e. the greater acid inhibition produced by the higher doses does not improve the therapeutic response (see Bardhan, 1978). Third, irrespective of the method by which a drug heals an ulcer, the proportions healed are similar, and no particular method has, in studies of sufficient size, resulted in healing in all patients in four to six weeks. Fourth, even in the same centre, the healing rate varies at different times (Cargill et al, 1978; Saunders et al, 1980). To me these observations suggest that once the balance between the attacking factors and mucosal defence is re-established, irrespective of method, healing starts and proceeds at a rate which varies between different individuals and in the same person at different times. In some individuals delayed healing may well be due to inadequate suppression of acid: however, in the majority, delayed healing seems to be more a part of the wide spectrum of ulcer healing rather than due to inadequate acid inhibition.

WHAT FACTORS INFLUENCE ULCER HEALING?

The factors examined have been age, sex, duration of history, smoking, drinking, bed-rest, ulcer morphology and gastric secretion. The evidence is conflicting and confusing.

Age

Three groups of investigators, one from the USA and two from Britain, found that the age of the patient has no bearing on ulcer healing (Binder et al, 1978; Wyllie, 1978; Martin et al, 1981). In contrast in Scotland it was found that healing in those patients whose symptoms started later in life was more frequent than in those whose disease started early (Hasan and Sircus, 1980); precisely the opposite has been found in Hong Kong (Shiu et al, 1979).

Sex

Most groups have found that this has little bearing, though in a study from Hong Kong healing was greater in men (Shiu et al, 1979). However, very recently data from Scotland have shown that whereas in 1975/1977 healing in men and women was similar (90 and 83 per cent at one month), in 1979/1980 healing in women was considerably less (79 and 52 per cent respectively) (Peden et al, 1981).

Duration of history

All three possibilities have been observed: in Britain it had no effect (Wyllie, 1978; Martin et al, 1981); in the USA, a long history was associated with reduced healing (Binder et al, 1978); in Hong Kong a long history favoured healing (Shiu et al, 1979).

Smoking

It was demonstrated several years ago that smoking retarded gastric ulcer healing and it has been suspected to interfere with duodenal ulcer healing as well. However, there was no firm evidence to support this. In studies on cimetidine and other anti-ulcer drugs the smoking habits of patients are commonly recorded. Some investigators found that healing was less in those who smoked (Shiu et al, 1979; Hasan and Sircus, 1980); however, others did not observe such an effect (Wyllie, 1978; Barbara et al, 1979; Cowen et al, 1980; Martin et al, 1981). A different approach was used in a recent study: at the outset, the patients were divided into smokers and non-smokers. Members of both groups were then randomly allocated to receive treatment with either antacids in large doses, or cimetidine. Amongst smokers, healing on antacids and on cimetidine was only 38 and 50 per cent respectively, whereas amongst non-smokers the corresponding figures were significantly higher: 80 and 100 per cent (Shaw et al, 1980). The mechanism by which smoking might interfere with ulcer healing remains unknown. There is evidence to show that in duodenal ulcer patients smoking might aggravate acid hypersecretion and has been demonstrated to increase the amount of pepsin 1 in the gastric juice (Walker and Taylor, 1979; Whitfield and Hobsley, 1979); however, it remains to be demonstrated whether these changes interfere with ulcer healing.

Drinking

There is no evidence that drinking influences ulcer healing (Wyllie, 1978; Martin et al, 1981). However, the evidence is indirect. To prove the point, formal studies would be required in which at the outset the patients would need to be divided into those who do drink and those who do not, and then treatment randomly allocated to patients in both groups.

Bed-rest

It is known that bed-rest increases gastric ulcer healing: it is also a common clinical observation that when patients with troublesome duodenal ulcer are put to bed, symptomatic improvement frequently follows. It is therefore presumed that this beneficial effect is perhaps because bed-rest increases ulcer healing. The matter has not been investigated directly but indirect evidence from two cimetidine studies on inpatients suggests that bed-rest might increase ulcer healing.

In the study from the USA, healing amongst inpatients after one week was: cimetidine, 35 per cent, placebo 24 per cent. Amongst three groups treated as outpatients, the corresponding values after one week's treatment were: 25 and 20 per cent, 32 and 22 per cent, 11 and 6 per cent, respectively. After treatment for two weeks, the inpatient group healing had increased: cimetidine, 56 per cent, placebo, 37 per cent. Only one out of the three groups treated as outpatients was assessed at this time: the healing was 46 and 26 per cent respectively. The data suggest that after two weeks (but not after one week) a higher proportion of inpatients heal both on cimetidine and on placebo than outpatients but it is difficult to know if this difference is entirely due to bed-rest (Binder et al, 1978). In a study from Germany, at two weeks the healing was significantly different: cimetidine, 49 per cent, placebo, 21 per cent. By four weeks, there was a marked increase in healing, particularly amongst those on placebo, so that the difference was no longer significant: cimetidine, 88 per cent, placebo, 79 per cent (Malchow et al, 1978).

A high spontaneous healing rate has been demonstrated amongst outpatients in some studies but not quite this high: it is therefore quite possible that the high healing rate in these two studies might at least in part be due to bed-rest.

Ulcer morphology

There is no difference in healing in those with single and multiple ulcers (Wyllie, 1978). Ulcers are said to heal by re-epithelialisation; therefore small ulcers should heal more quickly than larger ones. This has been observed to be the case by some investigators (Scheurer et al, 1977).

However, it is common clinical experience, as mentioned earlier, that the reverse is often observed; this has been confirmed in studies which have shown that the size of the ulcer has no bearing on the time taken to heal (Lenghel et al, 1980). In an earlier study from Japan, the shape of the ulcers was found to have a considerable bearing on the spontaneous healing rate. Single round ulcers healed quickly: 60 per cent in one month, and 76 per cent in two months. Irregular ulcers healed more slowly: 20 per cent in one month and 40 per cent in three months; and multiple ulcers healed about as slowly: 18 per cent in one month and 30 per cent in two months. But linear ulcers healed very slowly: only 7 per cent in one month and only 15 per cent at three months (Kohli et al, 1972).

In a more recent study on ulcer morphology, from Italy, the size and depth of the ulcers were found not to be the main determinant of healing rate: medium-sized ulcers were found to heal more quickly than large or small ulcers. As with the Japanese investigation, round and oval ulcers healed more quickly than linear ulcers. It is rather surprising that this should be the case for the area to be re-epithelialised in linear ulcers is generally very small. Also, cimetidine increased healing in ulcers in the mid-bulb rather than those close to the pylorus, and in ulcers located on the antero-superior wall rather than in the postero-inferior wall (Nava et al, 1979). These findings are unexpected; it suggests that the shape of the ulcer and its location are not chance occurrences without importance but they might affect the outcome. It would be interesting to know if the presence or absence of erosions had any bearing on healing; also, whether ulcers recurred in the same location or in different ones and whether this had any bearing on the rate of healing.

Gastric secretion
As expected, much emphasis has been placed on correlating acid secretion with rates of ulcer healing but no firm conclusion has emerged. Hypersecretion has been found to hinder healing in a Scottish population and to favour it in a Chinese one (Shiu et al, 1979; Hasan and Sircus, 1980). But others have observed that high pre-treatment acid secretion can be associated with delayed healing. In a study from Australia, of those patients who did not heal rapidly on cimetidine, several had higher basal and maximal acid secretion compared with those who did heal quickly (Hetzel et al, 1978). In the study from the USA, amongst outpatients maximal acid secretion was higher in the slow healers and lower in the rapid healers, albeit the basal secretion was similar in both groups. But the differences were not seen in the inpatients who as a group had a lower maximal secretion than outpatients (Binder et al, 1978).

In another study from Newcastle (UK) combined pentagastrin–insulin stimulation secretion tests were carried out and the output of acid and pepsin measured. Of 42 patients who were then treated with cimetidine, seven did not heal in 28 days. However, the output of acid and pepsin in response both to pentagastrin and to insulin was similar in those who did heal and in those who did not. The only difference found was in the ratio of acid secreted in response to pentagastrin compared with insulin: amongst the non-healers, this ratio was higher, i.e. those who failed to heal had a greater acid output when stimulated by pentagastrin than after vagal stimulation by insulin. However, the number of patients studied was small and the significance of this finding remains unexplained (Venables et al, 1978).

A different approach has been to examine whether the degree of acid inhibition produced by cimetidine has any predictive value or not. In a study from Haslar (UK) the reduction of nocturnal acidity in response to cimetidine was studied and found to fall into two groups. In 19 of 31 patients, the mean reduction was 88 per cent whilst in the remainder it was only 45 per cent. However, this did not correlate with ulcer healing (Hunt et al, 1980a). As mentioned earlier, in a study from Denmark, the blood levels of cimetidine and the degree of acid inhibition were compared. In those with a high acid secretion but with a low sensitivity to cimetidine, there was a suggestion that healing occurred more slowly (Rune et al, 1979).

In Leicester (UK) the volume of gastric secretion in response to insulin was measured after the patients had been on cimetidine for two weeks; treatment was then continued. Corrections were made for pyloric losses by using a marker; this step increases the discriminant value of the test when used to assess the completeness of vagotomy and, unlike the standard insulin test, it is the volume rather than the acid concentration of the gastric juice that is measured. Of 21 patients, in 8 cimetidine markedly suppressed secretion but in 13 it failed to do so. After four weeks treatment, four patients did not heal of whom in three cimetidine had failed to suppress secretion. It was therefore suggested that such a measure could be used to predict a slow healing response. However, this argument is considerably weakened by the fact that in the other 10 patients whose secretion was not adequately suppressed with cimetidine, ulcer healing occurred as quickly as it did in seven of the eight patients in whom secretion was suppressed (Maybury and Carr-Locke, 1980). (This test has given better results when used to predict those who are likely to relapse.)

In summary, acid secretion tends to be statistically higher in those who do not heal rapidly but the correlation is not a close one. Therefore, the measurement of basal or maximal acid secretion, or the assessment of inhibition by cimetidine, is unlikely to be of use in predicting healing rates in individual patients. The exception may be those who turn out to have a refractory ulcer; it remains to be seen whether the degree of acid inhibition produced by cimetidine in such patients is reduced or not (see below).

REFRACTORY ULCER: PERSONAL EXPERIENCE

In Rotherham, of 230 patients treated between September 1977 and March 1979, 80 per cent healed in one month. In 1980, of 245 patients, the cumulative healing at 1.5 months was 82 per cent; at two months 83 per cent; at 2.5 months, 92 per cent; and at three months 93 per cent, i.e. a small minority do not heal within three months. I have therefore defined a patient with a refractory ulcer as one that does not heal completely on cimetidine 1 g daily in three months; or, having started to heal breaks down again, and is associated with severe symptoms which require treatment with higher doses of cimetidine; or, having healed completely, recurs despite continuing full doses of cimetidine.

Preliminary analysis of the first 70 patients with refractory ulcer showed that when compared with patients with non-refractory ulcer there was no striking difference in age, sex, duration of history, smoking, previous treatment with cimetidine, acid and pepsin secretion and approximate ulcer size (graded as small, medium or large). However, the outcome was different. Overall, 41 patients healed — but only after a mean treatment period of 6.9 months; 28 patients did not heal even after an average treatment period of 9.4 months (and one patient defaulted). Severe symptoms caused 21 patients to be admitted on 27 occasions and, of these, 11 were eventually operated on because of severe pain. Further analysis shows that 62 patients were treated with cimetidine 1 g daily initially but that in 48 patients the dose had to be increased to 2 g daily. Of those who did not heal on this dose and were not operated, eight were put on cimetidine 3 g daily of whom healing has occurred in four.

It has been suggested that those who fail on medical treatment are also likely to do badly after surgery but others have not found this to be the case (Valleur et al, 1979; McWhinnie et al, 1980; Venables, 1980). In my experience, the results have been good.

ACID, ULCER HEALING AND REFRACTORY ULCER

The relation between acid and ulcer is enshrined in the phrase 'no acid, no ulcer'. Furthermore, unless the peak acid output is 15 mmol/hr or higher the chances of a duodenal ulcer occurring are slight (see Baron et al, 1980). Since much more is known about acid than about mucosal defence mechanisms, not surprisingly the main thrust of anti-ulcer treatment has been to reduce acid secretion; its success in turn has reinforced views about the role of acid in ulcer disease. But is ulcer healing proportional to the amount of acid reduced? Does acid secretion need to be reduced to a certain minimum before re-epithelialisation can occur? What is this level? Is it about the same for all patients? If this theory is correct, the high secretor is likely to be at a disadvantage for such a person will need a greater reduction of acid secretion than a person who secretes normal amounts. Alternatively, is the amount that needs to be reduced a proportion of the capacity to secrete acid? What is this proportion? Is it fixed? If so, since acid secretion varies between individuals, the absolute amount reduced will also vary. Or does the proportion vary between individuals and if so by how much? In other words, does each patient have his or her own ulcer threshold? From studies carried out on the relation between pretreatment acid secretion and ulcer healing, the evidence can be interpreted to support both views; perhaps both are correct but applicable to different populations.

Whilst acid is essential in ulcer development, is it the sole or the most important factor? The Zollinger–Ellison syndrome is usually cited as the best example to demonstrate the role of acid in duodenal ulcer disease but this is an extreme and quite unrepresentative of the usual patient with duodenal ulcer. Three well-known observations suggest that acid, though important in ulcer disease, may not be the crucial factor in determining ulceration and healing. First, when an ulcer heals spontaneously, acid levels do not change; this was observed in the cimetidine trials. Second, unless there is massive hypersecretion, as in the Zollinger–Ellison syndrome, for a given level of acid it cannot be predicted whether the person has an ulcer or not. Put another way, duodenal ulcer patients often happen to have high acid secretion but many normal people have similarly high levels as well. Third, drugs such as carbenoxolone and colloidal bismuth heal ulcers effectively without reducing acid secretion.

Presumably ulceration occurs because the mucosal defence for unknown reasons weakens and is unable to cope with existing levels of attacking factors; after a while, the defences strengthen, balance is re-established and healing occurs. Are some patients more sensitive to drugs that increase mucosal defence rather than reduce acid? There is no evidence to support this but in ulcer studies done so far the design would not allow such patients to be detected.

Why do some patients take many months to heal or fail to heal altogether? This is particularly surprising in those patients who in the past have responded swiftly to standard doses of cimetidine. Earlier studies have shown that intractability was often but not invariably associated with the development of ulcer complications. Thus in one study of 162 patients operated on for intractable symptoms confined perforations were found at laparotomy in 38 per cent and fibrous adhesions in 30 per cent; in the remainder these features were absent. Conversely, amongst patients found to have a confined perforation at operation, intractability of symptoms was the main indication for operation in 58 per cent of the patients (Haubrich, 1974). However, this cannot be the explanation in the patients I have studied for at laparotomy they did not have adhesions or confined perforations. Indeed on looking through the records of patients operated in my hospital during the last seven years because of intractable symptoms, a striking feature has been the absence of such findings, whereas surgeons who carried out operations many years ago recall such lesions as being common. Perhaps this reflects the changing natural history of the disease (Langman, 1979).

Since several of the patients I studied healed after the dose of cimetidine was increased it suggests that either the standard dose of cimetidine no longer reduces acid as effectively, or there has been a change such that greater degrees of acid inhibition are required to allow healing. Expressed differently, the ulcer may have become less sensitive to acid inhibition. This needs to be investigated by measuring the degree of acid inhibition in such patients during treatment. If confirmed, it would suggest that there has been a fundamental change in the nature of the disease which results in it becoming resistant to usual medical treatment. Therefore, the clinical importance of finding a patient with a refractory ulcer is that it generally indicates that the disease has become more virulent and that the prognosis is likely to worsen.

This paper is dedicated to Professor E. W. Gault, formerly Professor of Pathology at the Christian Medical College, Vellore, in India. I was fortunate to be his student: a great teacher, a great man.

REFERENCES

Awoke S, Lawrence G D 1980 Cimetidine and hyperparathyroidism. Lancet 1: 1134
Barbara L, Belsasso E, Bianchi Porro G, Blasi A, Caenazzo E, Chierichetti S M, Di Febo G, Di Mario F, Farini R, Giorgi-Conciato M, Grossi E, Mangiameli A, Miglioli M, Naccarato R, Petrillo M 1979 Pirenzipine in duodenal ulcer. A multi-centre double-blind controlled clinical trial. First two parts. Scandinavian Journal of Gastroenterology 14, Suppl 57:10-15

Bardhan K D 1978 Cimetidine in duodenal ulceration. In: Wastell C, Lance P (eds) Cimetidine. The Westminster Hospital Symposium. Churchill Livingstone, Edinburgh, p 31-56

Bardhan K D 1981 Medical treatment of duodenal ulcer: a review. Tropical Gastroenterology 2: 4-33

Baron J H, Langman M J S, Wastell C 1980 Stomach and duodenum. In: Bouchier I A D (ed) Recent advances in gastroenterology 4. Churchill Livingstone, Edinburgh, ch 2, p 23-86

Becker U, Faurschon P, Jensen J, Pedersen P B, Ranlov P J 1980 The efficacy of trimipramine and cimetidine in the treatment of duodenal ulcer. A double-blind comparison. Scandinavian Journal of Gastroenterology 15: A47

Binder H J, Cocco A, Crossley R J, Finkelstein W, Font R, Friedman G, Groarke J, Hughes W, Johnson A F, McGuigan J E, Summers R, Vlahcevic R, Wilson E C, Winship D H 1978 Cimetidine in the treatment of duodenal ulcer. A multicentre double-blind study. Gastroenterology 74 (part 2 of 2 parts): 380-388

Bodemar G, Norlander B, Walan A, Larsson R 1979 Short and long-term treatment with cimetidine in peptic ulcer disease and the pharmacokinetics of cimetidine. Scandinavian Journal of Gastroenterology 14: Supplement 55: 96-106

Bonfils S, Mignon M, Gratton J 1979 Cimetidine treatment of acute and chronic Zollinger–Ellison syndrome. World Journal of Surgery 3: 597-604

Cargill J M, Teden N, Saunders J H B, Wormsley K G 1978 Very long-term treatment of peptic ulcer with cimetidine. Lancet 2: 1113-1115

Cohen I A, Siepler J K, Nation R, Bombeck C T, Nyhus L M 1980 Relationship between cimetidine plasma levels and gastric acidity in acutely ill patients. American Journal of Hospital Pharmacy 37: 375-379

Collen M J, Hanan M B, Maher J A, Rent M, Stubrin S E, Arguello F, Gardner L 1980 Cimetidine vs. placebo in duodenal ulcer therapy. Digestive Diseases and Science 25: 744-749

Cowen A E, Pollard E J, Kemp R, Ward M 1980 A double-blind comparison of cimetidine and De-Nol in the treatment of chronic duodenal ulceration. Australian and New Zealand Journal of Medicine 10: 364-365

Dancygier H, Wurbs D, Classen M 1980 New method for endoscopic determination of ulcer size. Gut 21: A895

Domschke W, Domschke S, Demling L 1977 A double-blind study of cimetidine in patients with duodenal ulceration: clinical, kinetic and gastric and pancreatic secretory data. In: Burland W L, Simkins M A (eds) Cimetidine. Proceedings of the Second International Symposium on histamine H₂-receptor antagonists. Excerpta Medica, Amsterdam, Oxford, p 217-223

Fairclough P D 1980 An unusual form of peptic ulcer disease: the Zollinger–Ellison syndrome. Update 21: 1013-1020

Festen H P M, Lamers C B H, Tangerman A, Van Tongeren J H M 1980 Effect of treatment with cimetidine for one year on gastrin cell and parietal cell function and sensitivity to cimetidine in patients with duodenal or gastric ulcers. Postgraduate Medical Journal 56: 698-699

Graziani G, Aroldi A, Colussi G, Surian M, Benvenuti C, Ponticelli C 1980 Cimetidine and hyperparathyroidism. Lancet 1: 1134

Halter F, Barbezat G O, Van Hoorn-Hickman R, Van Hoorn W A 1980 Healing dynamics of traumatic gastric mucosal defects in the normal and hyperacid stomach. Digestive Diseases and Science 25: 916-920

Hasan M, Sircus W 1980 Clinical study of the features associated with failure and success of cimetidine in the treatment of peptic ulcer. Gut 21: A462

Haubrich W S 1974 Complications of peptic ulcer disease. In: Bockus H L (ed) Gastroenterology, 3rd edn. W B Saunders, Philadelphia, p 720-762

Heath H, MacGrevor G A 1980 Cimetidine in hyperparathyroidism. Lancet 1: 980-981

Hetzel D J, Hansky J, Shearman D J C, Korman M G, Hecker R, Taggart G J, Jackson R, Gabb B W 1978 Cimetidine treatment of duodenal ulceration. Short term clinical trial and maintenance study. Gastroenterology 74 (part 2 of 2 parts): 389-392

Hunt R H, Melvin M A, Mills J G 1980a Gastric function after treatment with cimetidine. In: Torsoli A, Luchelli P E, Brimblecombe R W (eds) H₂ Antagonists. H₂ receptor antagonists in peptic ulcer disease and progress in histamine research. Excerpta Medica, Amsterdam, Oxford, Princeton, p 119-129

Hunt R H, Vincent D, Kelly J M, Perry M, Milton-Thompson G J 1980b Comparison of medical and surgical reduction in intragastric acidity in duodenal ulcer. Gut 21: A455

Jacob A, Lanier D, Bourgoignie J 1980 Reduction by cimetidine of serum parathyroid hormone levels in uremic patients. New England Journal of Medicine 302: 671-674

Kohli Y, Misaki F, Kawai K 1972 Endoscopic follow-up observation of duodenal ulcer. Endoscopy 4: 202-208

Langman M J S 1979 The epidemiology of chronic digestive disease. Edward Arnold, London

Lanier D, Faure H, Jacob A I, Bourgoignie J J 1980 Cimetidine therapy for severe hypercalcemia in two chronic hemodialysis patients. Annals of Internal Medicine 93: 573-574

Lenghel A, Micle Tr., Cristea N 1980 Treatment of duodenal ulcer with carbonic anhydrase inhibitors. Hepatogastroenterology Supplement, XIth International Congress of Gastroenterology 257: 300, E32.7

Ljunghall S, Akerström G, Rudberg C, Wider L, Johansson H 1980 Cimetidine in primary hyperparathyroidism. Lancet 2: 480

Malchow H, Sewing K-F, Albinus M, Horn B, Schomerus H, Dolle W 1978 In patient treatment of peptic ulcer with cimetidine. 1. Effect on the healing of duodenal ulcer. Deutsche Medizinische Wochenschrift 103: 149-152

Marshall J B, Settles R H 1980 Zollinger–Ellison syndrome. A clinical update. Postgraduate Medicine 66: 38-50

Martin D F, Hollanders D, May S J, Ravenscroft M M, Tweedle D E F, Miller J P 1981 Differences in relapse rates of duodenal ulcer healing with cimetidine or tripotassium dicitrato bismuthate. Lancet 1: 7-10

Maybury N K, Carr-Locke D L 1980 The value of the new interpretation of the insulin test in predicting duodenal ulcer relapse after treatment with cimetidine. British Journal of Surgery 67: 315-317

McCarthy D M 1978 Report on the United States experience with cimetidine in Zollinger–Ellison syndrome and other hypersecretory states. Gastroenterology 74: 453-455

McCarthy D M 1980 The place of surgery in the Zollinger–Ellison syndrome. New England Journal of Medicine 302: 1344-1347

McCarthy D M, Peikin S R, Lopatin R N, Crossley R J, Harpel H S 1978 H_2-receptor antagonists in gastric hypersecretory states. In: Creutzfeldt W (ed) Cimetidine. Proceedings of an International Symposium on histamine H_2-receptor antagonists. Excerpta Medica, Amsterdam, Oxford, p 153-164

McCarthy D M, Peikin S R, Lopatin R N, Long B W, Spiegel A, Marx S, Brennan M 1979 Hyperparathyroidism — a reversible cause of cimetidine resistant gastric secretion. British Medical Journal 1: 1765-6

McWhinnie D L, Gray G R, Smith I S, Gillespie G Cimetidine or surgery for severe duodenal ulcer dyspepsia? Results of a three to four year follow-up. Gut 21: A 922

Mignon M, Vallot T, Galmiche J P, Dupas J L, Bonfils S 1980a Interest of a combined antisecretory treatment, cimetidine and pirenzipine, in the management of severe forms of Zollinger–Ellison syndrome. Digestion 20: 56-61

Mignon M, Vallot Th., Mayeur S, Bonfils S 1980b Ranitidine and cimetidine in Zollinger–Ellison syndrome. British Journal of Clinical Pharmacology 10: 173-174

Moshal M G, Spitaels J M, Khan F 1980 Bicitropeptide and cimetidine in the treatment of duodenal ulcer. South African Medical Journal 58: 631-633

Nava G, Pippa G, Ballanti R, Papi C 1979 Role of ulcer morphology in evaluating prognosis and therapeutic outcome in duodenal ulcer. Scandinavian Journal of Gastroenterology 14, Supplement 54: 41-43

Peden N R, Boyd E J S, Wormsley K G 1981 Women and duodenal ulcer. British Medical Journal 282: 866

Peter P, Gonvers J J, Pelloni S, Weber K, Sonnenberg A, Strohmeyer G, Hoffstetter J R, Blum A L 1978 Cimetidine in the treatment of duodenal ulcer. In: Creutzfeldt, W (ed) Cimetidine. Prodeedings of an International Symposium on histamine H_2-receptor antagonists. Excerpta Medica, Amsterdam, Oxford, p 190-198

Pettengell K E, Grayson M J 1980 Cimetidine and hyperparathyroidism. Lancet, 1: p 1134

Pounder R E, Williams J G, Hunt R H, Vincent S H, Milton-Thompson G J, Misiewicz J J 1977 The effects of oral cimetidine on food stimulated gastric acid secretion and 24-hour intragastric acidity. In: Burland W L, Simkins M A (eds) Cimetidine: Proceedings of the Second International Symposium on histamine H_2-receptor antagonists. Excerpta Medica, Amsterdam, Oxford, p 189-206

Richardson C T, Feldman M, McClelland R N, Dickerman R M, Kumpuris D, Fordtran J S 1979 Effect of vagotomy in Zollinger–Ellison syndrome. Gastroenterology 77: 682-686

Robinson M F, Hayles A B, Heath H 1980 Failure of cimetidine to affect calcium homeostasis in familial primary hyperparathyroidism (multiple endocrine neoplasia, type I). Journal of Clinical Endocrinology and Metabolism 51: 912

Rune S J, Hesselfeldt P H, Larsen N-E 1979 Clinical and pharmacological effectiveness of cimetidine in duodenal ulcer patients. Scandinavian Journal of Gastroenterology 14: 489-492

Saunders J H B, Peden N R, Boyd E J S, Wormsley K G 1980 Double-blind comparison of ranitidine and cimetidine in the treatment of duodenal ulceration. Gut 21: A455

Scheurer U, Witzel L, Halter F, Keller H-M, Huber R, Galeazzi R 1977 Gastric and duodenal ulcer healing under placebo treatment. Gastroenterology 72: 838-841

Shaw G, Korman M G, Hansky J, Schmidt G T, Stern A I 1980 Comparison of short term Mylanta II and cimetidine in healing of duodenal ulcers. Australian and New Zealand Journal of Medicine 10: 363

Sherwood J K, Ackroyd F W, Garcia M 1980a Cimetidine in hyperparathyroidism. Lancet 1: 1298

Sherwood J K, Ackroyd F W, Garcia M 1980b Effect of cimetidine on circulating parathyroid hormone in primary hyperparathyroidism. Lancet 1: 616-620

Shiu K L, Kui C L, Ching L L, Choi K Y, Yam L Y C, Woon S W 1979 Treatment of duodenal ulcer with antacid and sulpiride. Gastroenterology 76: 315-322

Sonnenberg A, Giger M, Kern I, Noll C, Stuby K, Weber K B, Blum A L 1979 How reliable is determination of ulcer size by endoscopy? British Medical Journal 2: 1322-1324

Stadil F, Stage J G 1978 Cimetidine and the Zollinger–Ellison (Z–E) syndrome. In: Wastell C, Lance P (eds) Cimetidine. The Westminster Hospital Symposium. Churchill Livingstone, Edinburgh, p 91-104

Valleur P, Adam M, Alasseur M, Bitoun A, Hautefeuille P 1979 Preliminary results in a series of thirty-three proximal vagotomies for duodenal ulcers not responding to cimetidine treatment. Chirurgie 105: 685-688

Vanherweghem J-L, Bourgeois N, Fuss M 1980 Cimetidine and parathyroid hormone levels. New England Journal of Medicine 303: 395-396

Venables C W 1980 Indications for surgery in duodenal ulcer non-responders to cimetidine. In: Torsoli A, Lucchelli P E, Brimblecombe R W (eds) H_2 Antagonists. H_2-receptor antagonists in peptic ulcer disease and progress in histamine research. Excerpta Medica, Amsterdam, Oxford, Princeton, p 16-23

Venables C W, Stephen J G, Blair E L, Reed J D, Saunders J D 1978 Cimetidine in the treatment of duodenal ulceration and the relationship of this therapy to surgical management. In: Wastell C, Lance P (eds) Cimetidine. The Westminster Hospital Symposium. Churchill Livingstone, Edinburgh, p 13-30

Walker V, Taylor W H 1979 Cigarette smoking, chronic peptic ulceration and pepsin secretion. Gut 20: 971-976

Webster J, Petrie J C, Griffiths R 1980 A combined clinical and pharmacokinetic study of cimetidine in patients with duodenal ulceration. Scottish Medical Journal 25: 81

Whitfield P F, Hobsley M 1979 Smoking and gastric hypersecretion in duodenal ulcer patients. Gut 20: A919

Wyllie J H 1978 Experience of controlled comparative trials in patients with duodenal ulcer. In: Creutzfeldt W (ed) Cimetidine. Proceedings of an International Symposium on histamine H_2-receptor antagonists. Excerpta Medica, Amsterdam, Oxford, p 202-216

8. Recurrent and stomal ulceration after partial gastrectomy

R. Gugler*, H.-G. Rohner, J. Kollmeier,
S. Miederer and W. Möckel
*Department of Medicine, University of Bonn, West Germany

Between 6 and 14 per cent of those undergoing partial gastrectomy for duodenal ulcer subsequently develop recurrent ulceration (Kennedy, 1978). Theoretical considerations support the concept of treatment of these ulcers with histamine H_2-receptor antagonists, since they occur only if gastric acid secretion is not eliminated by the gastrectomy procedure.

Evidence has been presented in a number of uncontrolled clinical trials that cimetidine promotes healing of ulcers recurring after gastric operations (Table 8.1). With very few exceptions the ulcers healed on a standard dose of cimetidine (usually 1 g daily) within a period of 4 to 12 weeks of treatment. Almost all patients in these open trials became symptom-free during the time of observation, whether the ulcer healed or not.

Table 8.1 Uncontrolled studies on cimetidine for recurrent ulcers after gastric operations.

Authors (dose)	No. of patients	Drop outs	Healing (wks) 4	6	8	12	Unhealed	Symp- tom-free
Delle Fave 1977 (1.6 g)	10	—	4	—	5	—	1	9
Hoare et al. 1978 (1.0 g)	20	1	—	17	—	2	—	20
Saunders et al. 1978 (1.0 g)	13	—	10	—	—	2	1	12
Wastell et al. 1978 (1.0 g)	8*	—	—	4 no follow-up			1	8

*Post-vagotomy patients.

When Kennedy and Spencer conducted a controlled clinical trial on the effectiveness of cimetidine postoperatively they failed to detect a significant difference between cimetidine and placebo, with 12 patients in each treatment group (Kennedy and Spencer, 1978). Their patients, however, had ulcers recurring after gastrectomy, vagotomy, vagotomy with pyloroplasty, and vagotomy with gastrojejunostomy, and the ulcer recurred in the stomach as well as in the duodenum and in the jejunum. Thus the patient group was not homogeneous.

A placebo-controlled, randomised double-blind trial was performed on the effect of cimetidine treatment on healing of anastomotic ulcers after partial gastrectomy in outpatients in three clinical centres (Gugler et al, 1979). The criteria for entrance into the study were:

1. A time interval of at least three months between operation and diagnosis of the anastomotic ulcer.

2. The ulcers had to be located at least in part within a range of 1 cm above and 1 cm below the anastomosis.

3. Visible sutures had to be removed endoscopically at least four weeks before entrance into the study. Exclusion criteria were: chronic liver disease, renal insufficiency, afferent loop syndrome, dumping syndrome, previous upper gastrointestinal bleeding.

METHOD

After patients had given informed consent basal and peak gastric acid were measured and a fasting serum gastrin level obtained to exclude Zollinger–Ellison syndrome. The duration of the study was eight weeks. All patients were seen once every week. Follow-up gastroscopies were performed after four weeks and after eight weeks of treatment. In randomised order patients received either cimetidine in the standard dose of 1.0 g (five tablets) or placebo. The size of the ulcer was determined during endoscopy by use of biopsy forceps; a minimum size in one diameter of 3 mm was required.

If at the first follow-up gastroscopy at 4 weeks the size of the ulcer had increased by more than 25 per cent the patient was considered a non-responder and was removed from the double-blind trial. If the ulcer had not changed its size, the patient remained in the study. Non-responders after four weeks or unhealed patients after eight weeks received open cimetidine treatment for eight weeks if they had been on placebo during the controlled study period.

For ethical reasons an intermediate evaluation by the statistician was planned after one year. This statistical analysis led to the termination of the trial: continuation would have been unethical because of the clear superiority of the cimetidine treatment. At that time 15 patients had completed the study. Not one patient had to be removed from the trial because of non-adherence to the protocol.

RESULTS

Eight patients had received placebo; 7 patients had received cimetidine. The two treatment groups were not significantly different with respect to age, sex, time interval since gastric surgery, number of patients with Billroth I and Billroth II gastrectomy, initial ulcer size, number of smokers or number of alcohol drinkers.

The difficulties of determining gastric acid secretion after partial gastrectomy are well known. However, all patients in this study produced gastric acid under stimulation, whereas BAO was not positive in all patients.

After four weeks treatment the ulcers in six out of the seven patients in the cimetidine group had healed whereas no ulcers had healed in the placebo-treated patients. After eight weeks ulcers had healed in all seven patients on cimetidine, but in only one patient in the placebo group. The differences are highly significant. All ulcers that did not heal under placebo did subsequently heal on open cimetidine treatment: four after four weeks, two after eight weeks, one after twelve weeks (Table 8.2).

Table 8.2 Cimetidine for anastomotic ulcers after partial gastrectomy**

Treatment	Number of patients	Healing		No healing	Healing open treatment
		4 wks	8 wks		
Cimetidine	7	6*	7*	0	—
Placebo	8	0	1	7	7
Total	15	6	8	7	7

*$P < 0.01$
**from Gugler et al. (1979) with kind permission of the Editor of the *New England Journal of Medicine.*

To determine the symptomatic response in the two treatment groups during the initial four weeks of the study, ulcer symptoms were recorded separately for day and night. Symptoms during the daytime showed a tendency to improve on cimetidine, but the difference was never significant during the four weeks. Symptoms at night were significantly less in those taking cimetidine than those taking placebo during the whole four weeks of treatment. It is of interest that even on cimetidine only four out of seven patients were completely asymptomatic (day and night) after four weeks, and also one placebo patient was asymptomatic.

Our results are in agreement with those of Festen et al (1979) who treated 21 patients with anastomotic ulcers after Billroth I and Billroth II partial gastrectomy over four weeks with cimetidine or placebo. From 12 patients of the cimetidine group the ulcer had healed in eight, in contrast to one healed ulcer in nine patients from the placebo group ($P < 0.05$). The double-blind part of the trial was followed by four weeks open cimetidine treatment of all treatment failures from the initial phase. During this treatment period three of the four cimetidine failures healed (total of 11 out of 12), and five of eight of the unhealed ulcers of the former placebo group healed.

DISCUSSION

The results of the two controlled trials are comparable and show a higher significance than most studies on cimetidine treatment of duodenal and gastric ulcers. The reasons for this may be:

1. The low tendency of anastomotic ulcer to heal spontaneously. In our study spontaneous healing occurred in only one out of eight patients in the placebo group. In duodenal ulcer we find a high spontaneous healing rate.

2. Good patient compliance, possibly because of the severity of symptoms and because the alternative treatment would be another operation.

Of particular interest is the question of long-term prophylaxis of anastomotic ulcers by histamine H_2-receptor antagonists, saving those patients from another surgical intervention. In the trial by Festen et al (1979) 19 of the 21 patients from the acute treatment study entered an open maintenance study with 400 mg cimetidine b.d. in the morning and at bedtime. Of 19 patients completing this one-year open trial three had a relapse confirmed by endoscopy ($\sim$ 15 per cent).

From our own acute treatment trial with cimetidine for anastomotic ulcers 15 patients entered placebo-controlled long-term prophylaxis with cimetidine over one year ago — however, with a 400 mg dose given only at bedtime. This dose is highly effective in preventing relapse of duodenal ulcer. One patient dropped out after six months but all the other patients have completed the full study period. Six of the remaining 14 patients received cimetidine, and eight were on placebo. Out of eight patients in the placebo group seven had a relapse during the one year study period, but also four out of the six cimetidine-treated patients relapsed, leaving only three patients without a relapse after one year (Table 8.3). When we look at the time of relapse we find no clear tendency to relapse earlier on placebo with this limited number of patients.

Table 8.3 One year cimetidine (400 mg) prophylaxis for anastomotic ulcers.

	No. of patients	Drop-outs	One year completed	No relapse	Relapse
Cimetidine	7	1 (6 months)	6	2	4
Placebo	8	—	8	1	7
Total	15	1	14	3	11

All patients who relapsed in the prophylactic treatment phase were subsequently placed on a full course of cimetidine treatment, 1 g daily, for eight weeks (Table 8.4). Ulcers healed in six patients on the former placebo and in three of the cimetidine group. Healing did not occur in one patient in each group. These two patients were operated on (extended resection plus vagotomy) and remained well.

Table 8.4 Open treatment with cimetidine (1 g) after relapse.

Relapsed under	Healing		No healing
	4 wks	8 wks	
Cimetidine (4)	2	1	1
Placebo (7)	5	1	1

CONCLUSION

Our tentative conclusion from these data is that despite excellent results in most studies with cimetidine in anastomotic ulcers after partial gastrectomy, the rationale for long-term prophylaxis is not established at the present time. It appears that 800 mg of cimetidine will prevent relapse in most patients, whereas our controlled study suggests that 400 mg cimetidine once daily (nocte) is not sufficient. If this hypothesis is confirmed by studies on larger numbers of patients, one would have to advise such patients to take 800 mg cimetidine for a life-time. Life-long treatment would be necessary since seven out of our eight patients relapsed on placebo.

Despite the small incidence of anastomotic ulcers after partial gastrectomy, and despite the trends in modern ulcer surgery towards selective vagotomy without gastric resection, these results may be important for the following reasons:

1. We have to treat patients who were operated on before the area of modern ulcer surgery.

2. In most countries more patients still undergo gastrectomy than selective vagotomy.

3. The alternative treatment is a second operation with a well-known high mortality rate.

ACKNOWLEDGEMENT

The work reported has been supported by the Deutsche Forschungsgemeinschaft.

REFERENCES

Delle Fave G F, Paoluzzi P, Bergonzi P, De Magistris L, Sparvoli C, Carrata R 1977 Cimetidine and post-gastrectomy recurrent ulcers. Rendiconti gastroenterologia 9: 150-151

Festen H P M, Lamers C B H, Driessen W M M, van Tongeren J H M 1979 Cimetidine in anastomotic ulceration after partial gastrectomy. Gastroenterology 76: 83-85

Gugler R, Lindstaedt H, Miederer S, Möckel W, Rohner H-G, Schmitz H, Székessy T 1979 Cimetidine for anastomotic ulcers after partial gastrectomy. New England Journal of Medicine 301: 1077-1080

Hoare A M, Jones E L, Hawkins C F 1978 Cimetidine for ulcers recurring after gastric surgery. British Medical Journal 1: 1325-1326

Kennedy T 1978 Recurrent ulcer after vagotomy or gastrectomy treated with cimetidine. In: Wastell C, Lance P (eds) Cimetidine. The Westminster Hospital Symposium, Churchill Livingstone, Edinburgh, p 79-83

Kennedy T, Spencer A 1978 Cimetidine for recurrent ulcer after vagotomy or gastrectomy: A randomized controlled trial. British Medical Journal 1: 1242-1243

Saunders J H B, Cargill J M, Peden N R, Wormsley K G 1978 Cimetidine for ulcers recurring after surgery. British Medical Journal 1: 1619

Wastell C, MacGregor G P, Hale J 1978 Treatment of recurrent duodenal ulcer after vagotomy with cimetidine. British Journal of Surgery 65: 367

9. Cimetidine and the Zollinger–Ellison syndrome

J. G. Stage* and F. Stadil

*Departments of Surgical Gastroenterology C, Rigshospitalet, and
D Herlev University Hospital, Copenhagen

All clinical features of the Zollinger–Ellison syndrome (ZES) can be attributed to the hypersecretion of gastrin from the gastrinoma. Hypergastrinaemia leads to hypersecretion of gastric hydrochloric acid and this hypersecretion in turn leads to the intractable ulcer diathesis which is the main clinical manifestation of the disease.

As the tumours are slow-growing and difficult to localize they usually remain silent for long periods of time, although normally they are malignant.

Because in the past survival depended primarily on the prevention of ulcer complications, the treatment of ZES was symptomatic by total gastrectomy. The development of histamine H_2-receptor antagonists has offered new possibilities for symptomatic control, and the first reports on the results of treatment with H_2-blockers were promising (Richardson and Walsh, 1976; Stage et al, 1977; Stadil and Stage, 1978). Since 1976 we have used cimetidine to treat all newly diagnosed patients with ZES, and the results are reported below.

THE PATIENTS

Between 1971 and 1981 we diagnosed a total of 40 patients with ZES. Early on the patients were treated by total gastrectomy (n = 18) but this treatment has not been used since 1976. A total of 21 consecutive patients diagnosed between March 1976 and January 1981 were treated with cimetidine. The distribution of sex and age appears in Figure 9.1 and the clinical data in Table 9.1.

In every patient diagnosis of ZES was based upon typical clinical findings in association with fasting hypergastrinaemia and hypersecretion of gastric acid. The diagnosis has subsequently been confirmed by one or more of the following criteria: histological confirmation of a gastrinoma, hypergastrinaemia in the veins draining the pancreas, and persisting hypergastrinaemia after total gastrectomy.

METHODS

After the diagnosis of ZES was established, cimetidine was started and treatment continued until the patient died or the tumours were removed.

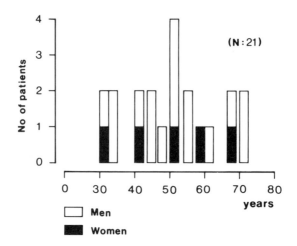

Figure 9.1 Distribution of sex and age in 21 consecutive ZES patients.

Table 9.1 Clinical data on Zollinger–Ellison patients on continuous cimetidine treatment

Patient	Sex	Age (years)	BAO	PAO	Gastrin pmol/l	Symptoms	Duration (years)	Diagnostic criteria
1.	F	31	75.8	120	2062	DV	3	2
2.	M	32	32.4	70	87	PV	10	2
3.	M	69	54.7	73	940	PDV	1/2	1
4.	M	57	32.0	43	223	P	10	2
5.	F	46	11.2	75	120	PV	9	1,2
6.	M	59	1.5	2	125	P	1	1
7	M	47	59.3	99	157	D	1/2	1,2
8.	M	72	31.0	59	768	PD	2	1
9.	F	51	11.5	60	66	PV	10	2
10.	M	57	33.0	85	85	PDV	40	1,2
11.	M	46	41.0	89	68	D	1/2	1,2
12.	M	70	20.3	75	99	PV	5	1
13.	M	60	23.3	51	2200	P	6	2
14.	M	51	102	131	527	PD	1	2
15.	M	32	43.0	106	114	PD	1/2	2
16.	F	59	34.3	48	142	D	1/2	2
17.	M	56	28.0	77	100	PD	5	1,2
18.	M	43	22.1	40	230	PD	2	2
19.	M	45	37.0	51.4	300	PDV	2/3	1
20.	F	69	8.4	32.4	195	PP	2	1
21.	M	32	37.4	119	117	PD	1/2	2
		51.6 ± 2.8	35.2 ± 5.1	71.7 ± 7.0	415.5 ± 134.5		5.2 ± 1.9	

P = pain. D = diarrhoea. V = vomiting.
Diagnostic criteria: 1. histology
2. hypergastrinaemia of pancreatic origin

The initial dose of cimetidine was 1.2 ± 0.1 g per 24 hours (mean ± SEM) varying from 1.0 to 1.6 g (Figure 9.2). During continuous treatment the dose of cimetidine was adjusted in most patients according to symptoms and findings, the aim being to keep the patient free of symptoms and ulcers.

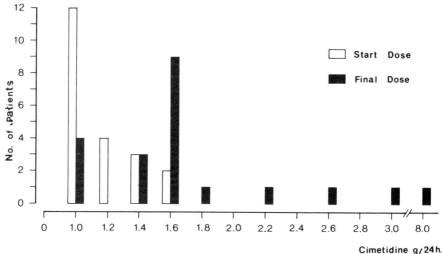

Figure 9.2 Initial dosage (open columns) and final dosage (black columns) of cimetidine in grams per 24 hours in 21 ZES patients receiving continuous cimetidine.

After discharge from hospital the patients kept a record of pain, vomiting, and diarrhoea, and they were seen frequently in the outpatient clinic or during control admissions to hospital.

In addition to X-ray of the stomach and endoscopy, gastric secretion of acid and serum concentration of gastrin were measured at frequent intervals. In seven patients the effect of discontinuation of cimetidine for three days after a long period of treatment was studied.

In order to monitor side-effects a number of standard haematological, endocrinological, or hepatological measurements were made.

For calculations of survival rates the logrank test was used. For statistical evaluation the Mann–Whitney or the Willcoxon test was used when appropriate.

RESULTS

Clinical course
As shown in Table 9.2 all symptoms rapidly disappeared in all patients after cimetidine treatment was started. About half the patients were relieved within a few days. During the course of treatment recurrences of symptoms were seen in most patients and required an increase in dose.

Two patients probably represent treatment failures. In the patient receiving 3 g cimetidine per 24 hours (Table 9.2) an unsuccessful Whipple's operation triggered

Table 9.2 Clinical data on 21 Zollinger–Ellison patients on continuous cimetidine treatment.

Patient	Start	Dose (g) Final	Duration (months)	Disappearance of: Symptoms (weeks)	Ulcers	Recur-rences	Status
1.	1.2	8.0	54	3	3	5	Maintained on cimetidine, metastases verified, cytostatics.
2.	1.0	3.0	54	4	4	4	Whipple's operation, no tumour removed, cimetidine continued.
3.	1.0	1.4	6	3	—	1	Died after 6 months from metastases.
4.	1.2	1.6	45	1	5	1	Maintained on cimetidine, gastrinoma located in the tail of pancreas.
5.	1.4	1.4	9	3	3	0	Whipple's operation, gastrinoma removed, cimetidine discontinued.
6.	1.0	1.6	40	1	1	3	Maintained on cimetidine, gastrinoma located in the tail of pancreas.
7.	1.0	1.6	39	1	3	1	Maintained on cimetidine, metastases verified, cytostatics.
8.	1.2	1.6	40	2	12	0	Maintained on cimetidine.
9.	1.2	1.6	39	1	2	3	Maintained on cimetidine, hypergastrinaemia of pancreatic origin.
10.	1.0	1.0	6	1	4	0	Whipple's operation, gastrinoma removed, cimetidine discontinued.
11.	1.0	1.0	17	1	1	0	Whipple's operation, gastrinoma removed, cimetidine discontinued.
12.	1.0	1.0	1/2	—	—	—	Died after 2 weeks from malignancy.
13.	1.0	1.4	18	1	12	1	Maintained on cimetidine, metastases verified, cytostatics, died from malignancy.
14.	1.6	1.6	34	4	12	0	Maintained on cimetidine, hypergastrinaemia of pancreatic origin.
15.	1.4	1.6	33	1	—	0	Maintained on cimetidine, hypergastrinaemia of pancreatic origin.
16.	1.0	1.0	37	1	1	0	Maintained on cimetidine, gastrinoma located in the pancreatic head, awaiting surgery.
17.	1.0	1.6	14	4		2	Whipple's operation, gastrinoma removed, died 2 months post op.
18.	1.0	2.2	11	2	2	1	Maintained on cimetidine.
19.	1.6	2.6	12	4	4	2	Maintained on cimetidine, metastases verified, cytostatics.
20.	1.0	1.6	24	2	2	1	Maintained on cimetidine, metastases verified.
21.	1.4	1.8	18	2	2	1	Maintained on cimetidine, hypergastrinaemia of pancreatic origin
	1.2 ± 0.1	1.9 ± 0.3	26.2 ± 3.6				

ulcer recurrences which required higher doses. He is presently suffering from a new recurrence and the effect of a still further increase in cimetidine dosage is being studied. The other patient receiving 8 g cimetidine per 24 hours is requiring additional treatment with antacids and anticholinergics and symptomatic control is still inadequate. She has been receiving this high dose for more than two years. A total gastrectomy has been offered, but she has refused.

Mortality

Four patients have died during cimetidine treatment: three from advanced malignant disease with widespread metastases and one from septicaemia after pancreatic surgery.

Secretory measurements

Initially, oral administration of 200 or 400 mg cimetidine markedly inhibited the spontaneous secretion of acid in all patients. Ultimately no discernible inhibition was seen in two of the patients mentioned earlier. Measurements of spontaneous secretion of gastric acid in the morning 10 to 12 hours after the last dose of cimetidine demonstrated a marked and significant decrease in the spontaneous secretion during treatment ($P < 0.05$, Figure 9.3).

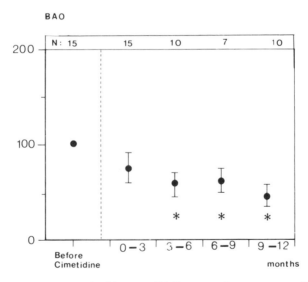

Figure 9.3 Measurements of basal acid output (BAO) expressed as percentage of basal secretion before and during continuous cimetidine treatment after various lengths of treatment. Measurements were carried out 10 to 12 hours after the last dose of cimetidine. The results are expressed as mean ± SEM*. $P < 0.05$.

In seven patients whose cimetidine was discontinued for three days, four had a marked prolonged inhibition and three had secretions of the same order of magnitude as before cimetidine treatment (Figure 9.4), with only a small change during the discontinuation period. Determination of plasma cimetidine concentration did not demonstrate any measurable amount of cimetidine in any of the patients during the experiment.

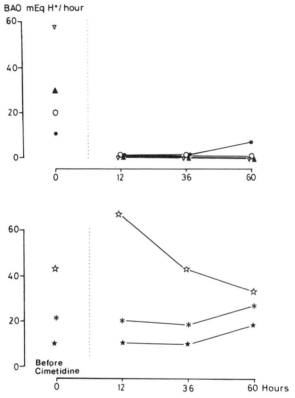

Figure 9.4   Effect of stopping cimetidine on BAO in seven ZES patients, measured 12, 36 and 60 hours after discontinuation.

Cimetidine treatment did not appear to influence gastrin concentrations in serum. The increasing concentrations in a few patients were probably due to acceleration of metastatic disease.

Side-effects

Two patients developed moderate gynaecomastia after three and nine months of treatment. No other clinical side-effects and no significant changes attributable to cimetidine were noted in any patient.

DISCUSSION

This study demonstrates that cimetidine is able to control all symptoms in ZES patients for long periods of time. However, during long-term treatment adjustment of dose was necessary in most patients in order to maintain complete relief. Endoscopy revealed that all ulcers could heal quickly after cimetidine treatment started, but 13 patients presented later recurrences. This might have been due to an insufficient dose of cimetidine, either because the patients did not take the tablets as instructed, or because the absorption of the drug had diminished. Decreased absorption was probable in one of the patients whose treatment is at present inadequate. The lack of response in the patient taking 8 g/24 hours remains unexplained.

In general these observations emphasize that cimetidine treatment of ZES patients is safe only if the patients are informed fully of the nature of the disease and treatment, and if they are closely supervised.

Apart from gynaecomastia no side-effects were observed, not even in the patients receiving high doses for prolonged periods. This agrees with other reports and emphasizes that cimetidine offers safe and reliable symptomatic control in almost all ZES patients (Bonfils et al, 1979; McCarty, 1978; Stadil and Stage, 1978).

The alternative therapeutic approach is total gastrectomy. Our experience comprises 18 Danish ZE patients treated with this operation from 1971 to 1976. There was only one operative death. In Figure 9.5 the two treatments are compared. The two groups of ZE patients do not differ with respect to age, duration of symptoms or survival, but considerations of side-effects and changes in working capacity and social status after the two treatments speak strongly in

SIDE EFFECTS	TOTAL GASTRECTOMY	CIMETIDINE
DYSPHAGIA	****	
REGURGITATION	********	
WEIGHT LOSS	*************	
MALABSORPTION	**	
DIARRHOEA	***	* *(***)
OSTEOMALACIA	*	
GASTRIC PAINS		**(**********)
GYNAECOMASTIA		**
MORTALITY	****	****
SOCIAL STATUS CHANGED	********	*

* No of Patients

( ) Intermittent

Figure 9.5 Comparison of the clinical outcome in 18 ZES patients treated with total gastrectomy and 21 treated with cimetidine. Each asterisk indicates one patient. The parentheses indicate that the symptoms were intermittent.

favour of cimetidine. However, as cimetidine was unable to control symptoms and ulcers indefinitely in all patients treated, total gastrectomy will probably still be required in occasional patients.

Treatment with cimetidine or with total gastrectomy is only symptomatic. Patients can be cured only if the gastrinomas are located and removed. The efficacy and safety of cimetidine treatment provide opportunities for careful preoperative localization of gastrinomas. We have depended on percutaneous transhepatic catheterization of portal tributaries from the pancreas with gastrin determinations (Burcharth et al, 1979). Using this investigation we have operated on a minority of the patients with a Whipple's procedure, and have been able to discontinue cimetidine in three out of five such patients. Improved procedures for localization of the gastrinomas during complete control of symptoms and ulcers with cimetidine may result in an increased number of ZE patients with curative resections in the future.

CONCLUSIONS

1. Cimetidine can replace total gastrectomy in the initial treatment of the ZES.

2. After long-term treatment with cimetidine the efficacy may decrease and total gastrectomy may still be required in some cases.

3. Long-term treatment with cimetidine in doses from one to two times the doses used in ordinary patients with duodenal ulcer is safe.

4. Cimetidine treatment permits an attempt at operation on the pancreas if tumours are adequately localized preoperatively.

REFERENCES

Bonfils S, Mignon M, Gratton J 1979 Cimetidine treatment of acute and chronic Zollinger–Ellison syndrome. World Journal of Surgery 3: 597-604
Burcharth F, Stage J G, Stadil F, Ingemann Jensen L, Fischerman K 1979 Localization of gastrinomas by transhepatic portal catheterization and gastrin assay. Gastroenterology 77: 444-450
McCarty D M 1978 Report of the United States experience with cimetidine in Zollinger–Ellison syndrome and other hypersecretory states. Gastroenterology 74: 453-458
Richardson C T, Walsh J H 1976 The value of a histamine H_2 receptor antagonist in the management of patients with the Zollinger–Ellison syndrome. New England Journal of Medicine 294: 133-135
Stadil F, Stage J G 1978 Cimetidine and the Zollinger-Ellison syndrome. In: Wastell C, Lance P (eds) Cimetidine. The Westminster Hospital Symposium. Churchill Livingstone, Edinburgh, p 91-100
Stage J G, Rune S, Stadil F, Worning H 1977 Treatment of Zollinger-Ellison patients with cimetidine. In: Burland W L, Simkins M A (eds) Cimetidine, Excerpta Medica, Amsterdam, p 306-310

Discussion on Duodenal Ulcer, part 1
Chairman: Dr J. H. Baron

Dr Kerr. Dr Stage had a very high number of Zollinger–Ellison patients. What was his catchment area, where did he get them from and what was his lower limit of gastrin level accepted as diagnostic of Zollinger–Ellison syndrome?

Dr Stage. Our catchment area is the kingdom of Denmark! In some of the patients whom we have studied the serum gastrin levels on some occasions have been at such a low level that it would be said that these patients could not have Zollinger–Ellison syndrome. It is therefore very important to emphasize that the diagnostic criteria in Zollinger–Ellison syndrome should not be based on a single measurement of serum gastrin: a series is necessary.

Dr Wormsley. Dr Stage, do you think that your Zollinger–Ellison syndromes have been converted into Werner–Morrison syndromes? Have they been biopsied and found to have normal parietal cells while they are achlorhydric?

Dr Stage. The 40 patients discussed here today have been characterized by means of every measurable and detectable hormone which could be analyzed in the gastrointestinal tract, brain and elsewhere. Therefore, if the Zollinger–Ellison syndrome is defined as a clinical syndrome in which the clinical features are related to hypersecretion of gastrin from a gastrin-producing tumour, then our patients are quite definite cases. If the tumours are studied histochemically, many other peptide-producing cells can be seen in some of them.

Professor Tytgat. Has Dr Stage taken into account the mortality of Whipple's operation and total gastrectomy?

Dr Stage. The threat of malignancy is real in gastrinoma, and sooner or later all tumours will become malignant. If there is an opportunity to cure the disease by removing the gastrinoma, I think that chance should be taken, rather than doing a total gastrectomy. If a 35-year-old active farmer has a total gastrectomy, he will have to change his job and will suffer from malabsorption and other side-effects. These are the results obtained in our studies and they are similar to the long-term results in the US register.

In both groups (cimetidine and total gastrectomy) four patients died. In the cimetidine group one patient died from septicaemia two months after a Whipple's procedure and in the gastrectomy group there was one operative death. I have not gone into details here on the treatment of tumours with streptozotocin or other compounds because I think this is outside the scope of the present discussion.

Dr Warnes. Friesen noted that metastases in the Zollinger–Ellison syndrome did regress after total gastrectomy. Has Dr Stage seen this, either following gastrectomy or cimetidine?

Dr Stage. Some years ago Friesen claimed that some patients, following a total gastrectomy, showed decreasing serum gastrin. He advocated the theory that total gastrectomy removed some kind of gastric factor and thus reduced metastases. However, if Friesen's data are carefully reviewed (and following some correspondence with him), it can be demonstrated that in some Zollinger–Ellison patients treated by total gastrectomy their serum gastrin levels do not indicate at all whether their disease is malignant. We have had a few patients with only slightly raised serum gastrin levels (about 200 pmol/l) who have been treated by total gastrectomy and have suddenly died four or five years later from advanced malignant disease.

Mr Elder. Has Dr Stage any views on the policy which Dr Fordtran has been advocating, that it is important to do a laparotomy? According to Dr Stage, it might be possible to do a partial pancreatectomy and remove a tumour. However, if the patient is being opened up, something should be done to decrease acid secretion. In a small series, Fordtran has been advocating the use of a proximal gastric vagotomy, followed by cimetidine. His early results are most encouraging.

Dr Stage. In our experiment in which we discontinued cimetidine there were four patients whose gastric acid secretion had decreased to almost achlorhydric levels. In those patients in whom a proximal gastric vagotomy has been performed in addition to cimetidine, gastric acid secretion has not been studied after stopping cimetidine for longer than 10 to 12 hours. If these patients had been studied one, two or three weeks after stopping cimetidine, I think the gastric acid secretion would have increased again, suggesting that proximal gastric vagotomy is inadequate.

Dr Baron. Let us now turn to the problems of healing duodenal ulcers, and why some of them do not heal. Dr Wormsley started off by suggesting that placebo is more powerful than no treatment at all. Would he elaborate on what he means by placebo as a drug, as opposed to placebo as a doctor? Do different doctors obtain different results in healing ulcers with placebo? Would this also not be true for different doctors obtaining different results even using the same pharmacological preparation, cimetidine?

Dr Wormsley. I did not point out precisely and specifically that the reason I use placebo is because placebo is a weak drug. There are all sorts of 'augmenting' and 'interfering' factors. All weakish drugs behave in this way, and show this more powerfully than the faster-healing drugs. I was talking about the rate of healing, not the completeness of healing. There are two different aspects to this. Placebo is a drug which does not heal all that quickly. The shape of the two types of curve means that the mechanism whereby the placebo/carbenoxolone type drug increases the rate of healing is different from that of cimetidine. Perhaps one promotes healing and the other interferes with factors that interfere with healing.

Dr Crean. We have heard a great deal about ulcers that did not heal. I would like to know what we are all talking about. First, it seems naive to suppose that any drug will heal all ulcers. Second, the methodology is not available to measure severe ulcers. What is meant by 'severe' ulcers? Does Dr Hunt mean by the term 'non-responders' patients who do not respond in terms of secretion? Is he referring to the effect of cimetidine on secretion? Dr Bardhan had patients with 'refractory' ulcers. There were many young people in this group — why? What are we talking about? Is it simply about up-market severe duodenal ulcers which will not heal whatever is done to them?

Dr Hunt. I share Dr Crean's dilemma. Our first observation was the one which I defined, i.e. the way in which the 36 patients on whom there was 24-hour data separated themselves very distinctly into two groups. An arbitrary discriminant of their inherent nocturnal intragastric acidity was used to define response and non-response.

For our current study we have, however, taken *clinical* criteria of non-response to determine whether the highly debatable clinical criteria which have been chosen are reflected retrospectively in the same type of changes in nocturnal intragastric acidity. This is so in the seven patients studied so far. The criteria which we have used for non-response are:

1. Those who failed to heal on a standard course of cimetidine, 1 g/day for six weeks.

2. Those who relapsed within one or two weeks of stopping treatment.

3. Those who have more than three relapses a year.

Dr Bardhan. The definition of severe ulcer is simply a clinical one. There is no other means of defining it. Size has nothing to do with it. About 20 years ago it used to be said that of those operated on because of intractable ulcers two-thirds would have a confined perforation or adhesions, but this is not true now and I am sure that there is a changing natural history. I happen to think that acid is much overrated in ulcer disease. This 'high acid' or 'low acid' business is neither here nor there in my view; people are just born with a certain amount of acid. Epidemiology suggests that some factor entered the human race at the turn of the century, it found a fertile soil and we are now having a hard time of it.

Dr Baron. May we now consider this topic of twice-daily cimetidine? The papers presented by Dr Kerr and Prof Eckardt on the UK and European multicentre studies showed consistency between Britain and the Continent of Europe on the advantages of twice-daily cimetidine. Can both Dr Kerr and Prof Eckardt tell me why it is not possible just to give 400 mg at night if it is true that 400 mg twice a day is as good as 1 g a day, particularly because the changes in acid shown by Dr Hunt seemed to be remarkably greater at night than during the day?

Dr Kerr. I suggested some time ago that such a trial should be done. However, it was thought that the present trial should be carried out first.

Dr Baron. Of course, the same applies to oxmetidine. Perhaps we need to use only one dose of oxmetidine, given at night.

Dr Russell. Are the side-effects of cimetidine different in those patients whose ulcers are refractory to treatment compared to those which heal readily? Are there any hormone profiles other than gastrin in the two groups of ulcers?

Dr Hunt. I cannot answer either of those questions.

Dr Baron. Why does everyone simply increase the dose of cimetidine for duodenal ulcers, recurrent ulcers, Zollinger–Ellison syndrome and indeed for intractable ulcers? Why not add something else instead, such as an anticholinergic drug in a synergic combination? Dr Wormsley, what is your attitude?

Dr Wormsley. My attitude varies: sometimes yes, sometimes no. It is easier to stick to one drug, from the patient compliance point of view, otherwise — at least in our population — patients get in a muddle.

Dr Bardhan. If a patient has a bad flare-up on cimetidine he is admitted to see whether it settles. If it does not settle, the dose of cimetidine is then increased, then about 250 ml of a powerful antacid is given and in some cases carbenoxolone is also given — but that does not really help. What else can we do? Anticholinergics are not used because they do not make much difference, other than producing side-effects.

Dr Wormsley. There are regional differences, of course, because we do not see this extraordinarily high proportion of resistant ulcers. Increasing the dose of cimetidine to 2 g/day is usually sufficient. It is very rare for an ulcer not to heal on that dose. Dr Bardhan's figures are quite extraordinary.

Professor Bianchi Porro. We have a small group of duodenal ulcer patients who are asymptomatic non-responders. What should we do with this small number of patients who do not respond to cimetidine after two, three or four months, but who are completely without any symptoms? We thought about this and decided to do nothing. Operation was suggested, but the patients did not want one because they said that they had no pain. We saw no clear alternative so we decided to think about it for a while. After six months they came back and were treated with cimetidine, 1 g/day, which healed their ulcers perfectly.

Dr Bardhan. By the time a decision was made in our 70 patients — that their ulcers were probably refractory — half of them were asymptomatic. It was just that their ulcers would not heal. However, in a number of patients outside this group of 70 many symptoms developed when an attempt was made to withdraw the cimetidine. The longest time we have continued to give cimetidine was 23 months. This woman healed only last week after being on cimetidine 3 g/day for four or five months — she just would not heal.

It used to be said that if only an erosion were present, it should be ignored. This is not true. If these patients are followed, continuous changes are seen in the duodenum. An ulcer will appear, disappear, other lesions occur and so on — cimetidine does not convert the duodenum into a stable duodenum.

10. Maintenance treatment, part 1 — length of therapy and indications

G. Bodemar*, R. Gotthard, M. Ström and A. Walan

*Linkoping University Hospital, Sweden

The inhibitory effect of cimetidine on gastric acid secretion is now widely used as a therapeutic tool in peptic ulcer disease both to induce healing of ulcers and to prevent recurrences. The results of most of the long-term trials comparing the effects of cimetidine and placebo in chronic duodenal ulcer disease are presented in Table 10.1.

CLINICAL OUTCOME AFTER SHORT-TERM TREATMENT WITH CIMETIDINE

Each patient, before entering these long-term trials, had healed an active peptic ulcer, in most cases after a short course of cimetidine treatment. After treatment with cimetidine between 50 and 100 per cent of the patients allocated to long-term treatment with placebo experienced an endoscopically proven relapse in ulceration within 6 to 12 months (Table 10.1).

Before cimetidine became available only a few trials had studied the relapse rate in peptic ulceration and none had used endoscopy.

INTERMITTENT TREATMENT WITH CIMETIDINE

In clinical practice probably most doctors give their patients short-term treatment with cimetidine when troublesome ulcer symptoms occur. Bardhan (1980) and Rune et al (1980) have studied, for two and one year periods respectively, intermittent treatment with short courses of cimetidine; 80 and 66 per cent respectively of their patients were considered suitable for this intermittent form of treatment. Because of frequent ulcer relapses, development of ulcer complications or abrupt development of severe ulcer pain 20 and 34 per cent respectively were considered by these authors to be candidates for either continuous treatment with cimetidine or operation.

The frequency of symptomatic and endoscopically proven asymptomatic recurrences of peptic ulcer is lower during treatment with cimetidine than with

Table 10.1 Summary of results of long-term trials of maintenance treatment with cimetidine

Reference	Number of patients		Cimetidine dosage	Duration of treatment	Relapse rate			
					Cimetidine		Placebo	
	Cimetidine	Placebo			with symptoms %	without symptoms %	with symptoms %	without symptoms %
Bardhan et al (1979)	29	31	400 mg × 2	6 months	14	7	58	10
Berstad et al (1979)	23	24	400 mg at night	12 months	9	0	58	8
Blackwood et al (1979)	21	24	800 mg at night	6 months	14	10	50	38
Bodemar and Walan (1978)	19	23	400 mg × 2	12 months	16	0	61	17
Dronfield et al (1979)	20	22	400 mg × 2	6 months	25	—[1]	73	—[1]
Gray et al (1978)	26	30	400 mg at night	6 months	27	0	80	0
Gudmand-Høyer et al (1978)	26[2]	25[2]	400 mg × 2	12 months	12[3]	—	80[3]	—[1]
Hansky et al (1979)	20	20	400 mg × 2	12 months	5	0	80	20
Mekel (1978)	26	14	400 mg × 2	12 months	8	8	100	0

[1] Endoscopy if symptoms appeared.
[2] X-ray proven ulcers.
[3] Relapse assessed symptomatically without X-ray or endoscopy.

placebo (Table 10.1). Thus new ulcers do occur after treatment with cimetidine is stopped; it is not only a case of reduced doses of cimetidine keeping patients symptom-free while their ulcers are allowed to recur. Although the relapse rate after stopping treatment seems to be high there is often no consistent pattern in the individual patient. A patient with an early relapse may experience a long remission period until the next relapse and vice versa (Bardhan, 1980; Rune et al, 1980).

Gastric acid secretion is of doubtful value in predicting which ulcers will recur early after withdrawal of short-term treatment with cimetidine. Long duration of disease, positive family history, smoking habits and slow healing of the active ulcer during the initial treatment have been reported to be more frequent among early relapsers although the prognostic value of these markers is limited (CURE, 1980; Rune et al, 1980).

CLINICAL OUTCOME AFTER SHORT-TERM TREATMENT WITH CIMETIDINE AND OTHER DRUGS

Treatment with frequent intake of high doses of antacids or with bismuth will accelerate the healing of peptic ulcers as effectively as cimetidine. The follow-up of patients in double-blind trials who have healed their ulcers during treatment with these drugs provides an opportunity to see if the drugs themselves influence the recurrence rate of new ulcers once treatment has been stopped. The CURE study reported in 1980 that 54 per cent of 41 patients who had healed their duodenal ulcers on cimetidine had recurred within six months compared to 60 per cent of 35 patients who had healed their duodenal ulcers on high-dose antacids. Hansky et al (1980) found that 17 of 18 cimetidine-treated patients had recurrences after a mean time of 2.8 months, and 9 of 13 patients treated with high-dose antacids after a mean time of 3.9 months during a follow-up period after the end of ulcer-healing treatment.

We have earlier reported our double-blind trial in which 71 patients with active duodenal (54 patients) or prepyloric (17 patients) ulcers were treated with cimetidine (23 patients), a combination of anticholinergic and high-dose antacids (24 patients) or placebo (24 patients).

We used a double-dummy technique, i.e. all patients received the same number of tablets and pads per day. The frequency of ulcer healing was not significantly different between the two actively treated groups (Table 10.2).

The endoscopically proven symptomatic recurrence rate in new ulcers during a one-year follow-up period after treatment was stopped is shown in Figure 10.1. The time taken for symptomatic relapses to occur was significantly shorter after treatment with cimetidine was stopped than after treatment with antacid/anticholinergic was stopped — a median time of 11 and 24 weeks respectively ($P < 0.05$).

Table 10.2 Ulcer healing on antacid/anticholinergic, cimetidine and placebo.

Treatment	Number of patients	Number of patients with healed ulcers at 6 weeks
Cimetidine 200 mg × 3 and 400 mg at night	23	19[1] (83%)
L-hyoscyamine 0.6 mg b.d and 10 ml antacid suspension (buffering 85 mmol) 7 doses per day	24	23[2] (96%)
Placebo	24	8[3] (33%)

[1] Three more patients were healed after 12 weeks treatment.
[2] The last patient was healed after 12 weeks treatment.
[3] 50% of the patients were healed after 12 weeks treatment.

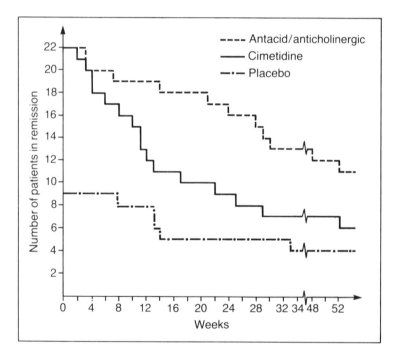

Figure 10.1 Following cessation of treatment with cimetidine, antacid/anticholinergic or placebo (at 0 weeks) patients were checked endoscopically for recurrence of ulcer during a one-year follow-up. From Ström et al (1981) with the permission of the Editor of *Scandinavian Journal of Gastroenterology.*

In Figure 10.2 the relapse rate after stopping ulcer-healing treatment with cimetidine or bismuth is shown (Martin et al, 1981); 85 and 89 per cent respectively had healed their duodenal ulcers during treatment with cimetidine or bismuth and 55 of the patients were followed for one year. Relapse was highly significantly more frequent ($P > 0.001$) in patients whose ulcers had initially been healed with cimetidine than in those whose ulcers had been healed with bismuth.

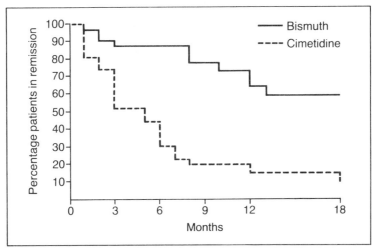

Figure 10.2   Relapse rates in patients whose ulcers healed while taking cimetidine or bismuth. From Martin et al (1981) with the permission of the Editor of *Lancet*.

CHANGES IN GASTRIC FUNCTION AFTER TREATMENT WITH CIMETIDINE

If it is true that the outcome of peptic ulcer disease is different after short-term cimetidine treatment than with antacids/anticholinergics or bismuth the question arises as to why this might be. Does treatment with cimetidine result in a change in gastric function that can explain such a development? Studies to date suggest no lasting effects on the regulation of gastric function after treatment with cimetidine.

Basal and maximal acid output are the same before and after both short and long-term treatment with cimetidine (Hunt et al, 1980). Aadland et al (1981) have shown an augmented acid secretory response after administration of submaximal doses of histamine in healthy volunteers but not in patients with duodenal ulcer after four weeks treatment with cimetidine. If this represents an increased sensitivity of the parietal cell to histamine and if it does occur in an individual patient it could influence the relapse rate after the end of treatment. However, there is a rapid renewal of parietal cells and the mean time to recurrence of ulceration is between three and five months after the end of a short course of cimetidine (Bodemar and Walan, 1978; Bardhan, 1980; Rune et al 1980).

Fasting gastrin as well as gastrin response to a peptone meal are unaffected by stopping treatment with cimetidine for at least two days (Hunt et al, 1980). Pepsin output is also the same before and after treatment (Aadland et al, 1981). No changes are seen in the ultrastructural appearance of the parietal cell after one year's treatment with cimetidine (Pillay et al, 1979).

RAPID SYMPTOMATIC RELIEF — POSITIVE OR NOT?

Little is known about the factors which lead to recurrence of duodenal ulcer. Both in the comparative trial with bismuth (Martin et al, 1981) and in that with antacid/anticholinergic (Ström et al, 1981) patients experienced more pronounced relief of pain during treatment with cimetidine than with the other drugs. This better symptomatic improvement might perhaps make the patients on cimetidine less prone to change their ulcerogenic habits such as smoking, intake of alcohol, coffee and acetylsalicylate-containing tablets. They may therefore continue with these habits after stopping treatment with cimetidine, possibly leading to early relapse.

CLINICAL OUTCOME AFTER LONG-TERM TREATMENT

A short course of cimetidine treatment does not seem to influence the outcome of chronic peptic ulcer disease once treatment is stopped. Gudmand-Hoyer et al (1978) reported that 20 of 25 patients, after 4 weeks treatment with cimetidine to heal their ulcers, suffered symptomatic relapses during one year's treatment with placebo; only 3 of 26 patients, who continued treatment with cimetidine, developed new symptoms. However, during the three months following the year's treatment with cimetidine a further 12 of these 26 patients had a symptomatic relapse.

In a group of 42 patients treated with a short course of cimetidine to heal their ulcers, Dronfield et al (1979) found that the clear difference in endoscopically proven recurrences in peptic ulcers were present only as long as cimetidine treatment was continued. During a six-month treatment period, 16 of the 22 placebo-treated patients relapsed compared to five of the 20 cimetidine-treated patients. The cumulative relapse rate eight months after completion of the trial was similar in the two groups — 75 per cent after cimetidine and 86 per cent after placebo.

As part of a long-term maintenance trial Hansky et al (1979) treated 40 patients with cimetidine 400 mg twice daily for one year. All patients remained free of symptoms and had no evidence of active duodenal ulcer at the end of this one-year trial. The patients were then allocated to either continued treatment with cimetidine 200 mg b.d. (15 patients) or placebo (25 patients) for a further six months. One of the 15 patients on cimetidine and 19 of the 25 placebo-treated patients had an endoscopically proven recurrence of ulceration during the six months.

The results of Gudmand-Hoyer et al (1978), Dronfield et al (1979) and Hansky et al (1979) suggest that longer periods of treatment with cimetidine do not influence the relapse rate once treatment is stopped. There was the same high rate of development of new ulcers after both short- and long-term treatment with cimetidine were stopped.

Our experience is, however, different. In Table 10.1 the results of our one-year maintenance trial in patients with proven recurrent duodenal ulcer are presented. We included 68 patients with chronic peptic ulcer disease localised in the prepyloric region and in the stomach. Most of these patients were first given a six to seven weeks cimetidine treatment to heal active ulcers and were then randomized to treatment either with cimetidine 400 mg twice daily (32 patients) or with placebo (36 patients) for one year (Bodemar and Walan, 1975). Six of the 32 patients on cimetidine (two without symptoms) and 30 of the 36 patients on placebo (seven without symptoms) experienced at least one endoscopically proven recurrence during the one-year trial.

Treatment with cimetidine or placebo was stopped at the end of the trial and all patients were then followed for two years. During follow-up repeat courses with cimetidine — or if it seemed necessary more prolonged courses — were restarted if troublesome ulcer symptoms recurred. Both during the one-year trial and during the two-year follow-up period patients were sent for elective operation because of frequent relapses, severe symptoms when recurrences occurred, development of ulcer complications or if operation was preferred to very long-term maintenance treatment. We reported earlier the results of this two-year follow-up study (Bodemar and Walan, 1980). Table 10.3 summarises the clinical outcome of the one-year trial and the two-year follow-up study.

Table 10.3 Clinical outcome of one year's treatment and two year follow-up

	Placebo n = 35[1]	Cimetidine n = 31[1]
Asymptomatic or with only mild symptoms during 3 years	6 (17%)	16 (52%)
Bleeding ulcers		
Before trial	11	17
During one-year trial	4	0
During two-year follow-up after trial	1[2]	1[2]
Referred for operation		
Candidates for surgery at start of trial	13	11
During trial	15	1
After trial	7	6[3]
Total number of patients operated on during one-year trial and two-year follow-up	22 (63%)	7 (23%)

[1] One patient from each treatment group stopped treatment during the trial.
[2] Both patients developed bleeding ulcers after they had been asymptomatic during one year after the end of the trial.
[3] Two patients were operated on; four were given continuous long-term treatment with cimetidine.

Our data suggest that the severity of chronic peptic ulcer is favourably influenced by one year's treatment with cimetidine compared with placebo and that this influence continues even after treatment is stopped. The difference in clinical outcome at the end of three years could not be explained by differences in the two treatment groups before the start of the trial: the sex ratio, age, number of smokers, duration of disease, acid secretion, number of pretrial complications to the peptic ulcer disease and number of pretrial candidates for surgery were not significantly different.

The mean ± SE of pretrial values of BAO was 4.4 ± 0.7 and 4.5 ± 0.7 mEq/h in the placebo and cimetidine groups respectively. In Figure 10.3 the values at the start of the one year trial are given as 100 per cent. It can be seen that the BAO rose during continuous treatment with placebo (a mean rise of 50 per cent at seven months, $P < 0.05$) but 2 days and 3.5 months after treatment with cimetidine was stopped the BAO was lower (n.s.) than at the start of the trial.

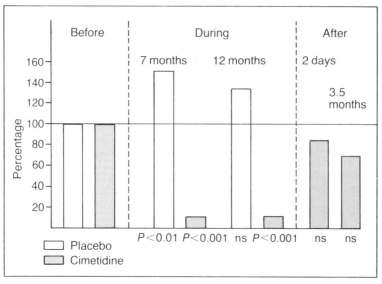

Figure 10.3   Basal acid output of 32 patients treated with cimetidine and of 36 patients treated with placebo for one year. Pre-trial BAO values are given as 100% in both groups. Mean BAO values during the one-year treatment period and 2 days and 3.5 months after the end of treatment are given as percentage changes compared with pre-trial values. P values are given for these differences. BAO was measured during the trial 1.5 and 2 hours after intake of either 200 mg cimetidine or placebo.

One of us (Walan, 1970) had found earlier that the same rise in BAO occurred with time during treatment with placebo. These results suggest that, during the years when patients have an active peptic ulcer disease, BAO rises steadily. This could explain the high recurrence rate in peptic ulcers in patients with chronic disease. Our data suggest that treatment with cimetidine might block this rise in BAO and favourably alter the course of the disease when maintenance treatment is stopped.

INFLUENCE OF ULCEROGENIC HABITS?

We tried to persuade our patients to stop smoking, reduce alcohol intake, coffee and acetylsalicylate-containing tablets and in a few instances suggested changes in the place of work. Whether these changes in habit had any influence on the different outcome compared with that reported by Hansky et al (1979), Dronfield et al (1979) and Gudmand-Hoyer et al (1978) can only be a matter for speculation. More studies need to be performed on the influence of such habits on the natural course of peptic ulcer disease.

In general practice there seems to be a peak in the severity of peptic ulcer disease, and 10 to 15 years after the start of the disease it seems to resolve, at least in those patients who have not been operated on (Fry, 1964; Greibe et al, 1977). Perhaps the great benefit of treatment with cimetidine is to keep patients in reasonably good health during the years the disease is active and perhaps surgery can then be avoided in many patients.

REFERENCES

Aadland E, Berstad A, Granerus G 1981 Augmented parietal cell sensitivity to histamine after cimetidine treatment in healthy subjects. Scandinavian Journal of Gastroenterology 16: 87-91
Bardhan K D, Saul D M, Edwards J L 1979 Double-blind comparison of cimetidine and placebo in the maintenance of healing of chronic duodenal ulceration. Gut 20: 158
Bardhan K D 1980 Intermittent treatment of duodenal ulcer with cimetidine. British Medical Journal 2: 20-22
Berstad A, Aadland E, Carlsen E 1979 Maintenance treatment of duodenal ulcer patients with a single bedtime dose of cimetidine. Scandinavian Journal of Gastroenterology 14: 827
Blackwood W S, Maudgal D P, Northfield T C 1978 Prevention by bedtime cimetidine of duodenal ulcer relapse. Lancet 1: 626
Bodemar G, Walan A 1978 Maintenance treatment of recurrent peptic ulcer by cimetidine. Lancet 2: 403-407
Bodemar G, Walan A 1980 Two-year follow-up after one year's treatment with cimetidine or placebo. Lancet 1: 38-39
CURE 1980 Is duodenal ulcer recurrence more common after cimetidine treatment? Gastroenterology 78 (5, part 2): 1152 (abstract)
Dronfield M W, Batchelor A J, Larkworthy W, Langman M J S 1979 Controlled trial of maintenance cimetidine treatment in healed duodenal ulcer: short and long-term effects. Gut 20: 526-530
Fry J 1964 Peptic ulcer: a profile. British Medical Journal 2: 809-812
Gray G R, Smith J S, Mackenzie J, Gillespie G 1978 Long term cimetidine in the management of severe duodenal ulcer dyspepsia. Gastroenterology 74: 397
Greibe J, Bugge P, Gjorup T, Lauritzen T, Bonnevie O, Wulff H R 1977 Long-term prognosis of duodenal ulcer; follow-up study and survey of doctors' estimates. British Medical Journal 2: 1572-1574
Gudmand-Hoyer E, Birger Jensen K, Krag E, Rask-Madsen J, Rahbek J 1978 Prophylactic effect of cimetidine in duodenal ulcer disease. British Medical Journal 1: 1095-1097
Hansky J, Korman M G, Hetzel D J, Shearman D J C 1979 Relapse rate after cessation of 12 months cimetidine in duodenal ulcer. Gastroenterology 76 (5, part 2): 1151 (abstract)
Hansky J, Korman M G, Schmidt G T, Stern A J, Shaw R G 1980 Relapse rate of duodenal ulcer after healing with cimetidine or Mylanta II. Gastroenterology 2 (5, part 2): 1179 (abstract)
Hunt R H, Melvin M A, Mills J G 1980 Gastric function after treatment with cimetidine. In: Torsoli A, Lucchelli P E, Brimblecombe R W (eds) Further experience with H$_2$-receptor antagonists. Excerpta Medica, Amsterdam, p 119-127

Martin D F, Hollanders D, May S J, Ravenscroft M M, Tweedle D E F, Miller J P 1981 Difference in relapse rates of duodenal ulcer after healing with cimetidine or tripotassium dicitrato bismuthate. Lancet 1: 7-10

Mekel R C P M 1978 Long-term treatment with cimetidine. African Medical Journal 54: 1089

Pillay C V, Moshal M G, Booyers J 1979 The effect of long-term use of cimetidine on the ultrastructure of gastric parietal cells in man. South African Medical Journal 55: 992-993

Rune S J, Mollman K M, Rahbek J 1980 Frequency of relapses in duodenal ulcer patients treated with cimetidine during symptomatic periods. Scandinavian Journal of Gastroenterology 15 (supplement 58): 85-92

Ström M, Gotthard R, Bodemar G, Walan A 1981 Antacid–anticholinergic, cimetidine and placebo in treatment of active peptic ulcers. Scandinavian Journal of Gastroenterology (in press).

Walan A 1970 Studies on peptic ulcer disease with special reference to the effect of L-hyoscyamine. Acta Medica Scandinavia. Supplement 516

11. Maintenance treatment, part 2 — surgery as an alternative

Michael W. L. Gear

Gloucestershire Royal Hospital, Gloucester.

The indications for surgery in duodenal ulcer have altered substantially since the advent of cimetidine.

The need for operation remains clear in patients with complications such as perforation, stenosis and massive bleeding. However, in uncomplicated chronic duodenal ulcer, a high percentage of patients on cimetidine are rapidly relieved of their pain and the ulcer heals. Operation is indicated for the small percentage whose pain persists or whose ulcer remains unhealed at check endoscopy.

The problem arises in those patients whose ulcer recurs after cimetidine treatment is stopped. Cimetidine may be given in maintenance doses over long periods or as intermittent courses as indicated by symptoms (Bardhan, 1980). At what point should cimetidine be abandoned and operation be offered to the patient?

RESULTS OF OPERATIONS FOR DUODENAL ULCER

Clearly before recommending surgery it is important to know the results of the most widely used operations. In the early days of gastric surgery, physicians were reluctant to refer patients because of the mortality and morbidity of gastrectomy. The patient had to 'earn' the operation (Small et al, 1969). Mortality rates were probably between two and five per cent, despite occasional reports of much better figures (Goligher, 1968).

In America, vagotomy and antrectomy became popular, because of the very low recurrent ulcer rate — below one per cent — but the mortality is similar to that from gastrectomy, at 1.6 per cent an unacceptable figure (Sawyers and Herrington 1977).

While vagotomy and pyloroplasty is safer there is, however, a morbidity from dumping and diarrhoea, and recurrent ulcer rates of about 10 per cent are reported in many series (Fawcett et al, 1969).

In contrast to gastrectomy and vagotomy and pyloroplasty, many large series have been reported for proximal gastric vagotomy (= highly selective) with a very low mortality and morbidity rate (Johnston, 1975; Kennedy, 1979). Early reports suggested a low rate of ulcer recurrence, but more recent assessment (Kennedy, 1979) has produced an average figure from several series of about nine per cent.

THE INTRODUCTION OF CIMETIDINE

Cimetidine was released for general use in November 1976 and rapidly became widely used. It had an immediate effect in Gloucestershire where the number of vagotomies carried out in 1977 dropped quite sharply.

Over the last three years there has been a steady decline in total operations for duodenal and gastric ulcers (and in vagotomies), the current totals being roughly half the average number carried out before 1976. In Gloucestershire epidemiological studies have shown a steady annual incidence of duodenal ulcer over the last five years (Gear and Barnes, 1980). There had been some evidence that the incidence of duodenal ulcer nationally was slowly decreasing between 1958 and 1972 (Brown et al, 1976).

It seems likely, however, that the number of operations for duodenal ulcer will increase again soon. The high relapse rate after treatment with cimetidine (whether short or long-term) demonstrated in many series is already resulting in increased referrals to surgical clinics. Patients are often symptom-free on the drug, but frequent relapses and return visits to the general practitioner for repeat prescriptions may lead to requests for surgical treatment. It is also possible that the incidence of stenosis will increase with the intermittent medication pattern frequently adopted by either the patient or doctor.

To compare the effectiveness of surgery and long-term maintenance cimetidine treatment, a long-term trial has been set up in Gloucestershire and is still in progress. Preliminary results are available.

METHOD

Patients with chronic duodenal ulcer at endoscopy were allocated either to full dosage cimetidine for three months followed by indefinite maintenance with 400 mg at night, or to proximal gastric vagotomy.

All patients fulfilled criteria used for selection for surgery prior to the advent of H_2 receptor blocking drugs and all accepted either continued medical treatment or surgery. Check endoscopy was carried out at three months and thereafter at approximately yearly intervals. All patients were reviewed in outpatients every three months. So far the length of follow-up has varied from one to three and a half years. The medical and surgical groups are similar for age and sex distribution and length of history.

RESULTS

The trial has not yet been completed, but preliminary results are available.

There has been one death from myocardial infarction in the medical group, the patient having been on maintenance cimetidine for almost two years. The ulcer had remained healed throughout.

Approximately half the patients in the cimetidine group have developed recurrent ulceration, either during maintenance or shortly after stopping treatment. There has been one serious complication of a probable allergic hepatitis, associated with eosinophilia and progressing to fibrosis, if not cirrhosis. Subsequent biochemical tests and liver biopsy indicated that the process is stationary or might even have regressed after stopping treatment.

In contrast, the patients in the surgical group have all had good results, most being graded as Visick I. There has been no mortality and, as yet, no reports of recurrent ulcer.

The patients with recurrent ulcers from the medical treatment group have also all been successfully treated surgically.

CONCLUSION

There seems to be little benefit from long-term maintenance therapy with cimetidine. The results so far suggest that at least half the patients have recurrences either while on treatment or soon after stopping the drug. Now that surgery has become much safer, the risks of duodenal ulceration over long periods (Bonnevie, 1978) are probably very similar to the risks of operation.

Patients can thus be treated with cimetidine to obtain rapid relief of symptoms and often short-term healing of the ulcer. If the ulcer recurs then operation provides a better guarantee of long-term freedom from symptoms and from the need for regular medication.

A frequent comment at follow-up of patients who have had years of medical treatment followed by proximal gastric vagotomy is: 'I wish I had had the operation years ago'.

ACKNOWLEDGEMENTS

I would like to acknowledge the help and support of Professor David Johnston of Leeds who originally suggested the idea of the randomised controlled trial. I would like to thank Mrs Jane Askew, my Research Secretary, who has administered the trial and carried out the secretarial work.

REFERENCES

Bardhan K D 1980 Intermittent treatment of duodenal ulcer with cimetidine. British Medical Journal 2: 20-22
Bonnevie O 1978 Survival in peptic ulcer. Gastroenterology 75: 1055-1060

Brown R C, Langman M J S, Lambert P H 1976 Hospital admissions for peptic ulcer during 1958-72. British Medical Journal 1: 35-37

Fawcett A N, Johnston D, Duthie H L 1969 Revagotomy for recurrent ulcer after vagotomy and drainage for duodenal ulcer. British Journal of Surgery 56: 111

Gear M W L, Barnes R J 1980 Endoscopic studies of dyspepsia in a general practice. British Medical Journal 2: 1136-1137

Goligher J C 1968 Five to eight year results of Leeds/York controlled trial of elective surgery for duodenal ulcer. British Medical Journal 2: 781-787

Johnston D 1975 Operative mortality and post operative morbidity of highly selective vagotomy. British Medical Journal 4: 545-547

Kennedy T 1979 A critical appraisal of surgical treatment In: Truelove S O, Willoughby C P (eds) Topics in Gastroenterology. Blackwell Scientific Publications, Oxford

Sawyers J L, Herrington J L 1977 In: Nyhus L M, Wastell C (eds) Surgery of stomach and duodenum, 3rd edn. Little Brown, Boston

Small W P, Cay E L, Dugard P, Sircus W, Falconer C W A, Smith A N, McManus J P A, Bruce J 1969 Peptic ulcer surgery: selection for operation by 'earning'. Gut 10: 996-1003

12. Maintenance treatment, part 3 — cost-effectiveness

Roy Pounder
Royal Free Hospital, London

When assessing any form of medical or surgical treatment, three aspects have to be reviewed: efficacy, cost and safety. The purpose of this contribution is to discuss whether maintenance treatment with cimetidine is more cost-effective than surgery for patients with chronic duodenal ulceration.

The State and individuals are prepared to pay for the treatment of duodenal ulceration not only because of the nuisance value of recurrent illness, but also because duodenal ulceration is a substantial cause of work-loss. Many patients with duodenal ulceration suffer only rare episodes of illness, respond promptly to cimetidine and are not candidates for maintenance treatment with the drug. Other patients suffer from recurrent illness and cimetidine maintenance treatment provides for this group a decisive reduction in the prevalence of active ulceration. Both cimetidine and surgery are effective for the long-term treatment of duodenal ulcer — are they worth the cost?

THE AVERAGE CHRONIC DUODENAL ULCER PATIENT

Perhaps the most up-to-date profile of patients needing maintenance treatment for duodenal ulceration is provided in the report of the international collaborative study involving 696 patients from 22 centres in Europe and South Africa (Burland et al, 1980). The ratio of men to women was three to one and the average age was 45 years. The life expectancy of an average British 45-year-old man is 27.4 years and for an average 45-year-old woman it is 32.9 years. The major question, which cannot be answered, is whether an average 45-year-old with a chronic duodenal ulcer will need to take cimetidine maintenance treatment until death. We have no idea, but for the purpose of cost analysis one must assume the answer is 'yes'. In practice I expect that this is not the correct answer.

A MODEL OF MEDICAL TREATMENT FOR DUODENAL ULCER

Most authors have considered that cimetidine fails when a patient develops recurrent or breakthrough ulceration. Such patients usually respond to a larger dose of the drug and then return to ulcer remission.

Before one can cost cimetidine treatment, one must assess how much of the drug an average patient consumes. In a recent discussion paper in *The Lancet*, I developed a model of medical treatment for chronic duodenal ulcer (Pounder 1981). This model uses the established healing and relapse rates for cimetidine and placebo, for both acute and maintenance treatment. The model predicts that with placebo treatment alone, one in six of the duodenal ulcer population will have an acute ulcer at any time (Figure 12.1). If cimetidine 1 g per day is used for

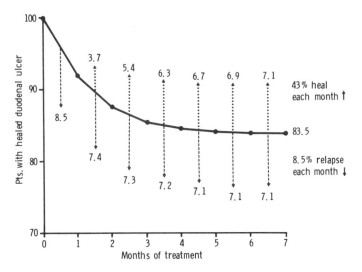

Figure 12.1   Effect of placebo for maintenance and for acute ulceration. Every month 8.5 per cent healthy patients relapse (downward pointing arrows) on placebo, and lesions in 43 per cent of the ulcer patients heal (upward pointing arrows) on placebo. The numbers at the tops and bottoms of the dotted lines represent the number of patients healing and relapsing respectively each month.

acute episodes, one in ten will have an acute ulcer at any one time (Figure 12.2). If maintenance treatment with cimetidine 400 mg at bed-time is given, changing to 1

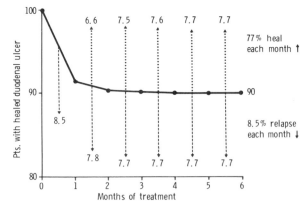

Figure 12.2   Effect of placebo for maintenance but cimetidine only for acute ulceration. Every month 8.5 per cent of patients relapse (downward pointing arrows) and 77 per cent heal (upward pointing arrows). The numbers at the tops and bottoms of the dotted lines represent the number of patients healing and relapsing respectively each month.

g per day at times of relapse, only one in 33 will have an ulcer at any time (Figure 12.3).

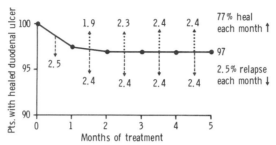

Figure 12.3 Effect of cimetidine for maintenance treatment and also for acute ulceration. Every month 2.5 per cent patients relapse (downward pointing arrows) and 77 per cent patients heal (upward pointing arrows). The numbers at the tops and bottoms of the dotted lines represent the number of patients healing and relapsing respectively each month.

THE COST OF MEDICAL TREATMENT

Using this model it can be calculated that maintenance cimetidine treatment will be needed on average for 50.4 weeks per year with, on average, 1.6 weeks per year of full-dose treatment. With present day British cimetidine prices, the drug cost alone will be approximately £100 per year. In Britain the cost of supervision of such treatment is negligible.

Can the State, or British individual, afford £100 per year for each patient with chronic duodenal ulceration? According to the Department of Employment's New Earnings Summary of Full-time Workers in Britain (April 1980), adjusted by the Average Earnings Monthly Index, the average duodenal ulcer patient in Britain is earning in March 1981 £113 per week, or £5876 per annum. Thus cimetidine maintenance treatment is equivalent to 1.6 per cent of the gross personal product of an average patient. There is one report which demonstrates that maintenance cimetidine does keep people at work (Bodemar and Walan, 1978); only a few days' work-loss would pay for a year's cimetidine.

THE COST OF SURGICAL TREATMENT

The only realistic long-term alternative to cimetidine is elective duodenal ulcer surgery. How much does a vagotomy cost? At the present time the average inpatient stay for a vagotomy is 15.1 days (Hospital Activity Analysis). In March 1981 an acute hospital bed in Britain cost approximately £75 per day. Thus the approximate hospital cost of a duodenal ulcer operation if £75 × 15.1 = £1133. To this must be added the inevitable work-loss during and after surgery. Mr Christopher Venables of the Royal Victoria Infirmary, Newcastle, has estimated that his patients lose 12 weeks from work — a fortnight in hospital and 10 weeks' convalescence at home. Twelve weeks' pay at £113 per week cost £1356. Thus the total immediate cost of a vagotomy must be approximately £1133 + 1356 =

£2489. This must be considered a low estimate, as it does not take into account either the 10 per cent recurrence rate of ulceration after surgery or the small risk of mortality which has devastating cost implications (Culyer and Maynard, 1981).

Thus, can one compare cimetidine costing £100 per year, perhaps for life, with a single immediate payment today of £2500? What interest is obtainable today for a similar capital investment? If one bought £2500-worth of Treasury 5½ per cent 2008-2012 (a British Government stock) in the second week of March 1981, it would yield an income of £282 per annum. In addition there would be a lump-sum repayment at par of £5133 sometime between the years 2008 and 2012, which coincides with the life expectancy of the average duodenal ulcer patient.

INFLATION AND THE COST OF DRUGS

If one is able to continue to buy cimetidine at today's price, it will clearly be more economical than surgery. However, one must compare surgery at today's price with cimetidine at an unknown price in the future.

In fact the price of cimetidine has dropped since it was introduced to Britain in November 1976 (Figure 12.4). From November 1976 to March 1981 the Retail Price Index has risen from 165.8 to 277.3 (corrected: 100 to 167). If the price of cimetidine had kept up with inflation its hospital cost should now be 24.3p rather than the present day price of 12.8p per tablet.

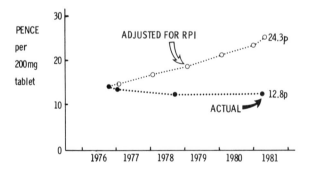

Figure 12.4   The actual cost of cimetidine, compared with its price in 1976, adjusted for inflation using the Retail Price Index.

Do other British drug prices reflect general inflation? Figure 12.5 demonstrates that there is a striking variation between the inflation rates for a number of new and old drugs used for gastrointestinal disease. British drug prices do not react solely to the forces of normal market competition. They are partly controlled by the near monopoly purchaser of drugs in Britain — the Department of Health and Social Security — and also the uniform pricing policies of international drug

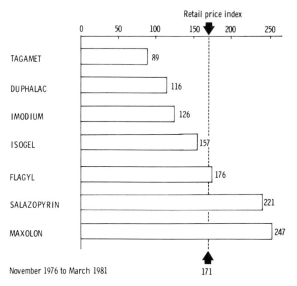

Figure 12.5   British drug prices since November 1976. The adjusted Retail Price Index has risen from 100 to 171. Tagamet is the only drug that has dropped in price.

corporations. Despite the imminent arrival of a competitive H_2-receptor antagonist, it is clear that one cannot expect cimetidine to continue indefinitely at its present price.

CONCLUSION

From the standpoint of an amateur economist, I believe that there is no decisive difference between the costs of long-term cimetidine or surgery for chronic duodenal ulceration. The present and future costs of both forms of treatment are so difficult to quantify that I believe that one cannot discriminate between them on that basis alone. One must assess efficacy and safety. I personally would rather be treated by a house physician writing his first cimetidine prescription than a surgical registrar performing any of his first 50 vagotomies.

REFERENCES

Bodemar G, Walan A 1978 Maintenance treatment of recurrent peptic ulcer by cimetidine. Lancet 1: 403-407
Burland W L, Hawkins B L, Beresford J 1980 Cimetidine treatment for the prevention of recurrence of duodenal ulcer: an international collaborative study. Postgraduate Medical Journal 56: 173-176
Culyer A J, Maynard A K 1981 Cost-effectiveness of duodenal ulcer treatment. Social Science and Medicine (in press)
Pounder R E 1981 Model of medical treatment for duodenal ulcer. Lancet 1: 29-30

FURTHER READING

Bodemar G, Gotthard R, Ström M, Walan A, Jönssen B, Bjurulf P 1980 Socioeconomic aspects of treatment with cimetidine in peptic ulcer disease. In: Torsoli A, Luccelli P E, Brimblecombe R W (eds) H₂-receptor antagonists. Excerpta Medica, Amsterdam, p 59-69
Fineberg H V, Pearlman L A 1980 Benefit-and-cost analysis of medical interventions: a case of cimetidine and peptic ulcer disease. Office of Technology Assessment, United States Congress
Geweke J, Weisbrod B A 1980 Some economic consequences of technological advance in medical care: the case of a new drug. Institute for Research on Poverty, University of Winsconsin — Madison, USA
Hertzman P, Jönssen B, Lindgren B 1979 The economics of ulcer disease. The Swedish Institute for Health Economics
Muttarini L 1980 A functional view of cost/benefit analysis in peptic ulcer disease. In: Torsoli A, Luccelli P E, Brimblecombe R W (eds) H₂-receptor antagonists. Excerpta Medica, Amsterdam, p 70-83
Rhode Island Health Services Research Inc. 1980 The effect of cimetidine on peptic ulcer disease in Rhode Island. Report to Smith, Kline & French
Ricardo-Campbell R, Eisman M M, Wardell W M, Cross R 1980 Preliminary methodology for controlled cost-benefit study of drug impact: the effect of cimetidine on days of work lost in a short term trial in duodenal ulcer. Journal of Clinical Gastroenterology 2: 37-41
Sonnenberg A, Hefti M L 1979 The cost of postsurgical syndromes (based on the example of duodenal ulcer treatment). Clinics in Gastroenterology 8: 235-248

13. Long-term management of duodenal ulcer — a physician's view

K. D. Bardhan

Rotherham District General Hospital, Rotherham

My views on the long-term management of duodenal ulcer are influenced by the following: the natural history of the disease and whether it can be altered by cimetidine; its severity; the options of treatment with cimetidine and when to use them; whether other drugs have more to offer than cimetidine; and a reconsideration of the role of surgery now that effective medical treatment is available.

THE NATURAL HISTORY OF DUODENAL ULCER

In his study carried out in the south of England, Fry (1964) showed that the natural history of duodenal ulcer is characterised by a progressive increase in the symptoms which reach a peak after five to ten years. Thereafter there is a strong tendency to remission and the disease gradually burns itself out. During this cycle, 16 per cent of the patients underwent elective surgery because of troublesome symptoms, 15 per cent to control haemorrhage, 7 per cent to repair a perforation and 1 per cent to relieve pyloric stenosis. A similar pattern has been observed in other parts of Britain (Watkinson, 1979) and in Denmark (Griebe et al, 1977).

However, when dealing with individual patients, it is virtually impossible to predict the course of the illness, the likely duration of the disease and indeed whether it will remit at all or last a lifetime, and whether complications will develop. In my experience, the pattern of past symptoms does not have as much predictive value as is often assumed to be the case. This is partly because the patient's memory of the frequency and pattern of past symptoms is often inaccurate, and partly because the pattern of symptoms is often erratic. Thus, it is not uncommon to see a short remission followed by a long one, and vice versa (see section on Intermittent Treatment). It is generally thought that ulcer symptoms steadily get more frequent, severe and last longer; however, not uncommonly the worsening is abrupt and unexpected. In others, the severity of symptoms remains unchanged over the years. At a time when the disease appears to be worsening, several patients find that they have an unexpectedly long remission. Finally, in others the pattern of symptoms is completely chaotic.

Duodenal ulceration is said to be getting less common and less severe, but it also affects an older age group (Langman, 1979). The mortality of ulcer disease arises principally because of complications occurring in the elderly, many of whom have associated illnesses (see section on Intermittent Treatment). Even though the disease overall seems to be less virulent than before, complications do occur. Therefore in the elderly, prophylactic treatment is probably preferable to intermittent treatment which could be used in a younger patient.

SEVERITY OF THE DISEASE

Contrary to popular opinion the majority of ulcer patients do not have severe symptoms. During their life several develop severe symptoms but at any one time in the community only a minority have a great deal of trouble. It is the patients in this small group who are seen in hospitals and about whom most is written; consequently a wrong impression is created that ulcer disease is generally severe and invariably requires vigorous treatment (Spiro, 1979). In fact many patients have mild symptoms which are controlled with occasional doses of antacids; unless there is evidence that active treatment alters the natural history of the disease there is little point in treating such patients with cimetidine (see below).

DOES CIMETIDINE ALTER THE NATURAL HISTORY OF THE DISEASE

In a study from Sweden, after ulcer healing the patients were put on either maintenance treatment with cimetidine or on placebo for a year. Treatment was then stopped and the patients followed up for another year. During the initial double-blind phase of the study, of 34 patients on placebo 15 (44 per cent) required surgery; in contrast, only 1 (3 per cent) of 30 patients on cimetidine was operated. During the year of follow-up, 7 (37 per cent) of 19 patients originally on placebo required surgery compared with only 2 (7 per cent) of 30 patients of those originally on cimetidine. In the two groups 54 and 41 per cent respectively had moderate or severe symptoms. The reduction in the number of patients operated in the group originally given cimetidine has been interpreted as indicating that the drug has a lasting beneficial effect (Bodemar and Walan, 1980). However, others have argued that by recalculating the data, 6 (20 per cent) of 30 rather than only 7 per cent required surgery and that statistically this was not different from the results in the placebo-treated group (Martin and Miller, 1980).

In a study from South Africa, 40 patients who healed on a short course of cimetidine were put on either maintenance treatment with cimetidine 0.8 g daily or on placebo for a year. At the end of this period, 21 (81 per cent) of 26 of those on cimetidine were still in remission whereas all 14 (100 per cent) of those on placebo had relapsed. Of those still in remission 20 received further treatment for a year — half on cimetidine and the other half on placebo. At the end of the second year, 8 (80 per cent) of the 10 on cimetidine were still in remission as were 6 (60 per cent) of those on placebo. The latter is in marked contrast to the high relapse rate in the first year and has been interpreted as indicating that the year's maintenance treatment had given lasting protection even after treatment was stopped (Mekel, 1980). But of the six said to be in remission, in fact four had silent ulcers or erosions, i.e. only two (20 per cent) patients were in true remission.

In contrast to these two studies all other studies have shown that, irrespective of the dose or duration of cimetidine treatment, once the drug is stopped there is a high relapse rate (Figure 13.1). In other words, cimetidine merely suppresses the disease: the natural history is unaltered (see Bardhan, 1981). This is illustrated by

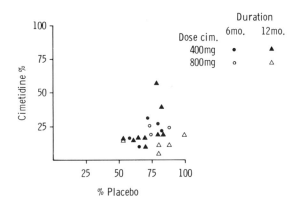

Figure 13.1   The results of 20 studies on maintenance treatment comparing cimetidine with placebo. The dose of cimetidine used and the duration of the studies are shown. Altogether there are 22 circles or triangles; the three extra symbols are from (a) the international collaborative study in which there are data on the efficacy of both the 400 mg and 800 mg dose (Burland et al, 1980); (b) from the Italian multicentre trial using cimetidine 400 mg in which data for relapse at both 6 months and 12 months are available (Salera et al, 1979). I have not included my own data since these are described in the text. This figure is taken from an article 'in press' with the permission of the Editor of *Tropical Gastroenterology*.

a study done in Rotherham. We divided into three groups 180 patients whose duodenal ulcer had healed within one month on cimetidine. The first group had no more cimetidine; the second group received cimetidine 1 g daily for another two months; and the third group for another five months. Thereafter they were given placebo and followed up for up to 25 months. During this time 69, 71 and 78 per cent respectively had a symptomatic relapse, and 81, 80 and 79 per cent respectively had either a silent or a symptomatic relapse. The rates of relapse in all three groups were similar. At 1, 3, 6, 12 and 24 months, the mean cumulative symptomatic relapse rate was: 12, 34, 55, 69 and 72 per cent. For either symptomatic or silent relapse, the corresponding figures were: 14, 46, 69, 79 and 80 per cent. Therefore the duration of cimetidine treatment did not influence the subsequent relapse rate (Bardhan et al, 1980).

But it remains to be seen whether very long-term treatment can alter the natural history; trials are in progress to examine this. A further unanswered question is whether starting treatment early in the disease affects the subsequent outcome. In most trials, the patients studied have had symptoms for several years. By this stage scarring and permanent deformity in the duodenal cap are common. It seems theoretically possible that if treatment were started early in the disease, before anatomical changes had occurred, the outcome could be different to that seen after treating patients when the condition was more established. This possibility has not been investigated; the difficulty is to find patients with early disease for at this stage symptoms are often trivial and most patients are not investigated.

CIMETIDINE: THE OPTIONS

There are two options for using cimetidine in long-term medical management: first, maintenance treatment may be used to try and prevent a relapse; second, intermittent treatment may be used to treat troublesome relapses as and when they occur.

Maintenance treatment
Several studies have confirmed that maintenance treatment markedly reduced the relapse rate (see Bardhan, 1981). Data pooled from 22 centres have shown that of 333 patients maintained on placebo after ulcer healing, 54 per cent had a symptomatic relapse within a year. In contrast, of 179 patients who received a single bedtime dose of cimetidine 400 mg nightly only 17 per cent relapsed; and of 184 patients who had 800 mg (400 mg at bedtime and 400 mg in the morning) only 15 per cent relapsed. A proportion of patients who were asymptomatic at the end of the study nevertheless had a check endoscopy: 83, 104 and 90 patients respectively, and 27, 10 and 16 per cent respectively were found to have silent re-ulceration (Burland et al, 1980). Therefore, without doubt maintenance treatment markedly reduces relapses. But there are several unanswered questions.

1. Will maintenance treatment remain effective?
Approximately one in seven patients on cimetidine relapse in the first year. Will similar proportions relapse in the following years? If so, cimetidine merely delays relapse rather than prevents it. Alternatively, will most recurrences occur early? If so, such 'treatment failures' could be selected for surgery. There are few data on the results of longer periods of treatment though recently some preliminary data have become available. Two studies by the same investigators in Milan have shown that on maintenance treatment with cimetidine 400 mg nightly, at the end of one year, 39 per cent (of 23 patients) and 42 per cent (of 31 patients) had relapsed. However, when treatment was extended for another year, only a further 12 per cent (of 36 patients) relapsed (Bianchi Porro et al, 1980). In Glasgow, a group of 47 patients on cimetidine 400 mg nightly has been followed up for three

to four years: 17 required surgery and had all relapsed within the first 14 months of treatment. Of the remaining 30 patients, only half took their treatment regularly but they remained asymptomatic. These early results suggest that the majority of relapses on maintenance treatment are likely to occur early (see below).

2. Should asymptomatic patients undergo periodic endoscopy to detect silent ulceration? (see below)

Is it important to know if the ulcer has recurred? Many feel that it is the symptoms that matter to the patient. The chances of ulcer complications such as bleeding and perforation are slight and since cimetidine does not alter the natural history of the disease, there is little point in undertaking the enormous effort of such periodic endoscopies. Others would argue that by finding a silent ulcer, early indication of treatment failure is detected and treatment can be changed if necessary. (There is a rough parallel with the treatment of hypertension. Even if asymptomatic, the blood pressure is generally checked to ensure good control. However, the consequences of a sustained rise in blood pressure, albeit silent, can be serious, and this is not the case with silent re-ulceration.)

3. What is the optimum dose of cimetidine?

The pooled data mentioned earlier showed that maintenance with 400 mg and with 800 mg gives similar results. But in individual studies this is not always the case. Thus, in two consecutive studies carried out in Milan by the same investigators, on maintenance with cimetidine 400 mg nightly, the relapse within one year was 39 per cent and 42 per cent. In the second study, the effect of an 800 mg dose was also investigated: only 19 per cent relapsed, suggesting that the higher dose is more effective (Bianchi Porro et al, 1980). In London, two consecutive trials of maintenance treatment were carried out by the same investigators. On both occasions the relapse on placebo was 66 per cent. On maintenance with cimetidine 800 mg, 24 per cent relapsed during six months. But in the second study on cimetidine 400 mg nightly, 66 per cent relapsed within six weeks.

A problem in assessing the effectiveness of different doses of cimetidine is that the relapse rate varies from centre to centre and even in the same centre at different times. Three examples are mentioned. In Dundee, after ulcer healing, four groups of patients were maintained on cimetidine 1 g daily for 3, 6, 9 and 12 months; the corresponding relapse rates were 12, 40, 23 and 50 per cent, average 30 per cent (Cargill et al, 1978). In London, maintenance treatment was given to three groups: 400 mg nightly for 6 and 12 months and 800 mg for 6 months; 55, 36 and 18 per cent respectively relapsed (Clark, 1979). In a multicentre study in which I was involved, during the six months on maintenance with cimetidine 800 mg, 19 per cent relapsed with symptoms and another 10 per cent had a silent recurrence (Bardhan et al, 1979). In contrast, in part of a recent study, two groups of patients were maintained on cimetidine 1 g daily for three months and for six months; only one and two patients respectively from each group relapsed with symptoms (3 per cent) and another five (8 per cent) from the second group had a silent ulcer; thus, in total, only 7 per cent had an ulcer recurrence (Bardhan et al, 1980).

4. Do all patients need maintenance treatment?
If cimetidine could'cure' ulcer disease, then most if not all patients would require such treatment; however, so far it appears that the drug only suppresses the disease. The indication for maintenance treatment has never been defined but the general view is that it is of value in those with frequent painful relapses. However, as mentioned earlier, in many the symptoms are mild or infrequent and there seems little point in putting them on prolonged treatment.

5. How long should treatment be continued?
As mentioned earlier, despite the strong tendency to remission, in individuals the course cannot be predicted and the disease may last a lifetime. Furthermore, if treatment were extended and remained effective, it would be difficult to know when the disease was burning itself out and therefore rendering further treatment unnecessary.

6. Is it safe?
There is the prospect of young or middle-age patients staying on the drug for many years: will it be safe? So far, cimetidine has proved to be remarkably safe but there are very few data available on any hazards associated with prolonged treatment.

My own experience on maintenance treatment is based on 261 patients who have been on cimetidine 400 mg nightly and followed up for up to two years. The cumulative symptomatic relapse at 6, 12, 18 and 24 months was 14, 18, 19 and 20 per cent. The patients had endoscopy whenever symptoms occurred but those who were asymptomatic had routine check examinations about every six months: the corresponding cumulative silent relapse was 19, 27, 32 and 34 per cent. Therefore, by combining both silent and symptomatic relapse the total, i.e. the true relapse, was 33, 45, 51 and 54 per cent. A further finding was the high rate of relapse in patients who had a refractory ulcer (which I have defined in my earlier chapter on non-responders to cimetidine). Of 201 patients whose ulcer healed quickly and were put on low-dose maintenance treatment, the total (symptomatic and silent) relapse rate at 6, 12, 18 and 24 months was 22, 33, 39 and 41 per cent. In contrast, of 61 patients whose refractory ulcer eventually healed, on maintenance treatment the corresponding relapse figures were 64, 82, 88 and 92 per cent.

There are several conclusions. First, relapses increase with the passage of time but the rate decreases; this is particularly noticeable when considering symptomatic relapse, the majority occurring within six months. Second, silent relapses occur more commonly than symptomatic relapse. Finally, those who had a refractory ulcer did not do well on maintenance treatment.

I find it difficult to understand why, if maintenance treatment prevents most relapses, it does not prevent all of them. Does the cimetidine no longer inhibit acid? Alternatively, does acid inhibition occur but the responsiveness to it is reduced? Do different attacks have varying responsiveness to acid inhibition? Does a relapse which occurs despite acid inhibition signify impaired 'defence mechanisms' and does this in turn indicate a change in the nature of the disease? If a patient relapses on maintenance treatment, is the chance of relapsing again increased? If so, it would be better not to repeat the treatment.

Intermittent treatment

An alternative approach is to treat intermittently, i.e. to treat individual symptomatic attacks as and when they occur (Bardhan, 1980). I have used this approach: patients with troublesome symptoms and with a proven ulcer were treated with short courses of cimetidine until healed and the drug was then stopped. If they developed minor symptoms, they were given antacids only; if their symptoms worsened and their ulcer was found to have recurred, they received a further course of cimetidine.

Of 125 patients treated, 83 (66 per cent) had a symptomatic relapse during the next 22 months; 38 per cent had relapsed within six months but 42 per cent had no significant symptoms for over a year. Of those who relapsed, 21 defaulted. The remaining 62 patients were re-treated but 36 (58 per cent) relapsed again. As before, the majority of relapses — 29 in all (47 per cent) — were within six months but another 29 (47 per cent) remained asymptomatic for over a year. Life-time analysis showed that such short courses of cimetidine did not alter the natural history of the disease (Figure 13.2). For the group of patients as a whole, after either one or after two short courses of cimetidine, the probability of staying

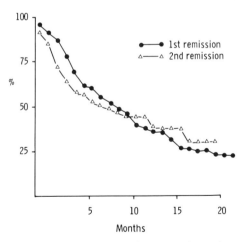

Figure 13.2 Probability of staying in remission after one and two short courses of cimetidine. The cumulative probability of relapse at one month or less is nine per cent; the corresponding figures for three and six months are 23 and 40 per cent. Conversely, 60 per cent of patients are likely to be in remission at six months, 48 per cent at nine months and 38 per cent at 12 months. Reproduced from the British Medical Journal with the permission of the Editor.

in remission fell with the passage of time, the rates of fall being similar on both occasions and greatest in the first six months. But in individual patients there was little correlation between the first and second remission periods. Some undoubtedly relapsed early each time treatment was stopped but in others, a long first remission could be followed by a short second remission and vice versa.

For the group of patients as a whole, the cumulative probability of relapse at one month or less was 9 per cent, and at three months and at six months 23 and 40 per cent respectively. Conversely, 60 per cent of the patients were likely to be in remission at six months, 48 per cent at nine months and 38 per cent at 12 months. In individual patients, I would expect that of 100 patients treated and then followed up for a year, only 7 would have 3 or more major attacks and 20 would have 2 attacks. In contrast, 37 would have only 1 attack while 36 would have none. These figures do not indicate the true ulcer relapse rate which is higher as it would include those with mild symptoms or with a silent relapse. Instead it indicates the frequency with which troublesome symptoms are likely to arise, which still remains the principal indication for treatment. Thus, the majority of patients do not have frequent attacks; as a short course of cimetidine rapidly relieves symptoms and accelerates healing in most instances, it is questionable whether they really need maintenance treatment.

Intermittent treatment is not suitable for all patients. Those who in the past have repeatedly started their attacks with haemorrhage or perforation or have developed severe symptoms abruptly cannot be treated in this manner. A major basis for intermittent treatment is that in most patients symptoms develop gradually and there is therefore enough time to intervene. However, this cannot be done if warning symptoms are absent. With every ulcer recurrence, there is a risk of haemorrhage or perforation. The chances of this occurring are very small but should it occur in the elderly or in those already ill with other problems, such as severe cardiorespiratory disease, the consequences could be serious; therefore, such patients are best not treated intermittently. By these criteria, about one-fifth of the patients are found unsuitable for this regime.

On the other hand, there are several advantages of intermittent treatment. First, it is simple. Once duodenal ulcer has been diagnosed, further treatment can be given without preliminary radiology or endoscopy. Recurrence of typical symptoms generally indicates re-ulceration and a one to two-month course of cimetidine will heal the ulcer in most instances (Bardhan et al, 1979). Endoscopy can be reserved for the few patients with either atypical symptoms or whose symptoms persist despite treatment. This regime therefore becomes suitable for use in general practice. Second, intermittent treatment is cheaper than maintenance treatment. The cost of treating a patient with the intermittent regime, taking into account the relapse rate mentioned earlier, is £55, while the cost for maintenance treatment of one patient is £126. Third, those who repeatedly relapse rapidly each time treatment is stopped are easily recognised; they can be selected for operation or for maintenance treatment.

Thus, for the majority of patients, intermittent treatment suffices for longer-term treatment.

A study from Copenhagen has given similar results (Rune et al, 1979): 65 patients were treated intermittently, and when treatment was stopped there was a high relapse rate. Many of those re-treated relapsed again but there was no correlation between the first and second remission period. During a one-year follow-up, 16 per cent had no further relapses; 32 per cent had one relapse and 23 per cent had two relapses; but 29 per cent had three or more relapses. The rate of relapse in this study was higher than the one I had observed. There are two likely explanations. First, the populations studied were different. Second, in the Danish study, the patients were seen at frequent intervals and therefore most if not all symptomatic attacks were detected. In contrast I asked my patients to return only when they felt their symptoms to be troublesome. Undoubtedly some did not do so because their symptoms were short-lived, resulting in an under-estimate of the number of relapses. Nevertheless there is agreement that the majority of patients have only up to two troublesome relapses a year.

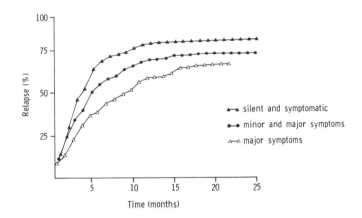

Figure13.3 The cumulative relapse rate of duodenal ulcer measured by three different criteria. The *open triangles* show relapse as judged by the recurrence of troublesome symptoms after ulcer healing with a short course of cimetidine. It is based on data from intermittent treatment and shows the outcome after the first short course of cimetidine (see Bardhan, 1980). The remainder of the data, shown by the other two symbols, shows the relapse rate on placebo, which was preceded by cimetidine treatment for variable lengths of time (Bardhan et al, 1980). In this study, the patients had a check endoscopy every three months if asymptomatic or earlier if symptoms developed. Because of the frequent attendance, silent and symptomatic recurrences were detected. The *closed circles* show relapse taking into account both minor and major symptoms. It is greater than those obtained with intermittent treatment in which the patients reported back only when they had sustained troublesome symptoms. The *closed triangles* show relapse, both symptomatic and silent; it is therefore a measure of the true relapse rate.
This illustration has been taken from a paper published in *Tropical Gastroenterology* and appears with the permission of the Editor.

The results of intermittent treatment will vary according to the proportion of patients seen with severe disease and the criteria used for judging relapse. In specialist units there will inevitably be a high proportion of patients with severe ulcer disease characterised by frequent disabling attacks; maintenance treatment would give better results than intermittent treatment here (Hetzel et al, 1980; Pounder, 1981). However, in general practice, a higher proportion of patients have milder disease: intermittent treatment is likely to give good results.

HOW DO OTHER DRUGS COMPARE WITH CIMETIDINE IN ULCER HEALING?

It is ironic that until six years ago no drug was found to be of proven benefit in duodenal ulceration; yet today several are available. The two new histamine H_2 receptor antagonists, ranitidine and oxmetidine are as effective as cimetidine. Several drugs of other classes are of proven effectiveness: antacids in large doses, carbenoxolone, colloidal bismuth, pirenzipine, tri-imipramine, sucralfate, prostaglandins, proglumide, thiopropamine (Di Mario, 1980), doxepin, sulglycotide, bicitropeptide (Moshal et al, 1980). Trithiozine and acetazolamide require special mention (see below) (see Bardhan 1981 for further details about these drugs).

The first six drugs have been compared with cimetidine in double-blind trials and found to be equally effective. But there are drawbacks: antacids in large doses are inconvenient and frequently cause diarrhoea; and carbenoxolone can be unsafe by causing fluid retention, hypokalaemia and high blood pressure. Colloidal bismuth is available as a liquid but its strong ammoniacal odour makes it unpleasant to take; but tablet preparations have been developed and found to be equally effective (Vantrappen et al, 1980; Hamilton and Axon, 1981). Pirenzipine can cause anticholinergic type side-effects; nevertheless it seems promising. The remaining drugs (with the two exceptions) have not been investigated to the same degree. Cimetidine remains one of the most thoroughly investigated drugs ever used in medicine and certainly the anti-ulcer drug studied in greatest detail; it is the standard against which other drugs will need to be compared.

Trithiozine inhibits acid secretion but its mechanism of action is unknown. In large studies carried out in Italy, it was found to be much superior to placebo and as effective as cimetidine. Yet little is known about this drug in the UK (Pellegrini, 1979).

The reports from Roumania on acetazolamide are astonishing; in both studies, the drug was compared with placebo. In the 'smaller' investigation of 49 patients on placebo, 18 per cent healed in 2 weeks and 31 per cent in 3 weeks. In contrast, of 385 patients on acetazolamide, 72 per cent healed in 10 days, 94 per cent in 2 weeks and 98 per cent in 3 weeks (Pascu and Búzás, 1980). In the larger study, of 568 patients on placebo 36 per cent healed in 2 weeks and 46 per cent in 3 weeks; at this stage, 53 per cent were pain-free. On the other hand, of 1211 patients on acetazolamide, the corresponding healing rates were 92 and 98 per cent; furthermore 97 per cent became pain-free within three to five days (Lenghel et al,

1980). The study and the results are all the more impressive because both were single-centre investigations. There is no other drug, including cimetidine, which has involved such large numbers of patients in double-blind trials or has produced such spectacular results. It is therefore surprising that virtually nothing has been heard of this achievement in the UK.

CAN SHORT-TERM TREATMENT INFLUENCE THE OUTCOME IN THE LONGER TERM?

As mentioned earlier, when cimetidine is withdrawn there is a high relapse rate and the disease continues its usual course. It therefore seems highly unlikely that any form of short-term treatment can produce a lasting effect on a disease with such a long natural history. Yet some reports suggest that with certain drugs the beneficial effects last, so that when treatment is stopped the subsequent relapse rate is less. These drugs are: carbenoxolone, colloidal bismuth, trithiozine, proglumide, antacid–anticholinergic combination and acetazolamide. These results are unexpected and as there are quite likely to be further developments in this area, further details are mentioned below.

A clue that the method of healing might have long-term consequences came from the pooled data on maintenance treatment. Of those who had healed on cimetidine and were then maintained on placebo 63 per cent (of 290 patients) had a symptomatic relapse within one year; in contrast, of those who healed on placebo and then continued on it, only 47 per cent (of 30 patients) relapsed. At the time it was felt that as the ulcer had healed on placebo the subsequent lower relapse rate reflected milder disease (Burland et al, 1980). However, it has also been suggested that the method of healing might have influenced these results (Baron et al, 1980).

In a study from Milan, treatment with carbenoxolone was apparently followed by a lower relapse rate than after treatment with cimetidine; the difference has been attributed to the different mechanisms of action of the drugs (Guslandi et al, 1980). However, the conclusion is not really supported by the evidence. Duodenal ulcer patients who healed on cimetidine 1 g daily in four to six weeks were then given further treatment with either cimetidine 400 mg nightly or carbenoxolone 150 mg daily for a further three months. At the end of this period, 22 per cent (of 27 patients) and 18 per cent (of 21 patients) respectively had relapsed. Those still in remission were given no further treatment. Three months later, 26 per cent of those previously on maintenance cimetidine had relapsed compared with only four per cent of those who were given carbenoxolone. The total proportions relapsed therefore were 48 and 21 per cent respectively. The 'muco-protective index' of gastric juice was measured and found to be low after cimetidine whereas it increased significantly after carbenoxolone. The most surprising part of these results is that during the maintenance phase the relapse rates were similar on both drugs: it would be expected that if carbenoxolone had a special protective action the relapse rate would be low whilst the patients were on the drug rather than off it. I also think it is questionable whether the 'mucoprotective index' is really a valid measurement of mucosal protection since spent mucus is used which is biologically inert and does not reflect the state of the active gel-forming mucus (Allen and Garner, 1980).

In a study from Manchester the outcome after ulcer healing with colloidal bismuth and cimetidine has been compared. Over the next 18 months, 89 per cent of 19 cimetidine-healed patients relapsed compared with 52 per cent of 23 patients healed on bismuth (Martin et al, 1981).

In a study from Belgium colloidal bismuth subcitrate tablets were shown to be as effective as cimetidine in healing ulcers. Of those who healed, 10 patients from each group were followed for the next three months; three treated with cimetidine relapsed compared with only one healed on bismuth (Vantrappen et al, 1980).

Proglumide is an unusual antisecretory compound which is said to be an anti-gastrin. In a study from Milan 12 patients who healed on cimetidine and 17 who healed on proglumide had no further treatment and were followed up over the next two years, endoscopy being carried out every three months (Galeone et al, 1980). Of the cimetidine-healed patients 15 (88 per cent) relapsed compared with only 4 (33 per cent) of those healed on proglumide. It was calculated that half the patients treated with cimetidine would relapse by five months compared with 31 months for those treated with proglumide.

Trithiozine is a new antisecretory agent whose mechanism of action is not understood. In a study from Spain 4 groups of 20 patients each were treated for 4 weeks with trithiozine or cimetidine (Guemes, 1980). In the first two groups, 80 and 95 per cent of the patients respectively healed. No further treatment was given. By six months, 19 and 53 per cent respectively of those healed on trithiozine and cimetidine had relapsed; at 12 months the corresponding figures were 44 and 58 per cent. In the other two groups, the healing was 80 and 85 per cent respectively. They were then continued on low-dose maintenance treatment with these drugs. At 6 months, 13 per cent of those on trithiozine and 35 per cent of those on cimetidine relapsed and at 12 months the corresponding figures were 25 and 41 per cent. Thus on maintenance treatment trithiozine appeared to give better results; also, after a short course, the early relapse rate after healing with this drug is lower than after healing with cimetidine.

In Sweden 54 patients with duodenal ulcer and 18 patients with pre-pyloric ulcer were treated with either cimetidine, an antacid–anticholinergic combination, or placebo; the corresponding healing rates were 96, 100 and 50 per cent respectively. The treatment was then stopped and the patients followed for up to a year. The total numbers relapsed were not significantly different: 73 per cent (of 22 patients), 50 per cent (of 22 patients) and 56 per cent (of nine patients) respectively. But the median time to relapse after healing on cimetidine was only 11 weeks compared with 24 weeks of those healed on the antacid–anticholinergic combination; these results are different (Ström et al, 1980).

In the study from Roumania referred to earlier, of those who healed on placebo, 51 per cent relapsed compared with only seven per cent of those healed on acetazolamide (Pascu and Búzás, 1980). No comparison was made with cimetidine; also, the duration of follow-up is not stated. However, the relapse after placebo healing is similar to that seen in other studies (Burland et al, 1980); also, the relapse rate after healing on acetazolamide is much lower than one would expect after healing with cimetidine.

The results of these studies are unexpected. If confirmed, it would suggest that the different pharmacological effects of the various drugs have an influence on the durability of healing. If these drugs are as safe as cimetidine, then it is quite likely that some of them will influence practical management, for short courses of treatment might be followed by longer periods of remission.

PRACTICAL MANAGEMENT: A PERSONAL PRACTICE

Briefly, I confirm the diagnosis, use intermittent treatment with cimetidine for the majority of patients and maintenance treatment for those with more troublesome disease; and reserve operation for those resistant to cimetidine. Further details are given below.

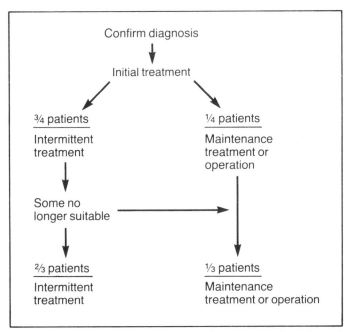

Figure 13.4 'The Rotherham plan': a flow diagram showing my personal practice. This approach serves for most patients. Management of those who do not heal or who relapse on maintenance treatment is discussed in the text.

Making an accurate diagnosis in the first place is essential: in my experience only about one in three patients referred with suspected ulcer disease turn out to have one. The main causes of 'non-ulcer dyspepsia' I find are irritable bowel syndrome and gastro-oesophageal reflux. Pain of musculoskeletal origin, gall stones and occasionally gastric cancer mimic ulcer disease. When there is a shortage of diagnostic facilities, there is a great temptation for hard-pressed practitioners to use cimetidine as a combined diagnostic and therapeutic measure; since the majority of patients with dyspepsia do not have an ulcer, it is hardly surprising that some patients appear resistant to cimetidine whilst others improve owing to a non-specific placebo response.

Endoscopy is the best diagnostic method, but the double-contrast barium meal can be nearly as accurate. With the latter, ideally an ulcer crater should be demonstrated before making the diagnosis of duodenal ulceration. However, quite commonly it is not possible to demonstrate this; in this case, if the duodenal cap is severely deformed, it indicates that there either is, or has been, an ulcer. But mild deformities of the duodenal cap, though compatible with ulceration, are certainly not diagnostic.

What about the patient whose symptoms have disappeared before investigations are carried out? This problem is not uncommon when waiting lists for investigations are long. If radiology fails to show an ulcer, only a deformed duodenal cap, it is not uncommon to find at endoscopy that there is still an ulcer remnant, or erosions or considerable duodenitis. But at times at endoscopy only a scar is seen. In this case it is difficult to know with certainty whether the recent symptoms were due to ulceration or not. In this case, I do not give cimetidine (unless the patient is old or has other major illnesses); instead, I arrange to carry out an endoscopy if and when symptoms recur, for the diagnostic yield then is at its greatest.

Having confirmed the diagnosis, I give cimetidine 1 g daily for about six weeks. The majority of patients are then treated intermittently, short courses of cimetidine being repeated when significant symptoms reappear (for research purposes, I carry out endoscopy to confirm ulceration and healing in each attack but as mentioned in the section on Intermittent Treatment, in the vast majority of patients, for practical management, this is unnecessary). In between, I advise patients to use antacids only for relief of minor symptoms; if heartburn is the main problem, I give an antacid–alginate combination. However, at the outset, between one-fifth and one-quarter of the patients are considered unsuitable for intermittent treatment; they are put on to low-dose maintenance treatment with cimetidine 400 mg nightly. With the passage of time, some patients are found no longer suitable for intermittent treatment, mainly because the attacks have become more frequent and severe or occasionally occur more abruptly; they too are transferred to maintenance treatment.

In the 'high-risk' group of patients (the elderly or those with other major illnesses) I have no hesitation in continuing them on cimetidine and plan to keep them on it permanently unless some hitherto unforeseen hazard with the drug is discovered. The reason for this approach is that the mortality and the morbidity of alternative treatment, namely operation, is greater than any theoretical risk of long-term treatment. Furthermore, several of such patients are in poor health and are unlikely to survive long; therefore there is little chance that they will experience any complication that might arise from long-term treatment.

The difficulty in deciding upon long-term management is in the young patient or the older person who is fit. Elective operation, particularly highly selective (proximal gastric) vagotomy, gives excellent results and the long-term consequences following operation are well known. In contrast, the long-term consequences of cimetidine treatment are not known. On the basis of present knowledge, it seems unlikely that there will be any long-term hazard but there is no certainty about this, a factor which needs to be remembered when treating patients for very long periods for a non-lethal disease when an alternative is available.

However, in Rotherham, there is a growing demand for maintenance treatment by the majority of patients and a reluctance to consider operation (see below). If they are unsuitable for intermittent treatment and provided they are willing to stay under close medical supervision, I put them on maintenance treatment. For the others with troublesome ulcer disease who cannot attend for periodic check-ups or who prefer surgery because it is a once-and-for-all treatment, I keep them on maintenance treatment until the operation: they stay asymptomatic and can lead normal lives until the operation, which therefore is no longer urgent.

In those on low-dose maintenance treatment, I carry out a check endoscopy every six to eight months if asymptomatic or earlier if symptoms recur. If ulcer recurrence is proven, then I give a short course of full-dose cimetidine and after healing put them back onto maintenance treatment. Those with symptomatic relapse clearly need a healing course of cimetidine. For those with a silent relapse, I give the same treatment on the grounds that, technically, maintenance treatment has failed. However, as mentioned earlier, even though in my experience silent relapse is more common than symptomatic relapse, it is not known whether this approach will make any difference in the long term. For those who relapse two or three times on low-dose maintenance treatment, I keep them on full dose (1 g) maintenance. But the result of this policy has not yet been assessed.

In my department, cimetidine is the mainstay of medical treatment. Apart from antacids (and occasionally carbenoxolone — see below) I do not use any other drugs, partly because some of the active agents are not available in the UK but largely because none of them has been as thoroughly researched as cimetidine. Mild symptoms, particularly heartburn, but without re-ulceration are not at all uncommon in those who are off cimetidine in the intermittent treatment regime, or are on low-dose maintenance treatment; I advise small amounts of antacids or an antacid/alginate combination.

The management of patients with a refractory duodenal ulcer is difficult. If the ulcer has not healed within three months and they remain asymptomatic, then arbitrarily I continue them on the same regime for a further three months or so. If, on the other hand, failure to heal is associated with much pain, or the ulcer has enlarged, then I increase the cimetidine to 2 g daily. If symptoms are severe, I admit them to hospital. Cimetidine 2 g daily is given and supplemented with large amounts of antacids: 25 ml one and three hours after meals, 50 ml at bedtime and another 50 ml whenever pain occurs (I use a mixture of equal parts of magnesium trisilicate and aluminium hydroxide though any antacid of high potency will do just as well). This regime provides relief in more than half the patients. In some of the patients where this has failed, I have tried adding carbenoxolone, 150 to 300 mg daily. But there is no clear evidence that this has really helped. Those with intractable symptoms at this stage are referred for operation. Occasionally at this stage I have tried the effect of a 3 g dose of cimetidine; it has helped in some patients.

When should operation be carried out? The indications remain unchanged: when medical treatment fails and when complications develop (and in many parts of the world when medical treatment proves too expensive). With cimetidine, medical treatment rarely fails. The problem is that the definition of failure varies from person to person. Thus, some would accept persistence of an ulcer on a standard dose of cimetidine as failure whereas others only if associated with troublesome symptoms. Many consider relapse, particularly symptomatic relapse on low-dose maintenance treatment, as failure. In contrast, I have tried to use cimetidine more vigorously as experience with the drug has increased. This practice has led to a considerable reduction in the number of patients undergoing elective operation. In contrast, the number of patients operated upon to repair a perforated duodenal ulcer has not changed; this is only to be expected as this complication occurs abruptly and none of the patients had been on cimetidine at the time of perforation (Table 13.1).

Table 13.1 Operations for duodenal ulcer in Rotherham before and after cimetidine.

Year	Number of patients undergoing elective vagotomy and drainage	Number of patients undergoing repair of perforation
1972	69	14
1973	52	17
1974	59	20
1975	61	16
Cimetidine introduced in April 1976		
1976	38	25
1977	43	15
1978	45	26
1979	8	24
Jan–June 1980	2	14

This paper is dedicated to Dr Sidney C. Truelove, Emeritus Consultant Physician at the Radcliffe Infirmary, Oxford, from whom I learned so much.

REFERENCES

Allen A, Garner A 1980 Mucus and bicarbonate secretion in the stomach and their possible role in mucosal protection. Gut 21: 249-262
Bardhan K D 1980 Intermittent treatment of duodenal ulcer. British Medical Journal 281: 20-22
Bardhan K D 1981 Medical treatment of duodenal ulcer: a review. Tropical Gastroenterology 2: 4-33
Bardhan K D, Cole D S, Hawkins B W, Sharpe P C 1980 Does extended cimetidine treatment after duodenal ulcer healing reduce the subsequent relapse rate? Gut 21: A898

*Bardhan K D, Saul D M, Edwards J L, Smith P M, Haggie S J, Wyllie J H, Duthie H L, Fussey I V 1979 A multicentre double-blind comparison of cimetidine and placebo in the maintenance of healing of chronic duodenal ulceration. Gut 20: 158-162

Baron J H, Langman M J S, Wastell C 1980 Stomach and duodenum. In: Bouchier I A D (ed) Recent advances in gastroenterology, 4. Churchill Livingstone, Edinburgh, p 23-86

Bianchi Porro G, Burland W L, Hawkins B W, Petrillo M 1980 Long-term treatment of duodenal ulcer with cimetidine: a review. In: Torsoli A, Lucchelli P E, Brimblecombe R W (eds) H₂-receptor antagonists in peptic ulcer disease and progress in histamine research. Excerpta Medica, Amsterdam, Oxford, Princeton, p 91-101

Bodemar G, Walan A 1980 Two-year follow-up after one year's treatment with cimetidine or placebo. Lancet 1: 38

Burland W L, Hawkins B W, Beresford J 1980 Cimetidine treatment for the prevention of recurrence of duodenal ulcer: an international collaborative study. Postgraduate Medical Journal 56: 173-176

Cargill J M, Teden N, Saunders J H B, Wormsley K G 1978 Very long-term treatment of peptic ulcer with cimetidine. Lancet 2: 1113-1115

Clark C G 1979 The influence of cimetidine on current surgical treatment of peptic ulceration. British Journal of Clinical Practice 33: 216-219

Di Mario F 1980 The value of thiopropamine (T) in the treatment of duodenal ulcer. Clinical Therapeutics 93: 389-400

Fry J 1964 Peptic ulcer: a profile. British Medical Journal 2: 809-812

Galeone M, Moise G, Casula P L, Bignamini A A 1980 Two year survey of ulcer relapses after proglumide: a comparative study. Hepatogastroenterology, Suppl, VI European Congress of Gastrointestinal Endoscopy, p 144, H3.1

Griebe J, Bugge P, Gjorup T, Lauritzen T, Bonnevie O, Wulff H R 1977 Long-term prognosis of duodenal ulcer: follow up study and survey of doctors' estimates. British Medical Journal 2: 1572-1574

Guemes F 1980 Short and long-term effects of trithiozine and cimetidine, followed or not by maintenance treatment in duodenal ulcer. Hepatogastroenterology, Suppl, XI International Congress of Gastroenterology, Hamburg 1980, p 49, F1.11

Guslandi M, Cambielli M, Tittobello A 1980 Carbenoxolone maintenance in cimetidine-healed patients. Scandinavian Journal of Gastroenterology 15: 369-371

Hamilton I, Axon A T R 1981 Controlled trial comparing De-Nol tablets with De-Nol liquid in treatment of duodenal ulcer. British Medical Journal 2: 362

Hetzel D J, Hecker R, Shearman D J C 1980 The long-term treatment of duodenal ulcer with cimetidine: intermittent or continuous therapy? Australian and New Zealand Journal of Medicine 10: 364

Langman M J S 1979 The epidemiology of chronic digestive disease. Edward Arnold, London

Lenghel A, Micle Tr, Cristea N 1980 Treatment of duodenal ulcer with carbonic anhydrase inhibitors. Hepatogastroenterology, Suppl, XI International Congress of Gastroenterology, 300, E36: 16

Martin D, Miller J P 1980 Cimetidine and course of peptic ulcer disease. Lancet 1; 307-308

Martin F 1980 Comparative healing capacity of sucralfate and cimetidine in short term treatment of duodenal ulcer: a double-blind randomised controlled study. American Journal of Gastroenterology 74: 85

Martin D F, Hollanders D, May S J, Ravenscroft M M, Tweedle D E F, Miller J P 1981 Differences in relapse rate of duodenal ulcer healing with cimetidine or tripotassium dicitrate bismuthate. Lancet 1: 7-10

Mekel R C P M 1980 Two-year maintenance treatment with cimetidine for duodenal ulcers. South African Medical Journal, 57: 293

Moshal M G, Spitaels J M, Khan F 1980 Bicitropeptide and cimetidine in the treatment of duodenal ulcer. South African Medical Journal 58: 631-633

Pascu O, Búzás Gh 1980 Endoscopic follow-up of duodenal ulcer scarring after treatment with carbonic anhydrase inhibitors. Hepatogastroenterology, Suppl, IV European Congress of Gastrointestinal Endoscopy 257: 43, E11.9

Pellegrini R 1979 Clinical effects of trithiozine, a newer gastric antisecretory agent. Journal of International Medical Research, 7: 452-457

Pounder R E 1981 Model of medical treatment for duodenal ulcer. Lancet 1: 29-30

Rune S J, Hesselfeldt P H, Larsen N-E 1979 Clinical and pharmacological effectiveness of cimetidine in duodenal ulcer patients. Scandinavian Journal of Gastroenterology 14: 489-492

Salera M, Taroni F, Miglioli M, Santini D, Di Febo G, Baldi F, Barbara L 1979 Long-term effects and after-effects of cimetidine in duodenal ulcer patients. Italian Journal of Gastroenterology 11: 49-52

Spiro H M 1979 Should we take duodenal ulcer so seriously? Journal of Clinical Gastroenterology 1: 199-201

Ström M, Gotthard R, Bodemar G, Walan A 1980 Symptomatic relapse after treatment for peptic ulcer with cimetidine or antacid/anticholinergic. Scandinavian Journal of Gastroenterology 15: A50

Vantrappen G, Rutgeerts P, Broeckaert L, Janssens J et al 1980 Randomised open controlled trial of colloidal bismuth subcitrate tablets and cimetidine in the treatment of duodenal ulcer. Gut 21: 329-333

Watkinson G 1979 Peptic ulcer: epidemiological aspects. In: Truelove S C, Willoughby C P (eds) Topics in Gastroenterology, 7. Blackwell Scientific Publications, Oxford, p 3-34

14. Long-term management of duodenal ulcer — a surgeon's view

Christopher Venables

Newcastle University Hospitals, Newcastle upon Tyne

Until the advent of histamine H_2 receptor antagonists surgery held the stage in the long-term control of duodenal ulcer when a patient had severe or rapidly recurrent symptoms. As a result surgeons became used to handling such patients and were able to recognise the problems of surgical management and to decide for whom it was the most appropriate form of therapy. The introduction of cimetidine (late in 1976) altered all this as it provided for the first time a medical means of controlling the ulcer and its associated symptoms over a long period. This has led to a major alteration in management of ulcer patients and a change in the pattern of hospital referral, the impact of which is still being evaluated. How then do surgeons view this change? There are three ways in which individual surgeons may and do react!

Reaction 1. That treatment with cimetidine only delays the need for operation and is therefore not justified
This reaction is based on the concept that all patients treated with cimetidine will eventually require surgical therapy and thus it is both a waste of money and the patient's time to delay this inevitable decision. If this were the case then one might expect to see evidence of this by examining the number of patients now coming to operation four years after the introduction of this drug. One would anticipate an immediate fall in the number of operations performed but this would be followed by a 'rebound' as those whose operations were initially delayed came to later operation. To investigate this point I have examined both the numbers of operations for duodenal ulcer performed in our Region and in my own surgical practice.

Figure 14.1 illustrates the results of our study for the Northern Region. Duodenal ulcer is a common problem in our area as is shown by the fact that the number of discharges with this final diagnosis remained fairly constant over the years 1971 to 1976 ($\bar{x}$ = 4700: range 4482–4935). Interestingly the number of such patients coming to operation was falling before cimetidine was introduced from a peak of 1757 in 1971 to a low of 1164 in 1975 — a fact which is difficult to explain. Cimetidine caused a further significant fall to a mean of 660 operations per year in the three years 1977 to 1979. Comparing the mean number of operations between 1971 and 1975 and between 1977 and 1979 there was an overall reduction in operations of 57 per cent.

113

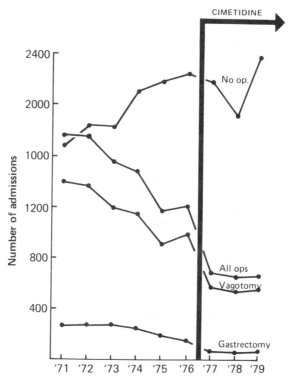

Figure 14.1   Admissions for duodenal ulcer in Northern Region, 1971–1979. Relationship to type and number of operations performed.

This is of considerable interest as it is very similar to the reduction which one might predict if a 'model' situation is constructed (Figure 14.2). If one were to assume that 100 patients were selected for surgery and 10 had to have it because of stenosis or drug intolerance one could estimate that 58 would avoid an operation if they were treated with cimetidine and placed on maintenance therapy (assuming 80 per cent ulcer healing and 80 per cent one-year control on maintenance).

These results (Figure 14.1) suggest that the number coming to operation in our Region has plateaued over the years since cimetidine was introduced. Certainly up to 1979 there has been no sign of a rebound. To investigate more recent trends I have examined my own surgical practice up to the end of 1980 (Figure 14.3). Through my known interest in both the medical and surgical therapy of duodenal ulcer I have a large referral practice in this condition, and local general practitioners tend to refer to me cases which have proved difficult to manage medically. It might be anticipated that my own practice would show evidence of a surgical 'rebound' long before it appeared in national or regional figures. In fact, whilst there has been a rise in operations since the initial trough, there is no evidence of the type of rebound one would anticipate if surgery were only being delayed!

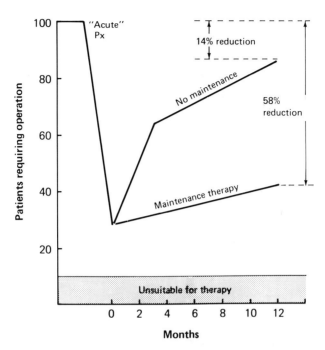

Figure 14.2   Theoretical effect of cimetidine therapy upon the number coming to operation whether a single or a maintenance course of therapy is used.

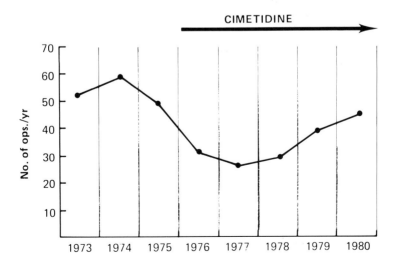

Figure 14.3   Operations for duodenal ulcer performed on our surgical unit 1973–1980.

Reaction 2. That cimetidine treatment would abolish the need for operation and this would be a surgical disaster.
This was certainly a fear amongst some surgeons when cimetidine was first introduced. However, this has not proved to be the case as can be seen in Figure 14.1. It might have been true had cimetidine treatment resulted in an alteration in either the incidence or natural history of the disease. As far as 'incidence' is concerned one of the best measures of this is the number of perforations. These occur usually without prior warning and probably represent a relatively stable proportion of all duodenal ulcers in the community. I have therefore examined the numbers of patients undergoing emergency surgery for peptic ulcer in our Northern Region (Figure 14.4). As can be seen, the number of perforations has

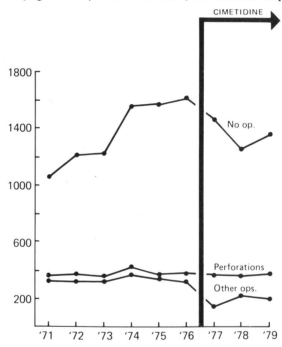

Figure 14.4   Emergency admissions for peptic ulcer disease 1971–1979.

remained remarkably stable over the past decade although there has been a fall in other 'emergency' operations since cimetidine was introduced. These figures would suggest that this drug has not altered the prevalence of duodenal ulcer in the community.

Has cimetidine altered the natural history of duodenal ulcer? So far, most studies set up to examine this topic have produced negative results (Gudmand-Hoyer et al, 1978: Dronfield et al, 1979: Salera et al, 1979: Cargill et al, 1978) but we must await longer-term assessment before we know the answer to this question. At the moment it certainly would appear that cimetidine does nothing more than control the disease whilst it is given. Thus the requirement for surgery should remain unless more effective agents are developed.

Reaction 3. That surgery and cimetidine therapy are complementary
This is the reaction which I believe is most appropriate. It is based on the concept that by using cimetidine one may avoid in some patients the need for operation. This is desirable because surgical side-effects are worse than those of medical therapy. I believe that one should examine this concept under a number of headings:

Effectiveness. Both surgery and cimetidine are effective in controlling duodenal ulcer disease. The former has the edge, as even with the least curative operation (probably proximal gastric vagotomy) one would expect to 'cure' the ulcer in at least 85 per cent, whilst cimetidine will produce long-term control in only about 58 per cent (Figure 14.2). However, this latter result is only true if further 'therapeutic' doses of cimetidine are not used and it is more likely that around 70 per cent could be controlled in the long term if repeat courses plus maintenance therapy were used when indicated.

The major disadvantage of cimetidine is that continued treatment is required even when the patient is asymptomatic. This can be difficult to achieve, and if the patient is not motivated to take the therapy then he is still exposed to the risks of complications of his disease.

Convenience. Clearly cimetidine scores over surgery from this point of view. Without doubt, it is more convenient to take pills than to come into hospital for an operation, even if the latter does eliminate the need for any further treatment in the future. Very few patients enjoy having an operation and it can seriously affect their social life and work.

Cost. Again cimetidine proves to be the 'better buy' as surgery involves considerable costs. The greatest cost of all is that of death which can occur after gastric surgery no matter how good or careful the surgeon is. Whilst large series of duodenal ulcer operations have been published without any reports of mortality (Goligher et al, 1968) the following mortality rates are generally expected: 0.8 per cent after vagotomy and 1.6 per cent after vagotomy plus gastrectomy (Cox et al, 1969). So far no one has died as a direct result of cimetidine therapy. The cost of just one death can vary from £37 500 to £3000 000 depending on the method one chooses to calculate cost (Culyer and Maynard, 1980).

There are inevitable costs involved in the operation itself such as the actual cost of performing the operation (£399 for a vagotomy in 1978) and loss of the patient's earnings whilst he is in hospital (average £600: 1978). Compared with these costs a 20-year outlay on cimetidine therapy (1 g/day for four weeks then 400 mg nocte for 20 years) of £884 is quite reasonable (Figure 14.5).

Side effects. Clearly this is the area of most controversy. It has been argued that it is reasonable to treat the elderly by long-term cimetidine therapy because the operative risks of surgery are greater but it is unreasonable to treat younger patients in this way because of the potential unknown long-term risks of such therapy. Whilst it behoves us all to continue to be vigilant during long-term therapy, so that any adverse events are spotted at an early stage, I do not believe that we have any reason to say that long-term maintenance therapy has

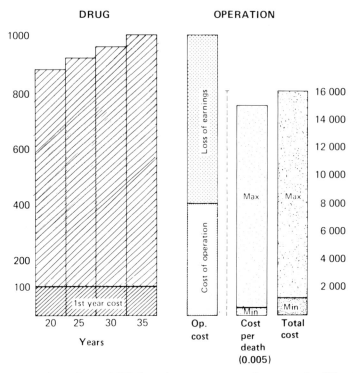

Figure 14.5 Comparison of costs (1978 figures): vagotomy versus long-term cimetidine. Right-hand columns are the estimated additional cost per patient if one patient per 200 dies from operation.

unacceptable risks. In contrast (Table 14.1) the medium and long-term risks of surgical treatment are well known and are neither completely predictable nor preventable. Furthermore, it is known that the younger the patient the greater the risk of side-effects occurring, as has been shown in the controlled trial of vagotomy plus pyloroplasty and vagotomy plus gastroenterostomy in Glasgow (Mackay et al, 1973).

Table 14.1 Complications of therapy for duodenal ulcer

	Cimetidine	Surgery
Short/ medium term	Skin rashes CNS side effects Hepatic toxicity Renal toxicity Drug interactions	Abdominal pain Heartburn Dumping Diarrhoea Vomiting
Long term	Gynaecomastia ? Immunological ? Gastric carcinoma ? Other unknown	Weight loss Anaemia Bone disease TB Gastric carcinoma

Thus it is my own belief that long-term cimetidine therapy is justified in any patient with rapid relapsing duodenal ulcer disease provided one is prepared to supervise and monitor progress on this treatment. It is undoubtedly easier to stop a 'pill' than it is to reverse the effects of an operation.

What about the question of whether carcinoma is induced by cimetidine therapy? Clearly we should continue to have an open mind regarding this possibility but there would appear to be no experimental or clinical grounds for believing this to be a possibility. Of course, surgery is not without this danger as Stalsberg and Taksdal (1971) showed that the incidence of cancer in the gastric remnant over 25 years after operation was six times that found in controls. Whether vagotomy is associated with such an increase has not, as yet, been shown but it remains a possible long-term problem.

WHEN SHOULD OPERATION BE PERFORMED?

The main danger of 'overenthusiastic' use of cimetidine is that surgery will not be used when it should be. Clearly no one would argue with the need for operation when a perforation has occurred, when stenosis is present, or if gastrointestinal bleeding cannot be controlled, but there is less agreement as to when it should be used in uncomplicated ulcers. In my own view the indications for operation are now as follows:

When the ulcer cannot be healed by any form of medical therapy
These patients are a risk to themselves and will usually continue to have symptoms that are incompletely controlled. They also offer a challenge to the surgeon as it is our impression that their ulcers have a greater tendency to recur after vagotomy than we would have expected (18 per cent at two years: Venables, 1980).

When 'long-term' control is impossible
In about 20 per cent of patients maintenance therapy is ineffective even when a therapeutic dose (1 g/day) has healed the ulcer. Personally I believe it is not reasonable to continue full-dose therapy for a prolonged period, except in the elderly or those on rheumatoid drugs, and I would therefore recommend operation in these patients. Our experience suggests that these patients respond very well to vagotomy.

When cimetidine produces side-effects or patient intolerance develops
Clearly these patients, if uncontrolled on any other therapy, will have to have surgical treatment.

If carcinoma is suspected
It is not reasonable to go on treating medically anyone who has an ulcer thought to be malignant. This is unlikely to be a problem with an uncomplicated duodenal

ulcer but sometimes there is a coexistent prepyloric or lesser curve gastric ulcer present. These latter ulcers are far more likely to undergo malignant change and therefore regular endoscopic and histological assessment is required.

How do these indications work in practice? Figure 14.6 shows all the patients who have come to operation on my unit since we started using cimetidine. As can be seen the major indication is 'failure to heal' which constitutes 62 per cent of my patients.

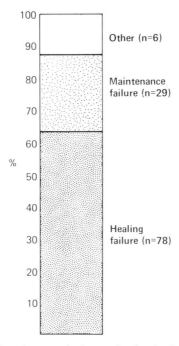

Figure 14.6   Reasons why patients have required operation for duodenal ulcer after treatment with cimetidine on our unit.

PROBLEMS RESULTING FROM REDUCED NEED FOR OPERATIONS

The most obvious problem resulting from a reduced need for operations is the impact upon training. Most operations for duodenal ulcer disease require skill and experience gained only by seeing and performing the operations many times under supervision. The reduced throughput of such operations has seriously reduced this experience, particularly on general surgical units without a major interest in gastroenterology. If this trend continues then surgical quality is threatened and the risks of emergency gastric surgery are increased. This effect should be recognised for the dangers it imposes. It may well lead to increased surgical specialisation in gastroenterology in an attempt to provide adequate experience in gastric surgery.

REFERENCES

Cargill J M, Peden N, Saunders J H B 1978 Very long term treatment of peptic ulcer with cimetidine. Lancet 2: 1113-1115

Cox D J, Spencer J, Tinker J 1969 Clinical results reviewed. In: Williams J A, Cox A G (eds) After vagotomy. Butterworths, London, p 119-130

Culyer A, Maynard A 1980 Treating ulcers with cimetidine can be more cost effective than surgery. Medeconomics 57: 12-14

Dronfield M W, Batchelor A J, Larkworthy W et al 1979 Controlled trial of maintenance cimetidine treatment in healed duodenal ulcer: short and long term effects. Gut 20: 526

Goligher J C, Pulvertaft C N, Dedombal F T et al (1968) Five to eight year results of Leeds/York controlled trial of elective surgery for duodenal ulcer. British Medical Journal 2: 781-787

Gudmand-Hoyer E, Birger J K, Krag E et al 1978 Prophylactic effect of cimetidine in duodenal ulcer disease. British Medical Journal 1: 1095

Mackay C, Kennedy F, Bedi B S et al 1973 Truncal vagotomy and drainage for duodenal ulcer. Gut 14: 425

Salera M, Taroni F, Miglioli M, Santini D, Di Febo G, Baldi F, Barbara L 1979 Long term effects and after effects of cimetidine in duodenal ulcer patients. Italian Journal of Gastroenterology 11: 49-52

Stalsberg H, Taksdal S 1971 Stomach cancer following gastric surgery for benign conditions. Lancet ii: 1175-1177

Venables C W 1980 Indications for surgery in duodenal ulcer non-responders to cimetidine. Excerpta Medica Int Congr Ser No. 521: 16-23

Discussion on Duodenal Ulcer, part 2
Chairman: Dr J. H. Baron

Dr Baron. It has been most interesting to hear three physicians and one surgeon coming down on the side of long-term cimetidine treatment rather than operation. The one surgeon who has done a controlled trial comes down heavily on the side of elective operation. There is at least one other series in the world in which a controlled trial is being done of medical treatment versus operation. Can Dr Bodemar tell us anything about this?

Dr Bodemar. Our trial includes about 90 patients who have been randomised to either maintenance treatment with cimetidine or operation. It is, however, too early to report any results.

(*Dr Baron* then asked if anybody else was doing a controlled trial on maintenance cimetidine versus operation. Two people indicated that they were but had insufficient data to comment. Dr Baron suggested that this would provide a good basis for another conference. He then asked Mr Gear to comment on the differences between his findings and those of the four other speakers.)

Mr Gear. It is important to remember that when our trial was set up the results of long-term maintenance treatment with cimetidine were not really known and certainly not for more than about six months. The study does not necessarily set out my philosophy or policy in treatment which would be closely in line with Dr Bardhan and Mr Venables. Our trial simply shows what is achieved when a group of patients who would otherwise have come to operation are randomised. That is the point of the trial. A trial is important because an awful lot of the discussion about 'physician versus surgeon' is time-wasting in the sense that different groups of patients are being compared.

Dr Schiller. Are Dr Bardhan's patients persuading him not to refer them to a surgeon, or is he persuading his patients not to go for operation? I wonder about keeping patients on maintenance treatment using very high doses of cimetidine for many months when they have already been categorised as refractory.

Dr Bardhan. I have no answer. There is a great demand for medical, as opposed to surgical, treatment. Most of those who have an operation self-select themselves out. When they feel they are having a hard time, when they are not healing and maintenance therapy keeps failing, then most of them opt for surgery. Most of these patients, of course, are being seen jointly by surgeons and myself and many of them are referred originally to the surgeons who send them to me for inclusion in series. We are thus dealing with a group of patients already with severe ulcer. I should make it quite clear that these are not patients with trivial disease who happen to be put on maintenance treatment to subserve a research programme. They have been referred because they have troublesome disease.

I suppose the reason we have fairly large numbers of patients is because we have open endoscopy. It is very much easier to do open endoscopy than to talk to a patient and also much quicker. The answer is obtained immediately. We are dealing here with virulent ulcers in a large number of people.

Dr Schiller. Dr Bardhan has not really answered my question, which was essentially about the ethics of using ever-increasing dosage of cimetidine in patients with virulent disease. Why not cut it short and let them be operated.

Dr Bardhan. We would certainly accept that, if Dr Schiller can demonstrate that surgery can do any better. This point has not been answered.

Dr Baron. This debate between surgery and maintenance cimetidine is unresolved and is hotly debated, for example, in France. Some doctors allege that anybody who heals well with cimetidine will also do well after operation and that those who do not heal with drugs will not do well with operation either. I do not happen to think that is true.

Dr Bardhan. We have already had two recurrences out of eleven operated.

Mr Venables. There is a real problem with the patient who cannot be healed — with what Dr Bardhan calls refractory ulcers. Some time ago we published the results of the first 42 patients treated in that way, and we had an 18 per cent recurrence rate in less than two years. We have certainly seen further recurrences since then. They form a resistant group, both to vagotomy and to cimetidine — I firmly believe this.

Dr Pounder. Rather than adding another drug why not change to De-Nol, for instance? I can understand scientifically why doubling the dose several times is attractive — it is nice and pure — or why operation might be done which, as far as is known, achieves the same result. Why not change to something completely different?

Dr Baron. I know of no controlled trials of refractory ulcers. Has anyone in the audience any data from controlled trials? (no response).

Section 2
GASTRIC ULCER

15. Gastric ulcer — short-term healing with cimetidine and other drugs

D. G. Colin-Jones
Queen Alexandra Hospital, Portsmouth

Any patient receiving treatment for gastric ulceration must be followed closely. All patients with gastric ulceration should be endoscoped and biopsies taken from the ulcer to ensure that it is benign. Since malignant ulcers can heal temporarily, healing of the ulcer is insufficient confirmation that the ulcer is benign.

At present the only way of influencing the dismal prognosis for gastric cancer is to diagnose the cancer very early. In Britain a gastric ulcer with a malignant area is the most likely way of picking up that cancer early. Furthermore, gastric ulceration itself tends to be dangerous. For example, haemorrhage from a gastric ulcer carries twice the mortality of haemorrhage from a duodenal ulcer, probably because the former is more likely to occur in older patients. But if the ulcer heals, the relapse rate is reduced and with it the risk of complications.

In this review a number of recently studied drugs for gastric ulcer will be briefly discussed and conclusions tentatively drawn. Not all drugs are discussed — more recent products were thought to be more appropriately reviewed than older products.

CIMETIDINE

In 1976 the preliminary studies by Pounder and his colleagues suggested that cimetidine would prove very valuable in the treatment of gastric ulceration, for in their uncontrolled study all 10 patients were healed of their ulcers. The results of controlled trials, therefore, were awaited with great interest and indeed the first two trials were very encouraging. In a study of 53 patients at a number of centres in France Bader and his colleagues (1977) reported a healing rate of 69 per cent which was significantly better than placebo. This was similar to the findings of Frost and his colleagues from Denmark (1978) who found a 78 per cent healing rate for cimetidine, which was a highly significant gain for the active treatment. The early promise shown by cimetidine in gastric ulcer disease was not borne out in all subsequent trials. Ciclitira et al (1979) in a four-week controlled study on 60 patients found no benefit for the cimetidine-treated group (Table 15.1).

In two major studies from the United States there was no significant gain when using cimetidine compared with placebo. Over a six-week period Dyck and his

Table 15.1 Controlled trials on the use of cimetidine in gastric ulcer

Author	No.	Cimetidine (% healed)	Placebo (% healed)	% Gain	P
Bader et al, 1977 (France)	53	69	37	32	< 0.02
Frost et al, 1977 (Denmark)	45	78	27	51	<0.002
Ciclitira et al, 1979 (UK)	60	66	52	14	NS
Dyck et al, 1978 (USA)	59	60	41	19	NS
Englert et al, 1978 (USA)					
Cimetidine	130	59	61	−2	NS
Cimetidine and antacid	60	70		9	NS

colleagues (1978) found a 60 per cent healing rate for cimetidine with a gain over placebo of 19 per cent which was not significant. Similar results were found by Englert et al (1978) in a large study with three groups containing 190 patients. They found no significant difference between cimetidine given with a dummy antacid, cimetidine given with an antacid, and an antacid given with a placebo tablet. As Table 15.1 shows there was a two per cent gain for placebo and a nine per cent gain for cimetidine plus antacid, i.e. no significant gain for any treatment group and none for hospitalization. The explanation for these last two trials may well lie in the amount of antacid consumed. In the French, Danish and English studies the daily intake of antacid appears to be very low, probably less than 15 mmol per day. However, in the American studies the daily intake has been computed at 279 mmol in the first trial and 345 mmol in the second.

No formal study of antacids in high dosage for gastric ulcers has been done. If one extrapolates from Petersen's studies (1977) in duodenal ulcer, then since antacids could promote healing in that situation, it is probable that they can also promote healing of gastric ulcer. Thus it may well be that antacids masked the therapeutic benefit of cimetidine. Further studies are needed on this point. In addition, it could well be that the American ulcer behaves differently from the European ulcer. Many studies, particularly of duodenal ulcer disease, suggest a much higher placebo healing rate in North America. The explanation, when resolved, could well be of great interest.

Other trials have been carried out in gastric ulcer disease (Table 15.2). Certain aspects of each of these trials left them open to criticism, and not too much

Table 15.2 Cimetidine in gastric ulcers, trials with problem in analysis

Author	No.	Cimetidine (% healed)	Healing rate in comparison group (%)	Problem
Landecker et al, 1979 (Australia)	48	84	Placebo: 56	Assessed on 90% healing
Cambielli et al, 1978 (Italy)	20	80	Gefarnate: 22	Low numbers
Turpini et al, 1979 (Italy)	22	63	Antacid: 45	Low numbers
Navert et al, 1980 (Canada)	31	95	Placebo: 20	Two doses cimetidine; ulcer size analysed

weight, therefore, should be put on their results. For example Landecker et al (1979) in a study from Australia confirmed that the gastric ulcers he saw were benign by endoscopy but he determined healing radiologically using 90 per cent healing as his criteria for analysis. This is different from the majority of other recent trials in gastric ulcer and makes comparison, therefore, rather difficult. Navert et al (1980) compared two doses of cimetidine (200 mg three times a day and 400 mg at night, and 300 mg four times a day) and a third group — placebo. He looked particularly at the reduction in ulcer size. Small numbers in each group make analysis difficult and his placebo healing rate was unexpectedly low at 20 per cent. Two recently published trials from Italy (Cambielli et al, 1978; Turpini, et al 1979) show therapeutic gain in the cimetidine group compared with antacid and gefarnate. The numbers in these trials were very small which reduces their value.

Cimetidine compared with carbenoxolone

The most widely studied drug for gastric ulcer prior to the advent of cimetidine was carbenoxolone. Carbenoxolone is a synthetic derivative of liquorice which is thought to work by improving the mucosal resistance to acid peptic digestion. It is thought to increase the production of mucus by the gastric mucosa and it reduces the permeability of the gastric mucosa to the passage of hydrogen ions from lumen to interstitial fluid.

The first results of the comparative trial of cimetidine against carbenoxolone were published in 1977 with final publication in 1980 by La Brooy et al. A therapeutic gain of 26 per cent was found for the cimetidine group but this was not significant. The reduction in frequency of attacks of abdominal pain was greater for the cimetidine group, and side-effects, notably fluid retention were appreciably higher in the carbenoxolone group. Thus there appeared to be some advantage for cimetidine but this was not confirmed by Bianchi Porro who in a similar sized study (Table 15.3) demonstrated only a four per cent gain for the cimetidine group (Bianchi Porro and Petrillo, 1979). This is a similar figure to

Table 15.3 Cimetidine and carbenoxolone in gastric ulcer.

Author	No.	Cimetidine (% healed)	Carbenoxolone (% healed)	% Gain	P
La Brooy et al, 1977 (UK)	54	78	52	26	NS
Bianchi Porro et al, 1979 (Italy)	51	76	72	4	NS
Morgan et al, 1978 (UK)	21	100	58	42	0.039
Coughlin et al, 1979 (Australia)	50	58	50	8	NS

Coughlin et al (1979) who published a communication in which there was an eight per cent gain in the cimetidine group. However, in the UK Morgan et al (1978), in a very small study comparing cimetidine and carbenoxolone in the under-sixties, demonstrated a 42 per cent gain for cimetidine which was significant. It is interesting that all nine of his cimetidine-treated patients healed their ulcers.

Overall analysis of the healing rate of carbenoxolone in gastric ulcer is surprisingly low, bearing in mind its reputation. Watkinson in a review in 1978 demonstrated from 13 studies that the overall healing rate was 49 per cent ($\pm$ 13 per cent S.D.) The results in the comparative studies quoted above fall very much in this range. Thus, bearing in mind that up to half the patients on carbenoxolone had side-effects and that it is contraindicated in the over-70s and in those with cardiac or renal disease, the role of carbenoxolone in gastric ulcer appears to be diminishing.

Cimetidine compared with tri-potassium di-citrato bismuthate (De-Nol)
Cimetidine has been compared with De-Nol by Tanner and his colleagues (1979) in a six-week trial which showed no significant difference (66 per cent complete healing with De-Nol and 63 per cent with cimetidine). This is a similar result to an earlier trial by Boyes et al (1974) who also used endoscopic assessment of ulcer healing and found that 91 per cent of the De-Nol treated group healed their ulcers compared to 36 per cent of the placebo group. Although there is a risk of bismuth toxicity, this is rare with a month's course and thus this compound appears to merit further investigation.

There has been much speculation as to whether the combination of an antisecretory drug with another drug supposed to heal by strengthening the mucosal barrier might lead to an improvement in the healing rate. The only study I have seen that attempts to clarify this is a very small one (17 patients) by Ward et al (1979) in which cimetidine and placebo are compared with cimetidine and De-Nol. There is no benefit from adding De-Nol to cimetidine (55 per cent healing compared with 75 per cent for cimetidine and placebo); indeed the preliminary figures show just the reverse. Nevertheless, it is interesting to speculate upon whether a drug combination might improve ulcer healing rates. There is no information on this topic at the present time.

Cimetidine compared with deglycyrrhizinised liquorice (Caved-S)
Of particular interest was a study by Morgan and his colleagues (1978) comparing cimetidine with Caved-S in patients over 60 years of age. Patients were followed for up to three months; the majority were endoscoped but some were assessed radiologically. There was a steady increase in the percentage of ulcers healing, with 85 per cent of cimetidine-treated ulcers healing at two months and 100 per cent healing at three months. Comparable figures for deglycyrrhizinised liquorice (Caved-S) were 79 and 90 per cent. There was, of course, no difference statistically between these two groups.

MacAdam in a personal communication (1981) has kindly released the results of his recently completed trial of cimetidine against Caved-S with 50 patients in each group. At six weeks 33 had healed with cimetidine and this rose to 47 (84 per cent) at three months. In the Caved-S group comparable figures were 30 and 44 (88 per cent). This enlarged trial confirms their earlier published study and emphasizes the need for further centres to repeat this work.

Deglycyrrhizinised liquorice is polypharmacy. It is an extract of liquorice from which glycyrrhizinic acid has been removed and with it various mineralocorticoid side-effects. It is thus a well-tolerated drug, is combined with frangula and antacid and is cheap. The therapeutic benefit reported in the literature shows wide variation from no benefit compared to placebo to nearly 100 per cent healing. This is illustrated by a study by Gutz et al (1979) who found a 69 per cent regression in ulcer size but only a 45 per cent actual healing of the ulcer crater at four weeks. The manufacturers of de-glycyrrhizinised liquorice claim that this variability is because until recently there have been two preparations of de-glycyrrhizinised liquorice on the market with very different dissolution characteristics (Glick L, personal communication, 1981). It is conceivable that this might have influenced the outcome of trials. Clearly other centres need to investigate Caved-S in view of its possible benefit.

OTHER DRUGS FOR GASTRIC ULCERATION

Sucralfate
Sucralfate is a sulphated disaccharide with antipeptic activity which appears to cause only minimal reduction in acidity. It is thought to work by producing a protective layer over the stomach and is poorly absorbed. It has been studied in South Africa and Japan, but is not yet available in Britain. Table 15.4 shows that the healing rate for sucralfate is between 50 and 70 per cent with doubtful benefit over placebo. The results of a study comparing it with cimetidine showed no significant advantage for cimetidine. Though widely used in certain parts of the World, further studies are needed for the efficacy of this drug must be regarded as unproven at the present.

Table 15.4 Sucralfate in gastric ulcers

Reference	No.	Sucralfate (% healed)	Healing rate in comparison group (%)	P
Mayberry et al (1978)	31	50	placebo: 13	NS
Fixa et al (1980)	44	70	placebo: 40	0.05
Lahtinen et al (1980)	38	68	placebo: 53	NS
Marks et al (1980a, b)	55	63	Cimetidine: 75	NS

Gefarnate
Gefarnate is derived from cabbage and is claimed to have an ulcer-healing effect. The satisfactory studies I have examined fail to show any obvious benefit for this drug, figures usually being comparable to those found with placebo.

Proglumide
Proglumide is claimed to be an antigastrin. It inhibits pentagastrin-induced acid secretion without any effect on the serum gastrin. The evidence that it works as a specific antigastrin, however, is poor. It has been studied in Japan with both open and double-blind studies which appear to confer some advantages for proglumide over placebo. The only European study is a very small one (16 patients) from

Germany (Miederer et al, 1979) in which a 75 per cent healing rate was reported for proglumide compared with 25 per cent for antacids. These results are very preliminary and of uncertain value.

Antidepressants
Since gastric ulcers have been claimed to be associated with an anxious personality and with stress, antidepressants have been used. Whilst no benefit was demonstrated for butriptyline, there was, however, a benefit for trimipramine (Valnes et al, 1978) but in this study only 60 per cent of the ulcers healed on the active compound and 20 per cent on placebo. This is an unexpectedly low figure for the placebo group. Drowsiness is a side-effect of many of these antidepressants and may make them poorly tolerated. Much more work is needed.

Newer compounds
Ranitidine is an H_2 receptor antagonist which has proven potency as an inhibitor of gastric secretion and has been compared with cimetidine both for its antisecretory effect and its ulcer healing properties in duodenal ulcer disease. To date no major published series are available. There was an open study by Barbier et al (1979) in which 11 of 16 ulcers healed on six weeks treatment. This 68 per cent healing rate would appear to be very similar to cimetidine. Apparently trials are in progress in Scandinavia and in Holland and results are awaited with interest.

Pirenzepine
Pirenzepine is an anticholinergic drug said to be relatively specific for muscarinic receptor sites within the stomach. It is claimed to inhibit acid secretion with minimal systemic side-effects. The very limited studies available at the present time show only marginal benefit for pirenzepine compared with placebo (Morelli et al, 1979) and no conclusions can be drawn regarding its effectiveness.

Prostaglandin E2 analogues
Despite much interest in prostaglandins and their possible cytoprotective effect, very little work appears to have been done in gastric ulceration. A very small study from Gibinski in Poland (1977) showed no obvious advantage for the prostaglandin analogue despite a reduction in acid secretion and increase in mucus production. The potential for this group of compounds and synthetic analogues may well be great, but at the present time investigations are at a very early stage.

DISCUSSION

Our ignorance of the best method of healing gastric ulceration is dismaying. Although circumstantial evidence suggests that antacids are of value, a formal endoscopically controlled trial even in this well-loved group of pharmaceutical products is still lacking.

In this review I have been comparing trials which have used different protocols. Usually endoscopy has been the method of assessment and I have only considered trials where ulcer healing has been the criteria of success. I find it extremely difficult to gauge the percentage reduction in ulcer size endoscopically, whilst radiological assessment of complete healing is very difficult. In addition to these problems there have been differences in concomitant treatment with antacids which vary in dose from less than 15 mmol per day to over 300 mmol per day. The duration of the trials is varied too: many run for six to eight weeks, but some trials have stopped at only four weeks. Thus, if one compares the overall percentage healing rate for different drugs, this is of limited value, but it does nonetheless give some indication as to the activity of a given drug.

Analysing the trials which I have indicated there was a 75 per cent healing rate for cimetidine ($\pm$ 12 per cent S.D.) If one eliminates any additional regime (such as antacid, De-Nol) the percentage healing rate remains very similar at 73.4 per cent ($\pm$ 12.7 per cent S.D.) It seems reasonable to conclude that cimetidine will heal approximately three-quarters of gastric ulcers over a six-week period. This percentage may well rise with continued treatment. Thus, provided the patient is fully investigated to ensure that the ulcer is benign and is monitored to ensure ulcer healing, cimetidine would appear to be the standard treatment for gastric ulcer against which any other compound has to be compared. Since only 75 per cent of the patients appear to heal their ulcers there is much room for therapeutic improvement but no other drug which I have reviewed appears to offer any major therapeutic advantage. A particular disappointment appears to be carbenoxolone which heals gastric ulcer in only half the patients who have received the drug and in whom there is a significant incidence of side-effects. De-glycyrrhizinised liquorice and tri-potassium di-citrato bismuthate look encouraging in a few studies, but these need to be repeated. The results of the trials published in the last three years or so have demonstrated that we are able to help the patients who have gastric ulceration, but by no means all of them are relieved and we still need a more potent drug for use in this condition.

REFERENCES

Bader J P, Morin T, Bernier J J, Bertrand J, Betourne C, Gastard J, Lambert R, Ribet A, Sarles H, Toulet J 1977 In: Burland W L, Simkins M A (eds) Cimetidine: Proceedings of the Second International Symposium on histamine H_2 receptor antagonists. Excerpta Medica, Amsterdam, p. 287-292

Barbier P, Dumont A, Adler M 1979 Evaluation en etude ouverte de la ranitidine dans la therapeutique de 40 ulcerations gastro-duodenales. Acta Gastroenterolica Belgica 42: 268-274 (Engl Abstr)

Boyes B E, Woolf I L, Wilson R, Cowley D J, Dymock I W 1974 Effective treatment of gastric ulceration with a bismuth preparation (De-Nol). Gut 15: 833

Cambielli M, Evangelista A, Fesce E, Grimoldi D, Guslandi M, Benvenuti C, Tittobelli A 1978 Cimetidine in benign gastric ulcer. Double blind study versus gefarnate. Acta Therapeutica 4: 207-218

Ciclitira P J, Machell R J, Farthing M J G, Dick A P, Hunter A 1979 Double-blind controlled trial of cimetidine in the healing of gastric ulcer. Gut 20: 730-734

Coughlin G P, Reiner R G, English E, Kerr Grant A 1979 Comparison of carbenoxolone and cimetidine in treating chronic gastric ulcer. Annual Scientific Meeting of the Gastroenterological Society of Australia, Brisbane, A8 (abstract)

Dyck W P, Belsito A, Fleshler T R, Liebermann P B, Dickinson M D, Wood J M 1978 Cimetidine and placebo in the treatment of benign gastric ulcer. A multicenter double blind study. Gastroenterology 74: 410-415

Englert Jr E, Freston J W, Graham D Y, Finkelstein W, Kruss D M, Priest R J, Raskin J B, Rhones B, Rogers A I, Winger J, Wilcox L L, Crossley R J 1978 Cimetidine, antacid, and hospitalisation in treatment of benign gastric ulcer. A multicenter double blind study. Gastroenterology 74: 416-425

Fixa B, Komarkova O 1980 Sucralfate in the treatment of peptic ulcer. Double blind trial. Abstracts of the XI International Congress of Gastroenterology

Frost F, Rahbek I, Rune S J, Birger Jensen K, Gudmand-Hoyer E, Krag E, Rask Madsen J, Wulff H R, Garbol J, Gotlieb Jensen K, Hojlund M, Nissen V R 1977 Cimetidine in patients with gastric ulcer. A multicentre controlled trial. British Medical Journal 2: 795

Gibinski K, Rybicka J, Mikos E, Nowak A 1977 Gastric ulcer healing with prostaglandin E_2 analogues. A double blind clinical trial. Gut 18: 636-639

Gutz H J, Berndt H, Jackson D 1979 The treatment of gastric ulcer. A comparative trial of four preparations. Practitioner 222: 849-853

La Brooy S J, Taylor R H, Hunt R H, Golding P L, Laidlow J M, Chapman R G, Pounder R E, Vincent S H, Colin-Jones D G, Milton-Thompson G J, Misiewicz J J, 1979 Controlled comparison of cimetidine and carbenoxolone sodium in gastric ulcer. British Medical Journal 1: 1308-1309

Lahtinen J, Ala-Kaila K, Aukee S, Hastaja M, Hajba A, Keyrilainen O, Maattanen J, Salmela J, Aarimas M 1980 Sucralphate and the antacid in the treatment of gastric and duodenal ulcer. A multicentre double blind trial. Abstracts of the XI International Congress of Gastroenterology

Landecker K D, Crawford B A, Hunt J H, Gillespie P, Piper D W 1979 Cimetidine and gastric ulcer healing. Medical Journal of Australia 2: 43-45

Marks I N, Lucke W, Wright J P 1980a Comparison of sucralfate with cimetidine in short-term treatment of chronic peptic ulcers. Hepatogastroenterology, Supplement, XI International Congress of Gastroenterology, p. 383

Marks I N, Wright J P, Denyer M, Garisch J A M, Lucke W, 1980b Comparison of sucralfate with cimetidine in the short-term treatment of chronic peptic ulcers. South African Medical Journal 51: 567-573

Mayberry J F, Williams R A, Thodes J, Lawrie B W 1978 A controlled clinical trial of sucralfate in the treatment of gastric ulcer. British Journal of Clinical Practice 32: 291-293

Miederer S E, Lindstaedt K, Kutz K, Mayershofer R 1979 Efficient treatment of gastric ulcer with proglumide in outpatients (double blind trial). Acta Hepato-Gastroenterologica 26: 314-318

Morelli A, Pelli A, Narducci F, Spadacini A 1979 Pirenzipine in the treatment of gastric ulcer. Scandinavian Journal of Gastroenterology 14 Suppl. 57: 51-56

Morgan A, McAdam W A F, Pacsoo C, Walker B E, Simmons A V 1978 Cimetidine: an advance in gastric ulcer treatment? British Medical Journal 2: 1323-1326

Navert H, Tetreault T, Wollin A, Beaudry R, Haddad H 1980 An evaluation of the therapeutic efficacy of cimetidine in gastric ulcer. Criteria for methods of analysis. In: Abstr. VI Asian Pacific Congress of Gastroenterology, Auckland, New Zealand

Petersen W L, Sturderant R A L, Frankl H D, Richardson C T, Isenberg J I, Elashoff J D, Sones J Q, Gross R A, McCullum R W, Fordtran J S 1977 Healing of duodenal ulcer with an antacid regime. New England Journal of Medicine 297: 341-345

Porro G B, Petrillo M 1979 A controlled trial comparing cimetidine with carbenoxolone sodium in gastric ulcer. Drugs in Experimental Research 5: 173-176

Porro G B, Petrillo M 1979 Short and long term treatment of gastric ulcer. A controlled trial comparing cimetidine and carbenoxolone sodium. In: Proceedings of the second national symposium, Brussels. Excerpta Medica, Amsterdam, p. 161

Pounder R E 1976 Healing of gastric ulcer during treatment with cimetidine. Lancet 1: 337

Tanner A R, Cowlishaw J L, Cowen A E, Ward M 1979 Efficacy of cimetidine and tri-potassium di-citrato bismuthate (De-Nol) in chronic gastric ulceration. Medical Journal of Australia 1: 1-2

Turpini R, Charalambakis A, Scotti A, Latella R 1979 Clinical trial with cimetidine versus antacid in the treatment of gastric ulcer. Drugs in Experimental and Clinical Research 5: 4-5, 97-102

Valnes K, Myren J, Ovigstad T 1978 Trimipramine in the treatment of gastric ulcer. Scandinavian Journal of Gastroenterology 13: 497-500

Ward M, Pollard E J, Kemp R, Cowen A E 1979 A double blind trial of the treatment of gastric ulcers with a combination of De-Nol and cimetidine. In: Gastroenterol Society of Australia, Adelaide Scientific Meeting 1979, p. A30 (abstract)

Watkinson G 1978 In: Avery Jones F, Langman M, Mann R (eds) Recent studies on Carbenoxolone. MTP, Lancaster

16. Gastric ulcer — long-term treatment with cimetidine

Richard J. Machell

West Cornwall Hospital, Penzance, Cornwall

Traditionally, the aims of peptic ulcer treatment have been in the short term to relieve symptoms and induce ulcer healing and in the long term to prevent recurrence. In the past, the emphasis in treatment has been directed at the acute exacerbations of the disease, neglecting the natural history of peptic ulceration with the propensity to relapse (Leading Article, 1977).

In gastric ulceration, as in duodenal ulcer disease, there is a high incidence of recurrence after initial successful treatment. In long-term follow-up studies in patients with healed gastric ulcers, recurrence rates of 40 to 60 per cent within two years have been reported (Gill, 1968; Kraus et al, 1976). These studies, however, were based on radiological follow-up and probably underestimate the true relapse rates. Since the likelihood of recurrence is unrelated to the age of the patient, length of ulcer history, size or location of the ulcer (Roth, 1971), it is impossible to predict which patients are at greatest risk.

There have been few studies to assess the efficacy of drug treatment in the prevention of gastric ulcer relapse. Carbenoxolone promotes healing of gastric ulcers, but the high incidence of side-effects with this drug precludes long-term treatment, particularly in elderly patients. Deglycyrrhizinised liquorice has proved ineffective in prophylaxis (Hollander et al, 1978). Maintenance treatment with cimetidine is effective in preventing duodenal ulcer relapse.

Gastric ulceration is less common than duodenal ulcer disease, although associated with a high morbidity and mortality. There is general agreement amongst clinicians that because of the risk of malignancy, all patients with radiologically demonstrated gastric ulcers should be referred for endoscopy, with biopsy and cytology, before commencing medical treatment. Close supervision of these patients is required during medical treatment because of this risk, with careful appraisal of healing, preferably by endoscopy.

There are few data on long-term treatment with cimetidine in gastric ulcers, but in this contribution I shall review the published literature available.

MAINTENANCE TRIALS WITH CIMETIDINE IN GASTRIC ULCER

Table 16.1 reviews three controlled trials of maintenance treatment with cimetidine in gastric ulcer. All these trials were double-blind and performed on ambulant patients on an outpatient basis.

Table 16.1 Results of maintenance trials of cimetidine in gastric ulceration

Author	Number of patients	Duration of treatment (months)	Daily dosage	Percentage remaining healed		Significance
				Cimetidine	Placebo	
Birger Jenson et al (1979)[1]	19	12	800 mg	100	44	$P < 0.025$
Machell et al (1979)	25	11	1000 mg	82	14	$P < 0.002$
Kang et al (1979)[2]	31	12	800 mg	100	56	$P < 0.02$

[1] Relapse defined on symptomatic grounds without endoscopic confirmation in all cases.
[2] Asymptomatic patients not submitted to follow-up radiology/endoscopy.

Trial 1 (Birger Jensen et al, 1979) was carried out at two centres in Denmark and followed on from an initial six-week controlled trial with cimetidine in gastric ulcer healing. Endoscopic confirmation of healing was obtained prior to entry into the long-term study and patients were treated either with cimetidine 400 mg b.d., or identical placebo. Antacid consumption was not encouraged. Relapse, however, was defined on symptomatic grounds and not all patients who relapsed clinically were subjected to endoscopic confirmation. Asymptomatic patients were not routinely endoscoped during, or at the end of, the twelve-month trial period, so that asymptomatic relapses would have been missed. Furthermore over half the patients included in this study originally had pre-pyloric ulcers.

Trial 2 (Machell et al, 1979) was a single-centre study from Cambridge and followed on from an initial four-week controlled trial with cimetidine in gastric ulcer healing. Following endoscopic evidence of complete healing, patients were entered into the study, receiving either cimetidine 1 g daily in divided doses or identical placebo tablets. Weak antacid tablets were permitted as required. Endoscopy was repeated routinely at 5 and 11 months, when the trial ended, or at any stage in the event of symptomatic recurrence. Patients were withdrawn from the trial if ulcer relapse was confirmed. Altogether 25 patients completed this study, of whom 24 originally had lesser curve ulcers and one a prepyloric ulcer. The two treatment groups were comparable with regard to age, sex, smoking habits and duration of ulcer disease. Gastric ulcers recurred during the trial period in 14 patients — 12 on placebo, 2 on cimetidine. In 11 patients (9 on cimetidine, 2 on placebo) the ulcers remained healed at the end of the trial ($P < 0.002$). The timing of relapse is shown in Figure 16.1. The mean time to relapse in the placebo group was 5.75 months.

Trial 3 (Kang et al, 1979) was also a single-centre study from Sydney, Australia and as yet has only been reported in abstract form. Initial healing on entry to this study was confirmed either by radiology or endoscopy and only patients with symptomatic relapse were routinely re-examined, either radiologically or by gastroscopy, although many of the asymptomatic cases were also checked. A significant result in favour of cimetidine emerged from this study ($P < 0.02$). In

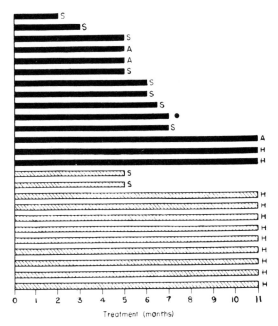

Figure 16.1   Progress of patients in trial. Solid bars represent the 14 placebo patients; hatched bars represent the 11 cimetidine patients.

S Recurrent symptomatic gastric ulcer
A Recurrent asymptomatic gastric ulcer
H Remains healed after 11 months
● Recurrent symptomatic gastric and duodenal ulcers

all these long-term studies no side-effects of note were observed and there were no significant alterations in the haematological and biochemical parameters assessed.

DISCUSSION

Gastric ulceration is principally a disease of the elderly and the morbidity associated with complications, such as haemorrhage and perforation, is high. Partial gastrectomy is a well-established procedure in the prevention of gastric ulcer relapse, but such surgery itself may be attended by significant risks in the elderly, especially those with intercurrent disease (Allan and Dykes, 1976). There is a clear need for a safe, effective medical treatment to prevent gastric ulcer relapse, particularly in these high risk patients. The results of these trials indicate that maintenance therapy with cimetidine may meet these requirements. The numbers of patients treated in these controlled trials, however, are so small that final judgement must be reserved until more data are available. Furthermore, the optimum dose of cimetidine required to prevent relapse needs to be determined.

On present evidence, long-term treatment with cimetidine is indicated in elderly and high-risk patients with gastric ulcers in whom surgery would be hazardous.

REFERENCES

Allan R, Dykes P 1976 A study of the factors influencing mortality rates from gastro-intestinal haemorrhage. Quarterly Journal of Medicine 180: 533-550

Birger Jensen K, Mollmann K M, Rahbek I, Rask-Madsen J, Rune S J, Wulff H R 1979 Prophylactic effect of cimetidine in gastric ulcer patients. Scandinavian Journal of Gastroenterology 14: 175-176

Gill A M, 1968 Gastric ulcer. British Medical Journal 3: 415-418

Hanscom D H, Buckman E 1971 Gastric ulcer, the follow-up period. Gastroenterology 61: 585-591

Hollander D, Green G, Woolf I L, Boyes B E, Wilson R J, Cauley D J, Dymock I W 1978 Prophylaxis with deglycyrrhizinised liquorice in patients with healed gastric ulcers. British Medical Journal 1: 148

Kang J Y, Canalese J, Piper D W, 1979 The use of long term cimetidine in the prevention of gastric ulcer relapse — double blind trial. In: Proceedings of the Annual Scientific Meeting of the Gastroenterological Society of Australia, Brisbane, May 14-15, A9 (Abstract)

Kraus M, Mendeloff G, Condon R E 1976 Prognosis of gastric ulcer. Annals of Surgery 184: 471-476

Leading Article 1977 Preventing recurrence of ulcers. British Medical Journal 2: 1440

Machell R J, Ciclitira P J, Farthing M J G, Dick A P, Hunter J O 1979 Cimetidine in the prevention of gastric ulcer relapse. Postgraduate Medical Journal 55: 393-395

Roth H P, 1971 Gastric ulcer healing of initial ulcers in relation to age and race. Gastroenterology 61: 570-575

17. Gastric ulcer — long-term management

John Alexander-Williams
The General Hospital, Birmingham

Before making a decision about the optimum long-term management of gastric ulcer, it is important to understand the natural history of the untreated disease. We must consider whether the statement made in 1956 by Doll and his colleagues still holds true; they said that 'the tendency to remission or cure (of gastric ulcer) is uninfluenced by medical treatment'.

NATURAL HISTORY

Gastric ulcer disease is not as common as duodenal ulcer disease and there have been relatively few long-term studies on a significant number of patients. In one of the earliest reliable reports Natvig et al (1943) from Norway reported 152 patients with gastric ulcer who were diagnosed on barium meal examination, followed for three years and then re-examined. The relationship between the continued presence of an ulcer crater and the presence or absence of symptoms is shown in Table 17.1. From their study it seems that even if the ulcer heals radiologically one in three of the patients still have dyspeptic symptoms, and that even if the symptoms disappear, one in six still have an ulcer crater demonstrated radiologically.

Table 17.1 152 patients with gastric ulcer followed for 3 years all had Ba. meal

	Still had symptoms	No symptoms
Those with ulcer crater on X-ray	51	7
Those with no ulcer	24	40

One of the longest follow-up series ever reported was from Aarhus in Denmark (Krag, 1966). From 1936 to 1945 inclusive, a total of 371 patients with confirmed peptic ulcer were admitted to the Department of Medicine. Of these, 347 were discharged after medical treatment, 58 of them had a radiological diagnosis of benign gastric ulcer and 9 of them (16 per cent) died during follow-up. It was known that none of these nine patients had required further hospital admission for dyspepsia and apparently none of them had developed a gastric cancer. The remaining 49 patients were all reviewed radiologically in 1963, i.e. 17 to 27 years

139

later. The long-term radiological findings in these patients are shown in Table 17.2. During this prolonged follow-up 21 per cent of the patients had to be admitted to hospital with further gastrointestinal bleeding.

Table 17.2 X-ray appearance of the ulcers in 58 patients who had gastric ulcer on first admission to hospital in 1936 – 1945

At follow-up in 1963	No	%
Gastric ulcer	23	40
Pyloric ulcer	2	3
Duodenal ulcer	3	5
Gastric and duodenal ulcer	2	3
No ulcer	18	31
Gastric cancer	1	2
No definite information	9	16
Total	58	100

In a much shorter follow-up study from the Veterans' Administration Trial (Hanscom and Buchman, 1971) 327 patients with gastric ulcer were observed for two years and reviewed. Although most of the patients were treated medically until the ulcer healed, 42 per cent of them recurred within two years; 42 per cent of the patients had to be treated surgically — 12 for bleeding. Within the two-year follow-up nine patients developed gastric cancer, six of them in the surgically treated group and three in the group treated by prolonged medical treatment. The high incidence of cancer in the short follow-up period suggests that the original diagnosis of simple gastric ulcer was incorrect. The relatively small number of cancers developing in the Aarhus long-term review suggests that the apparent risk of cancer in gastric ulcer is due to initial misdiagnosis and that the long-term risk is not great. Furthermore, Krag's figures (1966) suggest that in a prolonged follow-up there is a one in five chance of bleeding as a major complication. These studies and those from Norway suggest that the risk of bleeding during follow-up is no greater if the initial diagnosis was made at the time of a bleeding episode than if it was not.

In the comprehensive long-term review of the natural history of peptic ulcer disease in general practice, Fry (1964) emphasized that (i) the peak incidence of gastric ulcer disease is between 50 and 59, (ii) the prevalence of the disease in UK general practice was 27 per thousand per year between the ages of 70 and 79. Furthermore he made the important observations that (iii) the natural history of the severity of symptoms in gastric ulcer disease tends to be self-limited with a peak of severity about 6.5 years after the onset of symptoms and (iv) that if the disease is managed by symptomatic treatment, 15 years from the onset most patients have become symptom-free.

Our own study of 102 patients with a radiological and endoscopic diagnosis of gastric ulcer followed from two to eight years at the Birmingham General Hospital shows similar trends (Anselmi et al, 1981). There is a 60 per cent incidence of recurrence of symptoms, and 40 per cent of the patients who apparently had no recurrent ulceration at the time of review still have dyspeptic symptoms. Twenty per cent of the patients initially treated medically were readmitted during the follow-up period with a complication of bleeding.

These studies of the natural history of the disease suggest that gastric ulceration tends to affect older people and to produce intermittent symptoms for 15 or more years. They suggest that however well patients respond to medical treatment there is about a 50 per cent chance of recurrence in every two-year period of follow-up, that the risk of cancer developing is small (providing the original diagnosis was correct) and that the greatest risk to life is associated with the complication of bleeding.

HOW CAN WE ALTER THE NATURAL HISTORY OF THE DISEASE?

The logical approach in management should be directed towards altering some of the known causative factors of the disease. Although we do not know the precise cause of simple gastric ulcer certain well established factors are considered important:

1. Duodenogastric reflux
Patients with gastric ulceration have more bile in their stomach than normal patients and duodeno-gastric reflux is more frequent. The work of Fisher and Cohen (1973) indicates that in patients with gastric ulcer fasting serum gastrin levels were significantly higher than normal and pyloric pressure was significantly lower in response to intra-duodenal amino-acids or sodium oleate. These abnormal pyloric responses returned to normal following acidification of the stomach. Possibly then it is acid in the stomach that prevents duodenogastric reflux.

2. Gastric retention
Dragstedt and Woodwood (1947) produced some evidence in support of their hypothesis that gastric stasis was the principal cause of gastric ulceration. The hypothesis was supported by the good results seen following surgical drainage.

3. Acid/pepsin secretion
Patients cannot develop gastric ulcers unless the stomach pH falls below 3.5 to activate pepsinogen. Many patients who have been cured of their gastric ulcer by a Billroth I gastrectomy have much more duodenogastric reflux than patients with gastric ulcer. Furthermore, many of them have delayed gastric emptying, yet in the absence of acid peptic secretion they do not develop gastric ulcers.

4. Diminished mucosal resistance
As most patients with gastric ulcer have an acid secretory capacity the same or less than that of normal and as peptic ulceration is thought to be due to a breakdown of the normal balance between acid/peptic attack and resistance of the mucosa to digestion it is likely that the principal cause of gastric ulceration is

diminished resistance of the gastric mucosa. One of the contributing factors could well be the duodenal contents that reflux back into the stomach but many other factors have been implicated, such as the poor blood supply, poor nutrition and damage from drugs.

The first three of these aetiological factors have been studied extensively, and those studies that measure duodenogastric reflux, gastric retention or acid/pepsin secretory capacity show that there is no significant difference whether the ulcer is healed or in an active phase. Therefore, it seems that one of the measures we ought to consider when trying to change the tendency of gastric ulceration to relapse is improving mucosal resistance.

Drugs effective in healing

Although many drugs have been reported effective in the management of patients with gastric ulcers, it is only possible to consider seriously those drugs that have been subjected to properly controlled trials. In most of the controlled studies the effect of drugs has been compared with that of placebo but in some studies it has been compared with the effect of bed rest, hospital treatment or the use of simple antacids.

Antacids. There have been conflicting reports about the efficacy of antacids, particularly in long-term therapy. Some have considered antacid therapy ineffective (Baume and Hunt, 1969) whereas others have considered high doses of antacids as effective as cimetidine (Englert et al, 1978). The striking difference in the healing rate of placebo treatment has been largely due to the fact that in many they have allowed antacid therapy to be taken by the controls.

Bismuth compounds have been shown to be effective, particularly tripotassium dicitrato bismuthate which was apparently well tolerated by patients in medium-term studies (Bayes et al, 1975). Many of our patients have found it an unpalatable drug for long-term use.

Metoclopramide seems to be a logical drug to use if gastric retention is a factor in the genesis of ulcer. Hoskins (1973) and Kennedy (1973) have shown that metoclopramide gives as good results as carbenoxolone and better results than placebo. Their studies extended over a relatively short time. I have been unable to find any studies which indicate the long-term patient compliance and the efficacy of metoclopramide therapy.

Carbenoxolone. Extensive reports are available on the effects of carbenoxolone in patients with gastric ulcer; almost all show it to be more effective than placebo and as effective as bed rest. In all studies there is a significant incidence of long-term side-effects, particularly those associated with salt retention and with accompanying oedema and hypertension. Although many workers claim to be able to use the drug in the majority of their patients, others think that the complications limit its clinical efficacy, particularly in the long term (Hoskins, 1973; Freston, 1978). Some have claimed that long-term carbenoxolone reduces the recurrence rate in gastric ulcer disease (Bank and Marks, 1973).

Histamine H₂ receptor blockers, particularly cimetidine, have been the subject of recent extensive study. The immediate side-effects of cimetidine are of little consequence and do not limit its clinical usefulness to any significant degree. Generally it has been shown to be as effective in the healing of gastric ulcer in ambulant patients as carbenoxolone, proglumide or gefarnate. There are few studies to give positive proof of its long-term efficacy or to show whether a nocturnal dose is adequate in preventing recurrence of gastric ulceration as is the case with duodenal ulcer (Englert et al, 1978; Freston, 1978).

Anticholinergics. Glycopyrronium bromide has been shown to be more effective than simple bed rest and antacids in healing gastric ulcer. It is also claimed to reduce the risk of recurrence (Baume et al, 1972). However, the unpleasant side-effects of anticholinergics make them unattractive for long-term therapy.

Cholestyramine. If the damaging effect of bile refluxing into the stomach is important in the genesis of gastric ulceration one might expect bile salt-adsorbing drugs to be effective in long-term protection. However, long-term studies with cholestyramine in the treatment of gastric ulcer have shown no significant benefit (Black et al, 1971).

In all the drug studies on the rate of healing of gastric ulcers few of them have been shown to be more effective than bed rest or even hospital admission. Prolonged bed rest is obviously of no practical value in long-term management. However, in many elderly patients past retiring age the adoption of a life of leisure might be considered a practical prescription.

Although the group of drugs mentioned above is usually effective in speeding the healing rate of gastric ulcers little evidence has yet been produced that continuing treatment after healing conveys any benefit and protects against future recurrence. In other words, it is not possible to 'super heal' a gastric ulcer. Therefore, long-term therapy is not indicated. We must decide whether prophylaxis can reduce the risk of recurrence. We have learned already that simply healing the ulcer does not alter the environment of the stomach in these patients, does not decrease the amount of duodenogastric reflux, does not increase the rate of emptying or decrease acid/pepsin secretion. Furthermore, we have seen that the pyloric sphincter dysfunction found in patients with gastric ulcer is not reversible except by increasing the acidity of the stomach (Fisher and Cohen, 1973). Perhaps drugs that increase the acidity of the stomach might be effective in long-term prophylaxis! Claims that carbenoxolone prevents recurrence have been based on small numbers of patients followed for up to three years (Bank and Marks, 1973). However, it is a drug that offers some prophylactic promise. It acts without reducing gastric acidity.

IMPROVING MUCOSAL RESISTANCE

What are the causes of diminished mucosal resistance?

In patients with gastric ulcer, is poor mucosal resistance simply a function of age since the elderly are principally affected? Is it simply a function of general malnutrition which is why gastric ulcer disease affects the elderly and those in the poor socioeconomic groups? Is it related to specific deficiencies such as those vitamins known to affect epithelial health or intestinal motility, such as vitamins A, C, and E? The answers to these questions are not known. I feel that they warrant research and enquiry.

What can we achieve? We have no means of reducing a patient's age but the time may come when we understand more about rejuvenation. We can certainly correct general and specific malnutrition, and perhaps measures to this end, accompanied by tranquil retirement, might be attainable goals in prophylaxis. It seems to me that the logical approach to the long-term management of patients with gastric ulcer is to improve mucosal resistance rather than to attempt to reduce acid secretion. It seems illogical to attempt long-term suppression of an already low acid secretion by using antacids, histamine H_2 receptor blockers or anticholinergic drugs. The most logical drug to consider would be carbenoxolone, particularly if some of its practical disadvantages could be overcome in elderly patients and those with cardiovascular disease.

PRACTICAL CONSIDERATIONS

When considering the long-term management of patients with gastric ulcer it is important to bear in mind that many are elderly, many come from poor socioeconomic backgrounds and often are educationally underprivileged. Therefore, it is not surprising that in this group of patients there is poor compliance when attempting to administer regular long-term treatment. This is particularly so in patients who are in remission and asymptomatic.

When considering long-term surveillance to protect the patient against the possible risk of the development of cancer it is important to realise that the 'pay-off' of such surveillance for gastric cancer is poor in those countries with a relatively low incidence of gastric cancer. I feel that the long-term risk of cancer is not sufficiently great to warrant the introduction of expensive long-term surveillance.

Studies of the gastric contents of patients on long-term antacid therapy or those who have had operations that totally abolish gastric secretion, such as sub-total partial gastrectomy, suggest that they are heavily colonised with micro-organisms. Furthermore, there is some evidence to suggest that this state of achlorhydria and bacterial colonisation may increase the risk of gastric cancer. Therefore, perpetual anacidity may be a bad thing and is a poor goal for management.

Symptom-dictated treatment is much easier to enforce. The presence of unpleasant symptoms acts as a very efficient reminder to the patient to take treatment. In a symptomatic patient it may well be that nocturnal treatment is just as effective as 24-hour treatment, particularly if all we are aiming to do is to tip the gastric imbalance sufficiently to favour healing.

Some risk factors may well be avoided if the doctor has sufficient zeal and personality. Many patients can be frightened into giving up smoking and will usually accept advice to avoid oral anti-inflammatory drugs.

PRAGMATIC APPROACH

Our aims in the long-term management of gastric ulcer should be to control symptoms, to reduce risks and to conserve resources. When we prescribe any treatment or course of action we should always ask ourselves whether we are certain we are doing the patient any good. We should be sure that the community can afford what we are trying to do and we should be convinced that it is worthwhile bothering.

I will end with seven practical steps as guidelines in the management of patients with gastric ulcer:

1. Confirm diagnosis of simple ulcer by biopsy and cytology.

2. Treat the patient with an effective drug or drugs and re-endoscope after two months to ensure that the ulcer is healed and the lesion benign.

3. Frighten the patient to stop smoking.

4. Persuade the patient to avoid all oral anti-inflammatory drugs.

5. Prescribe no maintenance or prophylaxis; repeat treatment only if there are symptoms.

6. Treat recurrent symptoms in the simplest possible way.

7. Reinvestigate whenever recurrent symptoms remain unresponsive for two months.

No. 6 needs some explanation. My personal view — unsubstantiated as yet by scientific experiment — is that the following simple measures should be used in increasing order of complexity and decreasing order of enthusiasm:

1. Avoid aggravating factors such as fats and alcohol.

2. Instruct the patient to take the favoured antacid as required to control symptoms.

3. Prescribe 10 mg of metoclopramide each night.

   or

4. 400 mg of cimetidine each night.

   or

5. 150 mg of carbenoxolone per day.

I believe that, in the light of present evidence, there is nothing to justify a complicated or expensive regime of long-term management or surveillance of patients who have been proved to have a simple gastric ulcer.

REFERENCES

Anselmi M, Dykes P W, Alexander-Williams J 1981 An audit of management of gastric ulcer. Unpublished data

Bank S, Marks I N 1973 Evaluation of new drugs for peptic ulcer. Clinics in Gastroenterology 2: 379-395

Baume P E, Hunt J H 1969 Failure of potent antacid therapy to hasten healing of gastric ulcers. Australasian Annals of Medicine 18: 113-116

Baume P E, Hunt J H, Piper D W 1972 Glycopyrronium bromide in the treatment of chronic gastric ulcer. Gastroenterology 63: 399-406

Bayes B E, Woolf I L, Wilson R Y, Cowley D J, Dymock I W 1975 Treatment of gastric ulceration with a bismuth preparation. Postgraduate Medical Journal 51: 29-33

Black R B, Rhodes J, Davies G, Gravelle H, Sweetman P 1971 A controlled clinical trial of cholestyramine in the treatment of gastric ulcers. Gastroenterology 61: 821-825

Boyle J M, Hurwitz A L, Jones R S, Mansbach Ch M II 1977 Gastric ulcer effect of healing on gastric acid secretion and fasting serum gastrin levels. American Journal of Digestive Diseases 22: 1037-1039

Doll R, Price A V, Pygott F, Sanderson P H 1956 Continuous intragastric milk drip in the treatment of uncomplicated gastric ulcer. Lancet 1: 70-73

Dragstedt L R, Harper P V, Tovee E B, Woodward E R 1947 Section of vagus nerves to the stomach in the treatment of peptic ulcer: Complications and end results after four years. Annals of Surgery 126: 687

Englert E, Freston J W, Graham D Y, Finkelstein W, Krus D M, Priest R J, Raskin J B, Rhodes J B, Rogers A I, Wender J, Wilcox L L, Crossley R J 1978 Cimetidine, antacid and hospitalization in the treatment of benign gastric ulcer. A multi-centre double blind study. Gastroenterology 74: 416-425

Fenger C, Amdrys E, Christiansen P, Jensen H, Lindskov J, Nielson J, Nielsen S 1973 Gastric Ulcer 1. Analysis of 701 patients. Acta Chirurgica Scandinavica 139: 455

Fisher R S, Cohen S 1973 Pyloric-sphincter dysfunction in patients with gastric ulcer. New England Journal of Medicine 288: 273-276

Freston J W 1978 Cimetidine in the treatment of gastric ulcer. A review and commentary. Gastroenterology 74: 426-431

Fry J 1964 Peptic ulcer: a profile. British Medical Journal 2: 809

Hanscom D H, Buchman E 1971 The follow-up period from the Veterans Administration Cooperative Study on gastric ulcer. Gastroenterology 61: 585-591

Hoskins E O L 1973 Metoclopramide in benign gastric ulceration. Postgraduate Medical Journal, July Supplement: 95-98

Kennedy T 1973 Commenting on paper by Hoskins. Postgraduate Medical Journal 49: 98-99

Krag E 1966 Long-term prognosis in medically treated peptic ulcer. Acta Medica Scandinavica 180: 657

Natvig P, Romcke O, Swaar-Seljesaeter O 1943 Results of medical treatment of gastric and duodenal ulcer. Acta Medica Scandinavica 113: 444

Discussion on Gastric Ulcer
Chairman: Professor C. G. Clark

Professor Clark. I note that Mr Alexander-Williams has practically given up surgery for gastric ulcer. Can the three speakers say what they mean by 'gastric ulcer'? Are all forms of gastric ulcer included, or are we talking only about the lesser curve and not about prepyloric ulcers?

Mr Alexander-Williams. I am referring to type I lesser curve or posterior wall gastric ulcers, not combined ulcers and not pyloric channel ulcers.

Dr Colin-Jones. I agree. The nearer the ulcer is to the pylorus the more like a duodenal ulcer it behaves, with the difference that the prepyloric ulcer needs to be biopsied.

Dr Machell. I am in complete agreement.

Professor Clark. A paper published about a year ago suggested that the ulcers that responded well to cimetidine were the type I lesser curve ulcers, and paradoxically that prepyloric ulcers did not respond very well. Is that correct?

Dr Colin-Jones. I know of no detailed information on that point. The study referred to included several very small subgroups, including only three or four patients. Because of these small subgroups the authors could only comment on the results rather than provide any answers.

(*Professor Clark* asked whether any of the speakers had questions for the other speakers).

Dr Colin-Jones. For long-term treatment of gastric ulcers I tend to move towards operation for the younger patients. The chances of relapse with medical treatment have been demonstrated to be quite high so that, if the patients relapse and if they are young, I tend towards operation.

Dr M. E. Kitler. Sometimes patients say that they do not take anti-inflammatory drugs because they are thinking only of aspirin. What does the Panel think about paracetamol which is used extensively in the UK?

Professor Clark. Is there any evidence that paracetamol is ulcerogenic?

Dr Colin-Jones. Aspirin has been shown to have anti-inflammatory activity which paracetamol does not have, although they are both analgesics. Several studies on the mucosal permeability show damage from aspirin with impairment of the mucosal barrier. I can think of only one study in which this has been investigated for paracetamol, and such damage and impairment was not found. On that single objective study, paracetamol would appear to have less risk of damage to the patient with gastric ulcer.

147

Mr Alexander-Williams. Anti-inflammatory drugs are now used mainly for arthritis. Presumably indomethacin and ibuprofen are more common now than aspirin in this country.

Dr Colin-Jones. Yes — and they have been shown to increase the chances of a perforation. A couple of papers have shown that a gastric ulcer is more likely to perforate after one of these anti-inflammatory drugs. These drugs confer a risk, although it is still uncertain exactly how much.

Dr Wormsley. There have been one or two comments that have worried me. For example, although bed-rest may, *pace* Professor Doll, be as good as cabbage juice, it is unlikely that cimetidine will produce deep-vein thrombosis whereas, in the appropriate age groups, bed-rest will.

There is not much point trying to tell patients who have arthritis — and most of the patients with gastric ulcer in the older age groups have arthritis — not to take any anti-inflammatory drug because they will take it for their arthritis. We therefore have to protect these patients.

I agree with the American study that was quoted, about the danger of acute complications of gastric ulcer. Perforation and haemorrhage are dangerous in older patients. These complications occur, they do so unexpectedly and are extremely dangerous. It is for that reason that I think Dr Machell did his study a disservice by saying that he was not in favour of maintenance treatment. I am strongly in favour of maintenance treatment — that is, if we want to preserve elderly patients, a subject which we might discuss some time!

Dr Machell. Dr Wormsley misheard what I said. I was advocating maintenance treatment in elderly patients at high risk with surgery, that is, those patients with intercurrent disease, which so many of those patients have. However, on present evidence, I share the same reservations about offering maintenance treatment to younger gastric ulcer patients.

Mr Alexander-Williams. I cannot see, Dr Wormsley, that there is any reason for advocating maintenance therapy in asymptomatic patients who are not at high risk. Of course, it is an entirely different matter if someone has to take anti-inflammatory drugs because there is no alternative. However, the vast majority of people prescribed anti-inflammatory drugs in general practice are being so prescribed to keep them quiet rather than for a very specific medical reason. If anti-inflammatory drugs must be given because of severe arthritis which is not responsive to any other treatment, and if the patient has a gastric ulcer, I think there is probably a very good indication for surgical treatment. Indeed, that is one of our indications. There are not many indications for operation for gastric ulcer, but that is one of them.

Professor Clark. What do you actually do for your gastric ulcers, Mr Alexander-Williams?

Mr Alexander-Williams. We do a Billroth I gastrectomy which is a relatively simple and straightforward operation with a very good symptomatic follow-up. There is a very high proportion of asymptomatic patients after a Billroth I gastrectomy, so this is our standard practice.

Dr Wormsley. These elderly patients already have bone rot, and gastric surgery does not in the least improve that state of affairs. I am for medical treatment.

Professor Clark. That is something about which we could argue for a long time.

Dr Machell. I feel there is a place for treating asymptomatic elderly patients. It depends what is meant by 'asymptomatic'. They may present with a complication, they may heal on medical treatment and thereafter be asymptomatic. Nevertheless, these patients be they symptomatic or asymptomatic, remain at high risk of a complication, and this is a very strong indication for continuous maintenance treatment. All of us see many patients who present with their gastric ulcers initially with a complication. I think maintenance treatment should be considered in those patients.

Mr Alexander-Williams. But how many of the asymptomatic patients will take treatment? Even during the short period of the trial about 25 per cent of your patients gave up, even when they were being studied carefully and presumably being 'jollied' along.

Dr Machell. The same argument applies in duodenal ulcer disease. We can only do our best. If it is felt that cimetidine is a safer alternative to operation — as I believe it is — we must do our best to persuade patients to take the tablets.

Professor Clark. We have plenty of evidence that fewer operations are being done now for duodenal ulcer. That evidence combines both the elective operations and to some extent those for emergencies such as bleeding. I wonder what is happening with gastric ulcer?

Mr Venables. The national figures for gastric ulcer for 1977 and 1978, which I have looked up, show a 40 per cent reduction in gastric ulcer surgery by gastrectomy or by any other operation. There is a 42 per cent reduction in our Region.

Dr Bardhan. What about the small group of patients mentioned by Mr Alexander-Williams who have had a gastric ulcer that has healed but who continue to get intractable symptoms? We have had some experience of this group, and the patients have ended up having an operation which was completely unsatisfactory because there was no lesion present on which to operate!

Mr Alexander-Williams. Did the symptoms persist after operation?

Dr Bardhan. No — they improved.

Mr Alexander-Williams. Which operation was carried out?

Dr Bardhan. Two of the patients had a vagotomy/pyloroplasty, one had a highly selective vagotomy and one a Billroth I.

Mr Alexander-Williams. Did they have irritable bowel syndrome?

Dr Bardhan. Yes, they have had all that, but their symptoms were exactly the same as before their ulcer healed on cimetidine.

Mr Alexander-Williams. But when they had an ulcer their symptoms were still due to the irritable bowel syndrome.

Dr Bardhan. Their symptoms were not quite typical of that.

Professor Clark. I was just reflecting on some data, which I shall not show, on about half-a-dozen centres actively engaged in peptic ulcer studies. As far as duodenal ulcer operations are concerned, 1976 was a watershed, operations being reduced by about 38 to 40 per cent. But there was no consistency between Areas. In fact, the most inconsistent Area — which is carrying out exactly the same number of operations in 1980 as it was in 1971 — is in the Trent Region.

Mr Elder. When Dr Bardhan talks about operating for no lesion he is the most surgeon-like physician I have ever come across. Surely, this is the crux of the matter. I have always believed that a gastric ulcer is just an incident in a diseased mucosa, and that the patients have gastritis which does not change. As Mr Alexander-Williams has reassured us, scientific appraisal shows no measurable difference in the gastritis before and after ulcer healing. If the physicians in the Panel believe that there is sufficient evidence to treat an ulcer because of the healing that is thereby obtained, would they then say that the gastritis should be treated, because it is the gastritis that is the basis of the ulcer? Do they treat gastritis with drugs?

Dr Colin-Jones. No, there is no treatment for gastritis. Mr Elder is simplifying a complicated problem, and I am sure he does not believe that it is only gastritis that causes gastric ulcers.

Mr Alexander-Williams. Gastritis is not symptomatic either. Is not duodenogastric reflux the common factor? There is no hard evidence that duodenogastric reflux into the stomach causes any symptoms, but is it possible that symptoms occur when the bile gets into the oesophagus? Is that what produces the symptoms in these patients?

Dr Colin-Jones. Mr Alexander-Williams can of course answer his own question, perhaps indirectly, from his studies on bile reflux in the operated stomach. The relationship is bad with the gastritis, but there is perhaps some correlation with the bile itself. I do not think we know what causes ulcer disease as such. I must emphasise the fact that the endoscope is appreciably more accurate in picking up mucosal lesions, and we are having difficulty in interpreting some of those lesions. When I used to find erosions I sometimes tended to attribute symptoms to them. However, when the erosions went and the patients continued to have symptoms, I became sceptical.

Mr Alexander-Williams. I made my statement because we are currently investigating the question of where the bile has to be to produce symptoms? There may be much bile in the stomach but no symptoms, but once it goes into the oesophagus it seems to produce quite severe symptoms. The attractive hypothesis is that only bile in the oesophagus is bad. Bile enters the stomach much more readily in gastric ulcer disease and perhaps it produces symptoms when it goes even further up. Perhaps symptomatic patients are those with bile reflux.

Professor Clark. That final part of this discussion leads naturally into the first topic for the next session.

Section 3
OESOPHAGEAL REFLUX DISEASE

18. Assessment of the efficacy of cimetidine and other drugs in oesophageal reflux disease

Guido N. J. Tytgat
Department of Medicine, University of Amsterdam

It is of paramount importance in the design of rational management to understand the mechanisms that control lower oesophageal sphincter pressure (LESP) and reflux of irritating juices such as gastric acid and/or biliopancreatic secretions. The goals of medical or surgical therapy are to control the symptoms of reflux and to prevent the progression of oesophageal damage which may ultimately result in stricture formation, bleeding or the development of a Barrett-type oesophagus. In this contribution the value of the various pharmacological approaches is analysed.

CIMETIDINE

Rationale
Cimetidine inhibits basal and nocturnal gastric acid secretion as well as acid secretion stimulated by food, by numerous secretagogues (gastrin), and by vagal stimulation (sham feeding and fundic distension). Cimetidine also reduces pepsin secretion. Cimetidine has no clinically significant effect on LESP. Cimetidine's primary role in reflux disease is the reduction of gastric acidity and probably the reduction of acid volume available for reflux.

Results
The use of cimetidine has been reported in a substantial number of patients with reflux disease (Table 18.1). The severity of reflux disease in patients included in clinical trials varied considerably. At one end of the spectrum were patients with symptomatic reflux but without endoscopic signs of oesophagitis. At the other end were patients with severe oesophagitis, ulcerations and stricture. This variation must be taken into account when evaluating the effectiveness of cimetidine in the management of reflux disease.

In these controlled trials 468 patients, of whom at least 223 had endoscopic evidence of erosions and/or ulcerations, were usually treated for six to eight weeks (range 4 to 12 weeks). The dose of cimetidine varied from 1 to 2 g/day. In the majority of the European studies, a dose of 1.6 g/day was used (400 mg after each meal and at bedtime), in contrast to 1.2 g/day in the American trials. In all studies the patients had free access to antacids.

Table 18.1 Results of cimetidine treatment in reflux oesophagitis compared with placebo.

Reference	N	Erosive or ulcerative reflux oesophagitis	Dose (g/day)	Duration (weeks)	Symptomatic improvement	Antacid consumption	See footnote 3	Endoscopic improvement	Histologic improvement	Stricture improvement
Wesdorp et al (1978)	24	(24)	1.6	8	–	–	{– B, – Ma}	+	+	
Behar et al (1978)	84	(27)	1.2	8	+	+	+ B	–		
Powell-Jackson et al* (1978)	27	(?)	1.6	6	+	+	– B	–	–	
Lepsien et al (1979)	36 / 22	(36) / (22)	1.6 / 1.6	12 / 8	{+ / +}	{+ / +}		{– / +}		
Brown (1979)	20	(3)	1	8	+	+		+	+	
Druguet and Lambert (1980)	82	(49)	1.6	4	+	–		+	+	
Fiasse et al (1980)	34	(21)	1.6	8	+	+		–		
Festen et al (1980)	20	(20)	1.6	8	–	+		–		
Bright-Asare and El-Bassoussi (1980)	30	(?)	1.2	8	+	+	{– B, – Ma}	–		
Thanik et al[2] (1980)	43	(43)	1.2	4	+			+		
Bennett et al (1980)	68 / 18	(?) / (?)	1–2 / 1	6 / 12	{+ / –}	+	{+ pH 5, – pH}			
Ferguson et al* (1979) — Stricture	14		1.6	26	–			+	–	–
Petrokubi and Jeffries* (1979) — Scleroderma	15		1.2	8	+	+		+		–
Kothari et al[1] (1980) — Barrett-ulcer	7		1.2	8				+		–
Wesdorp et al[1] (1981) — Barrett-ulcer	9		1.6	104	+			+		–

+ = significant improvement over placebo.   * = cross-over.
– = non-significant difference from placebo.
[1] Open treatment.
[2] Comparison with bethanechol; treatment included standard amount of liquid antacid.
[3] B = acid perfusion test according to Bernstein.
pH = intra-oesophageal pH recording.
Ma = manometric analysis of LESP.

Significant symptomatic improvement with cimetidine was observed in 9 of 11 studies, usually for daytime pain as well as nighttime pain. In the two remaining studies (Wesdorp et al, 1978; Festen et al, 1980) an obvious trend towards symptomatic improvement was discernible but failed to reach statistical significance due to the small number of patients studied. This symptomatic improvement usually went parallel with a lower antacid consumption for relief of pain, which reached statistical significance in 8 out of 10 studies. Mucosal sensitivity, assessed with the acid perfusion test, according to Bernstein, was evaluated in four studies. A significant improvement was obtained only in the large-scale American trial (Behar et al, 1978). In that study there was no change in the mean time for appearance of heartburn following acid perfusion after 4 and 8 weeks of placebo treatment, the average time fluctuating around 6 min. In contrast, in the cimetidine-treated patients, a significant prolongation of 4 weeks was observed, pointing towards a diminished mucosal sensitivity. Throughout this study, a greater percentage of cimetidine-treated patients obtained a normal Bernstein test but the difference with placebo failed to reach significance. Overnight pH monitoring before and during the last week of the study was performed only by Bennett et al (1980). Those patients treated with 1 or 2 g cimetidine/day experienced a modest reduction in the amount of acid refluxed since the amount of time with a pH less than 5 was significantly reduced after 6 weeks of cimetidine treatment, compared with placebo, but not after 12 weeks.

Significant endoscopic improvement was obtained in 5 out of 10 studies. The overall endoscopic results are summarized in Table 18.2. Realizing all the restrictions inherent in combining different studies, there seems to be reasonable evidence that on the whole some 63 per cent of patients heal or markedly improve during six to eight weeks of cimetidine treatment compared to 35 per cent during

Table 18.2 Evaluation of endoscopic results in reflux oesophagitis after treatment with cimetidine.

	Cimetidine		Placebo	
	Healed/improved	Unchanged/worse	Healed/improved	Unchanged/worse
Wesdorp et al (1978)	8	4	0	12
Behar et al (1978)	18	22	13	22
Powell-Jackson et al (1978)	7	8	6	9
Lepsien et al (1979)	8	4	3	7
Brown (1979)	9	2	5	4
Druguet and Lambert (1980)	30	14	14	24
Fiasse et al (1980)	9	8	5	10
Bright-Asare and El-Bassoussi (1980)	15	5	7	2
Ferguson et al (1979)	10	6	5	11
Petrokubi and Jeffries (1979)	14	1	3	12
Total	128	74	61	113
Percentage	63%	36%	35%	65%

placebo. In two studies (Wesdorp et al, 1978; Lepsien et al, 1979), particularly stringent patient selection criteria were used in which only patients with erosive or ulcerative oesophagitis were included. The combined results of these studies show that 67 per cent of cimetidine-treated patients experienced healing or marked improvement compared to only 14 per cent of those who received placebo. It should be realized that in the Lepsien study this endoscopic improvement was seen only after 12 weeks. Finally significant histological improvement after cimetidine was seen in three out of four studies.

A few studies need to be discussed individually because selected subgroups of patients with reflux oesophagitis were studied. In a one-year crossover study, Ferguson et al (1979) compared cimetidine 1.6 g/day with placebo in 14 patients with reflux oesophagitis and a peptic stricture. The two treatment modalities did not produce significantly different symptomatic responses neither did they lessen the need for dilatation. The gross endoscopic appearance of the oesophageal mucosa, though not the grades of histopathologic change, improved significantly with cimetidine treatment.

Petrokubi and Jeffries (1979) compared the effectiveness of cimetidine with antacids in patients with reflux oesophagitis secondary to scleroderma. Cimetidine showed significantly greater symptomatic and endoscopic improvement. Also significantly less antacid was used during cimetidine. Neither of the two treatments had a discernible effect on the LESP. Neither treatment had any effect on mean stricture size. Dysphagia did not improve during either treatment period. Petrokubi and Jeffries (1980) continued their controlled study with a cimetidine dose of 1.2 g/day up to 12 months. Remission was obtained in 6 out of 19 patients, of whom 5 relapsed on a nighttime 400 mg cimetidine dose. The 13 other patients never went into remission because of persistent heartburn, oesophagitis or both. These authors conclude that the majority of symptomatic scleroderma patients require 1.2 g cimetidine/day indefinitely to minimize symptoms and to maintain remission. Data regarding the usefulness of cimetidine in patients with endobrachyoesophagus or Barrett oesophagus with inflammation and/or ulceration are limited but interesting. Kothari et al (1980) studied the effect of 1.2 g cimetidine/day in 7 patients with a Barrett ulcer. Repeated endoscopy at four and eight weeks showed complete healing of ulcers in six of the seven patients. Cimetidine had no effect on the strictures which still required dilatation. In another recent study by Wesdorp et al (1981) nine carefully selected patients with a Barrett's oesophagus received cimetidine 1.6 g/day, along with an aluminium hydroxide–magnesium carbonate antacid preparation taken every two hours. The study, which lasted two years, was conducted to determine whether it is possible to establish a regression of the squamocolumnar junction towards the cardia as a means of reducing the premalignant disposition of Barrett's oesophagus. The intensive cimetidine–antacid regimen had a favourable effect on symptoms with healing of endoscopically verified oesophagitis and Barrett ulcers. However, re-establishment of the squamocolumnar junction at the level of the cardia was not observed. This long-term therapy did not produce any clinically significant side-effects.

Comments

Overall, cimetidine appears to be effective in the pharmacological management of gastro-oesophageal reflux disease. Symptomatic response to cimetidine therapy is usually favourable and rapid and patients with all grades of the disease seem to respond. Cimetidine facilitates improvement and healing of endoscopically established oesophagitis and oesophageal lesions in a substantial number of patients. Response to therapy is also present in the more severe forms of erosive or ulcerative oesophagitis. The cimetidine treatment may need to be continued beyond six weeks for more complete endoscopic healing. Also in patients with a Barrett oesophagus, cimetidine has a beneficial effect upon symptoms, oesophagitis and ulceration. Patients with an established fibrous peptic stricture cannot be expected to respond favourably to drug therapy. Failure of reflux oesophagitis to respond to therapy with cimetidine may perhaps indicate that there are some patients in whom biliopancreatic reflux is the primary causative factor but, at this time, there is no easy way to confirm or to refute this hypothesis.

ANTACIDS

Rationale

The pharmacological action of antacids is based upon the neutralisation of acid gastric contents, thereby reducing the hydrogen ion concentration in the refluxed material, and perhaps also upon the elevation of LESP following gastric alkalinization up to a pH of 6 (Castell and Levine, 1971; Higgs et al, 1974).

Results

In uncontrolled studies, antacids seem to be effective in controlling the symptoms of reflux, particularly heartburn, in 60 to 70 per cent of patients and, to a certain extent, prevent the recurrence of heartburn during the day. Serebro et al (1973) compared in 19 patients the beneficial effect of a continuous intra-oesophageal drip of a liquid antacid with a drip of water and hourly oral administration of antacids. Both continuous intra-oesophageal antacid drip therapy as well as hourly oral antacid administration significantly improved the patients' response to acid perfusion while reflux symptoms treated with continuous water perfusion therapy remained unchanged. The overall antacid drip therapy results were significantly better than those obtained after hourly oral antacid therapy. Olesh (1976) also studied the efficacy of a continuous antacid drip in 26 patients with rather refractory reflux oesophagitis. After 10 to 12 days of treatment all patients improved subjectively and endoscopically. There is very little information regarding the overall effect of oral antacid therapy on the course of reflux oesophagitis. It is not known whether antacids prevent stricture formation and induce complete healing of the oesophageal inflammation. A controlled trial comparing surgical versus medical therapy showed that antacids were able to control symptoms in only 17 per cent of patients followed for three years or longer, but were not very effective in patients with severe reflux symptoms, gross endoscopic oesophagitis and severe sphincter incompetence (Behar et al, 1975).

Comments

Although antacid treatment is still considered by many physicians as the mainstay of the therapy in reflux oesophagitis, objective proof of its efficacy is scanty. The difficulty in view of antacids' transient neutralizing effect is to maintain a gastric pH above 3.5 throughout the 24-hour period. The action of antacids is far fromadequate, especially during the night when the oesophagus is maximally exposed because of the patient's recumbent position, the diurnal rise in basal acid secretion and the impairment of oesophageal acid clearance. Preferably antacids of high buffering capacity should be given in a liquid form, at frequent intervals for adequate suppression of gastric acid.

ALGINATE/ANTACID

Rationale
Alginate/antacid creates a viscous foamy raft which floats on the stomach fluid in the erect position (Beckloff et al, 1972). The antacid component is incorporated in this gel-like layer. Therefore, if reflux does occur, the material which contacts the oesophageal mucosa is presumably not acidic.

Results
In two of three controlled studies, symptoms of both postprandial and nocturnal heartburn and acid regurgitation were significantly relieved by Gaviscon, compared to alginate or antacid alone (Table 18.3). Stanciu and Bennett (1974) showed that both the number of reflux episodes and the percentage of time with an acidic oesophageal pH were also significantly reduced by Gaviscon. In three further studies (Scobie, 1976; Graham et al, 1977; McHardy, 1977) Gaviscon was compared to standard antacid therapy. In all three, both drugs appeared to be equally effective in relieving symptoms and in improving the endoscopically documented lesions.

Comments
From the rather limited number of patients studied in these controlled trials, it seems reasonable to conclude that alginate/antacid may improve patient symptomatology and perhaps reduce the number of reflux episodes. This effect cannot be explained by neutralization of gastric contents. However, this drug has not been shown to be superior to standard antacid therapy. Whether Gaviscon accelerates endoscopic healing of oesophageal lesions is uncertain due to lack of appropriate placebo controls and needs further investigation.

Table 18.3 Results of alginate/antacid and carbenoxolone in reflux oesophagitis.

	N	Erosive or ulcerative reflux oesophagitis	Dose per day	Duration (weeks)	Symptomatic improvement	Antacid consumption	See footnote 3, table 18.1	Endoscopic improvement	Histological improvement	Stricture improvement
Alginate–antacid[3] versus placebo										
Beeley and Warner (1972)[1]	28	(?)	8 tab	2	+					
Stanciu and Bennett (1974)	40	(10)	8 tab	2	–		+ pH			
Barnardo et al (1975)[1]	26	(?)	4 tab	6	+					
Scobie (1976)[2]	20	(12)	8 tab	3	–			–		
Graham et al (1977)[2]	41	(?)	8 tab	4	–			–		
McHardy (1978)[2]	133	(28)	8 tab	4	–			–		
Carbenoxolone										
McAndrew and Foote (1970)[1]	12	(?)	80 mg	12	+					
Atkinson et al (1970)	27	(18)	120 mg	6	–			–		
Carbenoxolone–alginate[4]										
Reed and Davies (1978)	37	(?)	100 mg	8	+			+	–	

[1] Crossover.
[2] Comparison to standard antacid therapy.
[3] Gaviscon (260 mg alginic acid, 260 mg sodium alginate, 260 mg magnesium trisilicate, 104 mg colloidal aluminium hydroxide, 88.5 mg sodium bicarbonate.
[4] Pyrogastrone.
+ = Significant improvement over placebo or weak antacid.
– = Non-significant difference from placebo or weak antacid.

CARBENOXOLONE ± ALGINATE

Rationale
The rationale upon which carbenoxolone therapy in reflux disease is based is rather ill defined. Speculations centre around those factors which have been invoked in explaining its healing properties in peptic ulcer disease.

Results
McAndrew and Foote (1970) were able to demonstrate significant symptomatic and endoscopic improvement but this was not confirmed by Atkinson et al (1970). In these two studies, in which only a small number of patients was investigated, a liquid preparation was employed (Table 18.3). Reed and Davies (1978) found that the addition of carbenoxolone to an alginate/antacid compound as a chewable tablet significantly enhanced symptomatic improvement and increased endoscopic healing of reflux oesophagitis, including all oesophageal ulcers, when compared to the alginate antacid compound alone.

More recently these authors analysed their clinical experience in 104 patients treated openly with pyrogastrone during a 3.5-year period (Markham and Reed, 1980). Significant symptomatic improvement was achieved in 85 per cent and endoscopic healing in 76 per cent after treatment for four to eight weeks. Besides the well-known side-effects of carbenoxolone, palatability was occasionally a problem.

Comments
The efficacy of carbenoxolone as single agent therapy in reflux disease is dubious; when combined with alginate/antacid, the healing and symptom-relieving action is more convincing, but needs confirmation by other investigators. Why carbenoxolone should be efficacious is still a matter of speculation (alteration of mucus secretion? cell-kinetics? prostaglandin content? or other mechanisms?).

Finally one should keep in mind the mineralocorticoid side-effect, especially in elderly patients.

BETHANECHOL

Rationale
Bethanechol is a cholinergic muscarinic drug which increases LESP in normal subjects and in patients with reflux oesophagitis. In addition bethanechol may increase oesophageal clearance and gastric emptying.

Results
Oral bethanechol 25 mg q.i.d. has been evaluated by Farrell et al (1974). Patients receiving bethanechol fared significantly better than during either the pretreatment or the placebo period (Table 18.4). In addition there was a significant reduction in the amount of antacid consumed during bethanechol

Table 18.4 Results of bethanechol, metoclopramide and domperidone in reflux oesophagitis.

	N	Erosive or ulcerative reflux oesophagitis	Dose (mg)	Duration (weeks)	Symptomatic improvement	Antacid consumption	See footnote 3 in table 18.1	Endoscopic improvement
Bethanechol								
Farrell et al (1974)[1]	20	(?)	4 × 25	8	+	+		
Thanik et al (1978)[2]	28	(28)	4 × 25	4	-			+
Thanik et al (1980)[3]	43	(43)	4 × 25	4	+			+
Metoclopramide								
Venables et al (1973)[1]	15	(?)	3 × 10	8	-	-		
Paull & Kerr Grant (1974)	31	(?)	4 × 10	6	-			
McCallum et al (1977)[1]	31	(?)	4 × 10	8	+	-	– Ma	
Bright-Asare and El-Bassoussi (1980)	30	(?)	4 × 10	8	+	+	{ – B, – Ma }	-
Domperidone								
Valenzuela (1980)	23	(?)	4 × 20	8	+			
Blackwell et al (1980)[4]	22	(?)	4 × 20	2	-	-	{ – B, – pH, – Ma }	-
Gordon & Joseph (1980)[5]	12	(?)	4 × 20	4	+			

[1] Crossover.
[2] Treatment included standard amount of liquid antacid.
[3] Comparison with cimetidine; treatment included standard amount of liquid antacid.
[4] Treatment included standard alginate/antacid regimen.
[5] Patient in remission after open treatment.
+ Significant improvement.
– No significant difference.

therapy. Rather similar results were obtained by Thanik et al (1980) when bethanechol was combined with a liquid antacid. When compared to cimetidine, the symptomatic and endoscopic improvement after bethanechol was indistinguishable from that after cimetidine.

Comments
Bethanechol may be a useful addition to the therapeutic measures for chronic heartburn although the number of patients studied is limited. Also more information is needed regarding the changes in the LESP during bethanechol treatment. A disadvantage of the drug is that gastric acid secretion is stimulated. Routine combination with antacids or H_2-histamine receptor blockers may prove to be useful in clinical practice in this regard.

METOCLOPRAMIDE

Rationale
Metoclopramide is a dopamine antagonist which increases the amplitude of oesophageal contractions and of LESP and stimulates gastric emptying and pyloric sphincter competence (Stanciu and Bennett, 1973; Cohen et al, 1976; Valenzuela et al, 1976). Metoclopramide does not affect gastric acid secretion.

Results
Two initial studies (Table 18.4) in patients with symptomatic gastro-oesophageal reflux did not show a significant effect of metoclopramide. In Venables et al's study (1973) the negative results could have been due to inappropriate timing of the medication since LESP does not rise until about 30 minutes after ingestion. In Paull and Kerr Grant's study (1974), more patients improved with metoclopramide but the difference was not significant. In contrast McCallum et al (1977) showed that metoclopramide 10 mg q.i.d. over eight weeks produced improvement in both frequency and severity of heartburn attacks, the percentage symptomatic improvement being 57 ± 10 for metoclopramide compared to 33 ± 6 for placebo. This improvement was, however, not associated with a significant rise in LESP. Rather similar results were obtained by Bright-Asare and El-Bassoussi (1980). A significant number of patients taking metoclopramide had less pain than before, which resulted in concomitant lower antacid usage. Also in that study, however, there was no significant change in mucosal sensitivity, LESP or endoscopic improvement. Furthermore, metoclopramide was attended by significant side-effects.

Comments
There is some evidence that metoclopramide may improve the symptomatology of patients with reflux disease. The absence of a significant rise in LESP in these studies suggests that other mechanisms, such as accelerated oesophageal acid clearing and gastric emptying, may be more important. A disadvantage of

metoclopramide is the appreciable number of neurologic and psychotropic side-effects which may occur at the customary dosage level.

DOMPERIDONE

Rationale
Domperidone is another peripheral dopamine receptor antagonist which has been shown to exert a stimulatory effect on the LESP and upon oesophageal peristalsis (Weihrauch et al, 1979).

Results
In Valenzuela's study (1980) domperidone caused significant improvement in the symptoms of gastro-oesophageal reflux, but when compared to placebo did not promote the healing of the oesophageal mucosa. In addition, no significant changes in LESP or oesophageal motility were observed. Blackwell et al (1980) added domperidone or placebo to a standard alginate/antacid regimen. They were also unable to demonstrate any benefit from the addition of domperidone. On the other hand, Gordon and Joseph (1980) compared domperidone with placebo in patients who responded well to previous open domperidone treatment and found persistent improvement of symptoms during domperidone in contrast to symptomatic relapse during placebo.

Comments
Results with domperidone therapy in reflux disease are still preliminary but overall rather similar to those obtained with metoclopramide. Compared to metoclopramide domperidone has the theoretical advantage of passing the blood–brain barrier with difficulty, suggesting that a low incidence of extrapyramidal side-effects is to be expected. Oral domperidone has not been shown to raise the LESP. One wonders, therefore, whether the potential beneficial action of domperidone in reflux disease is not related to other mechanisms such as accelerated gastric emptying, reduced duodenal–gastric reflux or other undetermined actions.

DISCUSSION

The three most important goals in the treatment of reflux oesophagitis are: to neutralise gastric acidity, to increase the lower oesophageal sphincter pressure, and to facilitate acid clearance by enhancing oesophageal peristalsis and accelerating gastric emptying. In all three areas, considerable pharmacological progress has been made recently although our pharmacological possibilities are still far from ideal. Of the drugs which have been studied in a controlled way, cimetidine has been investigated most extensively and most adequately.

Cimetidine's primary role in reflux therapy is the reduction of gastric acidity and probably the reduction of acid volume available for reflux. Presumably the most damaging reflux episodes occur at night in recumbency as many intraluminal pH measurement studies have indicated. In particular, reduction of nocturnal acid secretion by cimetidine should therefore be beneficial.

At present cimetidine therapy, in addition to standard antireflux measures, should be used only in patients with objectively (endoscopically) documented moderate to severe (erosive–ulcerative) reflux oesophagitis and exceptionally in patients with severe heartburn and acid regurgitation not controlled by antireflux measures and antacids. In most experimental studies a rather high dose (4 × 400 mg cimetidine/day) has been used for six to eight weeks. It is, however, conceivable that the usual dose of 1 g cimetidine/day may prove to be equally effective. When after six to eight weeks therapy no objective improvement is obtained, the cimetidine treatment should be prolonged for another six to eight weeks, either at the same dose of 1 g/day or at a higher dose.

It seems reasonable to allow free access to antacids or alginate/antacid for symptomatic control of persistent heartburn or regurgitation when not controlled by cimetidine. Although no experimental data are available as yet, one may also try to combine cimetidine with drugs (domperidone or metoclopramide) which tighten the lower oesophageal sphincter pressure, in particular in severe rather intractable cases. Domperidone should perhaps be the first choice in view of the lower incidence of side-effects. These drugs should be preferred to bethanechol because additional stimulation of acid secretion, as seen with the latter, is avoided.

If no substantial improvement occurs after three months of intensive medical therapy, one should consider surgical correction of the sphincteric area. If objective improvement occurs and healing of the epithelial lesions is obtained, the patient should be eligible for maintenance therapy because severe forms of reflux oesophagitis tend to relapse. How and for how long such maintenance therapy should be conducted is unknown at present due to lack of appropriate studies. One of the various possibilities could be to combine postprandial antacids with either 400 mg cimetidine at night or with a morning and evening dose of 400 mg cimetidine for several months. The duration of such maintenance therapy should depend greatly upon the clinical situation. Patients with scleroderma or with achalasia after Heller operations, for example, with a permanently impaired oesophageal muscle function leading to permanent symptomatic reflux, may require indefinite maintenance therapy once remission has been obtained. Also patients with Barrett's oesophagus may need prolonged maintenance therapy to prevent relapse when surgery is contraindicated. In other patients, the duration of maintenance therapy will be determined by eventual correction of aggravating factors such as weight reduction in severe obesity, (permanent!) cure of peptic ulcer disease, permanent avoidance of excessive alcohol, cessation of smoking, etc. The clinician has to decide at which point maintenance therapy with cimetidine can be stopped, to be continued only with anti-reflux measures and perhaps antacids for intermittent control of heartburn.

REFERENCES

Atkinson M, Cuming J H, Majekodumni A E 1970 A trial of carbenoxolone electuary in the treatment of reflux oesophagitis. In: Baron J H, Sullivan F M (eds) Symposium on carbenoloxone sodium. Butterworths, London, p 123-127

Barnardo D E, Lancaster-Smith M, Strickland I D, Wright J T 1975 A double-blind controlled trial of 'Gaviscon' in patients with symptomatic gastro-oesophageal reflux. Current Medical Research and Opinion 3: 388-391

Beckloff G L, Chapman J H, Shiverdecker P 1972 Objective evaluation of an antacid with unusual properties. Journal of Clinical Pharmacology 12: 11-21

Beeley M, Warner J O 1972 Medical treatment of symptomatic hiatus hernia with low-density compounds. Current Medical Research and Opinion 1: 63-69

Behar J, Sheahan D G, Biancani P, Spiro H M, Storer E H 1975 Medical and surgical management of reflux oesophagitis. New England Journal of Medicine 293: 263-268

Behar J, Brand D L, Brown F C, Castell D O, Cohen S, Crossley R J, Pope C E, Winans C S 1975 Cimetidine in the treatment of symptomatic gastroesophageal reflux. Gastroenterology 74: 441-448

Bennett J R, Martin H D, Buckton G 1980 Cimetidine in reflux oesophagitis. In: Hepato-Gastroenterology Supplement. Abstracts of the XI International Congress of Gastroenterology, Hamburg, June 8-13, 1980, p. 30

Blackwell J N, Heading R C, Fettes M R 1980 Effects of domperidone on lower oesophageal sphincter pressure and gastro-oesophageal reflux in patients with peptic oesophagitis. In: Progress with Domperidone, A Gastrokinetic and Antiemetic Agent: Proceedings of a meeting at the Royal Society of Medicine. International Congress and Symposium Series No. 36. Academic Press, London, p 57-61

Bright-Asare P, El-Bassoussi M 1980 Cimetidine, metoclopramide or placebo in the treatment of symptomatic gastro-oesophageal reflux. Journal of Clinical Gastroenterology 2: 149-156

Brown P 1979 Cimetidine in the treatment of reflux oesophagitis. Medical Journal of Australia 2: 96-97

Castell D O, Levine S M 1971 Lower oesophageal sphincter response to gastric alkalinization. A new mechanism for treatment of heartburn with antacids. Annals of Internal Medicine 74: 223-227

Cohen S, Morris D W, Schoen H J, DiMarino A J 1976 The effect of oral and intravenous metoclopramide on human lower oesophageal sphincter pressure. Gastroenterology 70: 484-487

Druguet M, Lambert R 1980 Oral cimetidine in reflux oesophagitis: a double-blind controlled trial. In: Dress A, Barbier F, Harvengt C, Tytgat G N (eds) Cimetidine/Tagamet. Proceedings of the Second National Symposium, Brussels, 27 October 1979. Excerpta Medica, Amsterdam, Oxford, Princeton, p 30-36

Farrell R L, Roling G T, Castell D O 1974 Cholinergic therapy of chronic heartburn. Annals of Internal Medicine 8: 573-576

Ferguson R, Dronfield M W, Atkinson M 1979 Cimetidine in treatment of reflux oesophagitis with peptic stricture. British Medical Journal 2: 472-474

Festen H P M, Driessen W M M, Lamers C B H, van Tongeren J H M 1980 Cimetidine in the treatment of severe ulcerative reflux oesophagitis: results of an 8-week double-blind study and of subsequent long-term maintenance treatment. Netherlands Journal of Medicine 23: 237-240

Fiasse R, Hanin Ch, Lepot A, Descamps Ch, Lamy F, Dive Ch 1980 Controlled trial of cimetidine in reflux oesophagitis. Digestive Diseases and Sciences 25: 750-755

Gordon S J, Joseph R E 1980 Domperidone in patients with postprandial upper gastrointestinal distress. In: Progress with domperidone, a gastrokinetic and anti-emetic agent: Proceedings of a meeting at the Royal Society of Medicine, International Congress Symposium Series No. 36. Academic Press, London, p 67-75

Graham D Y, Lanza F, Dorsch E R 1977 Symptomatic reflux oesophagitis: a double-blind controlled comparison of antacids and alginate. Current Therapeutic Research 22: 653-658

Higgs R H, Smith R D, Castell D O 1974 Gastric alkalinization: effect on lower oesophageal sphincter pressure and serum gastrin. New England Journal of Medicine 291: 486-490

Kothari T, Mangla I C, Kalra T M S 1980 Barrett's ulcer and treatment with cimetidine. Archives of Internal Medicine140: 475-477

Lepsien G, Sonnenberg A, Berges W, Weber K B, Wienbeck M, Siewert J R, Blum A L 1979 Die Behandlung der Refluxösophagitis mit Cimetidin. Deutsche Medizinische Wochenschrift 104: 901-906

McAndrew G M, Foote A V 1970 Carbenoxolone sodium treatment of peptic oesophagitis: a preliminary report. In: Baron J H, Sullivan F M (eds) Symposium on carbenoxolone sodium. Butterworths, London, p 117-112

McCallum R W, Ippoliti A F, Cooney C, Sturdevant R A L 1977 A controlled trial of metoclopramide in symptomatic gastroesophageal reflux. New England Journal of Medicine 296: 354-357

McHardy G 1978 A multicentric, randomized clinical trial of Gaviscon in reflux. Southern Medical Journal 71: 16-21

Markham C, Reed P I 1980 Pyrogastrone treatment of peptic oesophagitis: analysis of 104 patients treated during a 3.5 year period. Scandinavian Journal of Gastroenterology 15, Supplement 65: 73-79

Olesh K 1976 Therapie der Refluxösophagitis mittels Sondeninfusion. Leber Magen Darm 6: 185-187

Paull A, Kerr Grant A 1974 A controlled trial of metoclopramide in reflux oesophagitis. Medical Journal of Australia 2: 627-629

Petrokubi R J, Jeffries G H 1979 Cimetidine versus antacid in scleroderma with reflux oesophagitis. Gastroenterology 77: 691-695

Petrokubi R J, Jeffries G H 1980 Chronic cimetidine therapy for reflux oesophagitis in scleroderma. Gastroenterology 78: 1236

Powell-Jackson P, Barkley H, Northfield T C 1978 Effect of cimetidine in symptomatic gastroesophageal reflux. Lancet ii: 1068-1069

Reed P I, Davies W A 1978 Controlled trial for a new dosage form of carbenoxolone (Pyrogastrone) in the treatment of reflux oesophagitis. American Journal of Digestive Diseases 23: 161-165

Scobie B A 1976 Endoscopically controlled trial of alginate and antacid in reflux oesophagitis. Medical Journal of Australia 1: 627-628

Serebro H A, Friedman M, Beck I T 1973 Efficacy of continuous intra-oesophageal antacid drip therapy in the treatment of reflux oesophagitis. South African Medical Journal 47: 1656-1659

Stanciu C, Bennett J R 1973 Metoclopramide in gastroesophageal reflux. Gut 14: 275-279

Stanciu C, Bennett J R 1974 Alginate/antacid in the reduction of gastro-oesophageal reflux. Lancet i: 109-111

Thanik K D, Chey W Y, Shah A S, Gutierrez J G 1980 Reflux esophagitis: effect of oral bethanechol on symptoms and endoscopic findings. Annals of Internal Medicine 93: 805-808

Thanik K D, Chey W Y, Shah A N, Hamilton D L, Nadelson N W 1980 Comparative studies on effects of cimetidine and bethanechol in the treatment of reflux esophagitis. Gastroenterology 78: 1277

Valenzuela J E, Defilippi C, Csendes A 1976 Manometric studies on the human pyloric sphincter: effect of cigarette smoking, metoclopramide, and atropine. Gastroenterology 70: 481-483

Valenzuela J E 1980 Effects of domperidone on the symptoms of reflux oesophagitis. In: Progress with domperidone, a gastrokinetic and anti-emetic agent: Proceedings of a meeting at the Royal Society of Medicine, International Congress and Symposium Series No. 36. Academic Press, London, p 51-56

Venables C W, Bell D, Eccleston D 1973 A double-blind study of metoclopramide in symptomatic peptic oesophagitis. Postgraduate Medical Journal 49, supplement 4: 73-76

Weihrauch T R, Förster Ch F, Krieglstein I J 1979 Evaluation of the effect of domperidone on human oesophageal and gastroduodenal motility by intraluminal manometry. Postgraduate Medical Journal 55, supplement 1: 7-10

Wesdorp E, Bartelsman J, Pape K, Dekker W, Tytgat G N 1978 Oral cimetidine in reflux oesophagitis: a double-blind controlled trial. Gastroenterology 74: 821-824

Wesdorp I C E, Bartelsman J, Schipper M E I, Tytgat G N 1981 Effect of long-term treatment with cimetidine and antacids in Barrett oesophagus. Gut, in press

19. Gastro-oesophageal reflux and bronchial asthma – a relationship?

Alan Bernstein and John G. Temple

Department of Thoracic Medicine and University Department of Surgery, Hope Hospital, Salford

A variety of oesophageal lesions may be complicated by pulmonary problems including repeated pulmonary infections, lung abscess, pulmonary fibrosis and haemoptysis. In many cases the patient may present with respiratory symptoms only (Urschel and Paulson, 1967). The mechanism in many of these situations is thought to be repeated aspiration into the lungs of gastric contents (Mays et al, 1976).

A relationship between gastro-oesophageal reflux, with or without hiatus hernia, and bronchial asthma has been suggested for a number of years, but is far less easy to demonstrate. The mechanism for this remains to be proven. A number of investigators have demonstrated an increased incidence of gastro-oesophageal reflux in asthmatic patients compared with the normal population (Clemencon and Osterman, 1961; Mays, 1976). Other studies have yielded a high incidence of asthma in groups of patients undergoing investigation for gastro-oesophageal reflux (Davis, 1969). Finally, an improvement in asthmatic symptoms has been reported in patients in whom gastro-oesophageal reflux has been treated, either surgically (Overholt and Ashraf, 1966; Urschel and Paulson, 1967) or medically (Mays, 1976).

In this study we have attempted to show an improvement in symptoms and respiratory function in asthmatic patients with well-documented gastro-oesophageal reflux by controlling this reflux with cimetidine in a double-blind cross-over trial.

MATERIALS AND METHODS

Twenty patients, thirteen male and seven female, with proven bronchial asthma and symptomatic gastro-oesophageal reflux were included in the study. The mean age was 54 years (range 30–65 years). Asthma had been diagnosed in these patients on clinical grounds with particular emphasis upon nocturnal wheezing, the response to treatment with disodium cromoglycate and oral or inhaled steroids, a personal or family history of allergy, blood or sputum eosinophilia and evidence of reversible airways obstruction (Table 19.1). Seventeen of the patients were considered to have late onset asthma. Gastro-oesophageal reflux was investigated by barium studies, oesophagoscopy, lower oesophageal manometry, overnight pH monitoring and an acid infusion (Bernstein) test (Table 19.1).

Table 19.1 Characteristics of 20 patients with asthma and gastro-oesophageal reflux.

Asthma	No. of patients	Gastro-oesophageal reflux	No. of patients
Nocturnal wheezing	20	Symptoms	19
Previous and/or family history of atopy	17	Hiatus hernia/reflux on X-ray	19
		Endoscopic abnormalities	11
Good response to disodium cromoglycate	12	Gastro-oesophageal sphincter pressure low	8
Good response to steroids	15	Abnormal prolonged pH test	8
Reversible airways obstruction	11	Positive acid infusion test	11
Blood or sputum eosinophilia	15		
Positive skin testing (common allergens)	10		

Full lung function tests were performed initially and the patients were treated in a randomised double-blind cross-over fashion with cimetidine or placebo at six-week intervals, with the oesophageal and full lung function tests being repeated at six and twelve-week intervals. In addition all patients recorded on a diary card a score of their day and night-time asthmatic symptoms (Table 19.2) and also recorded peak flow rate on a regular basis each day. At the same time the patients recorded on a daily basis their symptom scores for heartburn and regurgitation (Table 19.2). The analysis of the data was performed by a non-parametric method for crossover trials using a Mann–Whitney U test.

Table 19.2 Results of patient records of day and night-time asthmatic symptoms and symptom scores for heartburn and regurgitation

Asthma

Day time
0 — Good day, no wheezing
1 — Wheezy for 1-2 hours
2 — Wheezy for much of the day
3 — Wheezy all day

Night time
0 — Good night
1 — Slept well but slightly wheezy
2 — Woken 2-3 times because of wheezing
3 — Bad night awake most of the time

Reflux

Heartburn
0 — No heartburn
1 — Occasional heartburn
2 — Heartburn requiring antacids or medical advice
3 — Heartburn constantly interfering with activities

Regurgitation
0 — No regurgitation
1 — Occasional regurgitation on straining or position change
2 — Predictable regurgitation on straining or position change
3 — Occurrence of pulmonary aspiration

Table 19.3 Reflux symptom score, asthma score and peak flow readings after cimetidine and after placebo. Median values and range given.

		After placebo		After cimetidine
Reflux symptom score		2.8 (0-5)	P<0.02	1.1 (0-5)
Asthma score: day		1.2 (0-2.3)	NS	0.9 (0-2.6)
night		1.1 (0-1.7)	P<0.05	0.7 (0-1.8)
Peak flow readings (l/min)	1	295 (105-480)	NS	305 (135-465)
	2	320 (145-515)	NS	330 (190-510)
	3	335 (175-515)	NS	350 (225-525)
	4	310 (170-485)	P<0.05	335 (210-505)

RESULTS (Table 19.3)

Eighteen patients completed the study. After cimetidine the gastro-oesophageal reflux score improved in 14 patients, and the improvement in the median values for reflux symptom scores was significant ($P < 0.02$). Upon completion of the trial the patients were asked to state which of the two treatment periods had produced greater relief of the respiratory symptoms. In 14 patients this was the cimetidine period. Cimetidine produced a significant improvement in the night-time asthmatic scores ($P < 0.05$) but there was no measurable difference during the day time. The peak flow values all showed a trend towards improvement while the patient was taking cimetidine but only the improvement in the last reading of the day was significant. The full pulmonary function tests showed no significant change after either treatment period. There was no relationship between improvement in asthma symptoms and bronchodilator usage. In addition computer analysis of the data revealed that during the period of placebo tablets there was a correlation between the severity of both the reflux and asthmatic symptoms during the day (r = 0.46, $P < 0.05$) and during the night (r = 0.45, $P < 0.05$). During cimetidine therapy there was no such correlation.

DISCUSSION

A relationship between bronchial asthma and gastro-oesophageal reflux is not clearly defined. However, a high incidence of reflux in adults with bronchial asthma has been reported elsewhere. In this study 20 asthmatic patients with gastro-oesophageal reflux were easily found on routine questioning in a short period of time.

A review of the histories showed that in nine patients the reflux symptoms preceded the onset of asthma. In ten patients the asthmatic attack was usually preceded by severe reflux symptoms, while in eight patients there was no such relationship. Finally, one patient reported that the reflux symptoms often developed as a result of the asthmatic attack.

Cimetidine was used in this study to control the gastro-oesophageal reflux because it has been shown to be a potent inhibitor of gastric acid secretion, reducing both the volume and the hydrogen ion concentration. It is, however, unlikely that cimetidine has any direct effect upon bronchial smooth muscle by virtue of H_2 receptor antagonism. No studies so far have shown any significant bronchodilator effect which could be attributed to cimetidine in either healthy or asthmatic subjects (Maconochie et al, 1979).

This study has shown that cimetidine was very effective in alleviating the symptoms of gastro-oesophageal reflux in most patients. Cimetidine also appeared to be associated with an improvement in the asthmatic symptoms. The fact that this occurred particularly at night might be anticipated if nocturnal gastro-oesophageal reflux either precipitates or aggravates respiratory symptoms. Furthermore, three of the patients noted such a dramatic improvement in their respiratory symptoms, albeit subjectively, while they were taking cimetidine, that they received a more prolonged course of this therapy with apparent benefit.

The disappointing feature of this study was that there was no concomitant, dramatic, objectively demonstrable improvement in respiratory function. Comprehensive pulmonary tests were performed, but only the daily peak flow rates showed a trend towards improvement, and furthermore, only one of these reached statistical significance. However, the subjective improvement experienced by most patients should not be ignored.

That gastro-oesophageal reflux can influence bronchial asthma has been suggested by series in which the asthma has been improved or completely relieved by surgical correction of the reflux. If gastro-oesophageal reflux can actually initiate bronchial asthma, is the mechanism simply one of intrapulmonary aspiration of reflux gastric contents? Such evidence is entirely lacking at the present time (Ghaed and Stein, 1979). A more acceptable theory relating the two problems has been suggested by Mansfield and Stein (1978). They showed evidence of demonstrable airways obstruction during and after infusion of dilute hydrochloric acid into the distal oesophagus. These authors postulate a vagal reflex mediated by oesophageal receptors which is responsible for the association between gastro-oesophageal reflux and asthma.

The present study does not reveal which of these two mechanisms is responsible for the relationship. Cimetidine, by reducing the volume and acidity of the refluxed material into the body of the oesophagus, could have influenced either of these two mechanisms. Further study is necessary in a similar group of patients with gastro-oesophageal reflux and asthma to evaluate the reflex hypothesis, perhaps by assessing airways obstruction following the intra-oesophageal installation of dilute hydrochloric acid. Should this be the case, then topical anaesthesia administered to the distal oesophagus should abolish this reflex.

CONCLUSIONS

The results of this study have shown that in a group of patients with asthma and gastro-oesophageal reflux, objective control of the latter produced subjective improvement in the former. However, the exact mechanism for this improvement is still not clear and further work is necessary.

REFERENCES

Clemencon G H, Osterman P O 1961 Hiatal hernia in bronchial asthma — the importance of concomitant pulmonary emphysema. Gastroenterologia 95: 110-120

Davis M V 1969 Evolving concepts regarding hiatal hernia and gastro-oesophageal reflux. Annals of Thoracic Surgery 7: 120-133

Ghaed N, Stein M R 1979 Assessment of technique for scintographic monitoring of pulmonary aspiration of gastric contents in asthmatics with gastro-oesophageal reflux. Annals of Allergy 42: 306-308

Maconochie J G, Woodings E P, Richards D A 1979 Effects of H1 and H2 receptor blocking agents on histamine-induced bronchoconstriction in non-asthmatic subjects. British Journal of Clinical Pharmacology 7: 231-236

Mansfield L E, Stein M R 1978 Gastro-oesophageal reflux and asthma. Annals of Allergy 41: 224-226

Mays E E 1976 Intrinsic asthma in adults. Association with gastro-oesophageal reflux. Journal of the American Medical Association 236: 2626-2628

Mays E E, Dubois J J, Hamilton G B 1976 Pulmonary fibrosis associated with tracheo-bronchial aspiration. Chest 69: 512-515

Overholt R H, Ashraf M M 1966 Esophageal reflux as a trigger in asthma. New York State Journal of Medicine 66: 3030-3032

Urschel H C J R, Paulson D L 1967 Gastro-oesophageal reflux and hiatal hernia. Journal of Thoracic and Cardiovascular Surgery 53: 21-32

20. Long-term management of reflux patients

Robert C Heading*, John N Blackwell and Evan W J Cameron
*Department of Therapeutics and Clinical Pharmacology, Royal Infirmary of Edinburgh

Assessment of long-term treatment for any chronic condition requires long-term follow-up and observation. For this reason we do not yet know what impact modern agents such as cimetidine or carbenoxolone–antacid–alginate preparations are going to have on the eventual outcome of patients suffering from gastro-oesophageal reflux. Indeed very little information about any specific treatment regime relates to a period of more than a few months. In consequence, the clinician must make decisions on the management of individual patients by interpreting and extrapolating the available short-term information and by rejecting it where it seems to run counter to his own experience and intuition. This situation will of course permit the emergence of passionately held opinion, conviction and even prejudice in some clinicians, but more important for the majority is the risk of an inadequate overall view of the condition. In this contribution an attempt is made to answer some questions which seem relevant to the maintenance of a proper perspective.

WHAT IS THE CLINICAL ENTITY WE ARE DEALING WITH?

In a prospective study of more than 1000 patients, Palmer (1968) observed that sub-xiphoid pain and various complex dyspepsias were twice as frequent as the classical symptoms of pyrosis, substernal pain and regurgitation in the presentation of oesophagitis. In contrast, however, Price and Castell (1978) declared that the presentation of oesophagitis with non-specific symptoms was a myth. We have examined retrospectively the case records of 50 patients presenting during the year 1977, in whom oesophagitis and/or a benign stricture was considered to be responsible for upper gastrointestinal symptoms. The diagnosis was established in all cases by endoscopy and biopsy. Patients who at the time of endoscopy had peptic ulceration of the stomach or duodenum or who had bled from oesophagitis associated with varices were excluded. The further management of approximately half the patients was carried out by staff associated with the Gastrointestinal Service of the Royal Infirmary of Edinburgh; the remainder were under the care of other physicians and surgeons in the hospital.

Details of the 50 patients are given in Table 20.1. Although classical symptoms of gastro-oesophageal reflux were recorded in 30 patients, it seems unlikely that a confident clinical diagnosis of oesophagitis or reflux could have been made from the clinical history in the remainder. Dysphagia was a common presenting symptom as it was in the study of Palmer (1968). Five of our 21 patients with dysphagia did not have an oesophageal stricture. Anaemia was a feature in seven patients, including one presenting with haematemesis and melaena.

Table 20.1 Clinical features in 50 patients with oesophagitis

	No. of patients
Principal symptoms	
Heartburn, waterbrash, regurgitation, retrosternal discomfort	30
Vague dyspepsia, epigastric pain/discomfort	13
Dysphagia	21
Anaemia	7
Severe concomitant disease	15
Cardiovascular disease	9
Diabetes with complications	4
Alcohol abuse	2
Psychiatric illness	2
Rheumatoid arthritis	1
Requiring long-term geriatric hospital care	2

All these patients had problems which appeared attributable to gastro-oesophageal reflux. However, it is important to realise that not all were suffering incapacitating or intolerable symptoms. Such patients, and their family doctors, had been concerned about the possible cause of these symptoms, especially the possibility of malignancy. The diagnosis and the reassurance which followed presumably did nothing for the gastro-oesophageal reflux, but nevertheless represented a satisfactory outcome in the patient's view. For such patients, further therapy of the simplest kind may then reduce the symptoms to a level where the patient will subsequently declare that he is 'much better'. This is indeed true, but the improvement owes more to the fact that he is no longer worried by the symptoms than to the suppression of reflux. This sort of improvement is not to be discerned from clinical trials of drugs being developed for oesophagitis but it is nevertheless a part of the clinical spectrum of gastro-oesophageal reflux.

One other aspect of the clinical presentation of gastro-oesophageal reflux merits comment. It is common knowledge that many patients with oesophagitis are elderly and have other medical problems. In our group of 50 patients (16 men and 34 women) the mean age was 61 years and 12 were over the age of 75. Fifteen patients had one or more medical conditions besides oesophagitis which had a continuing major impact on their lives (Table 20.1). In addition, other patients exhibited the general frailty of old age, which is not readily quantified. Thus from the group of 50 patients with oesophagitis, it would seem that for ethical and practical reasons at least 15 would probably not have been suitable for inclusion in the usual sort of clinical trial of antireflux therapy. If other clinicians share our view, the corollary is that such trials report on patient groups which represent no more than two-thirds of the clinical problem as a whole. Possibly the two-thirds is representative of the whole but it is not certain.

The severity of oesophagitis in the 50 patients is given in Table 20.2. The categorisation is admittedly approximate and arbitrary, being based on the extent of friability, erosion and ulceration of the oesophageal mucosa as judged by the endoscopist. Two patients included in the 'mild' category were considered normal by the endoscopist, but oesophagitis was apparent on the biopsy. Two patients with strictures had not complained of dysphagia.

Table 20.2 Principal endoscopic findings in 50 patients with oesophagitis.

	No. of patients
Oesophagitis: Mild	19
Moderate	16
Severe	15
Stricture	18
(Previous gastric surgery	3)

WHAT IS THE RESPONSE TO TREATMENT?

The treatment given to the 50 patients is summarised in Table 20.3. We assume, but do not know for certain, that general advice was also given, including stopping smoking, elevating the head of the bed, the avoidance of large meals in the late evening and weight reduction where appropriate. Six patients underwent operation at some time during the three to four-year follow-up. Four of these were elective antireflux operations combined with stricture dilatation, and a further patient underwent a resection for a stricture associated with a Barrett ulcer. The sixth patient developed a prepyloric gastric ulcer two years after

Table 20.3 Treatment of 50 patients with oesophagitis.

Treatment	No. of patients	
Operation	6	⎰ 4 elective antireflux operations for oesophagitis + stricture 1 resection for Barrett ulcer + stricture 1 fundoplication carried out with vagotomy and pyloroplasty for gastric ulcer
Stricture dilatation(s) + medical therapy	7	
Medical therapy alone	37	

oesophagitis had been recognised and underwent vagotomy and pyloroplasty for this reason. A Nissen fundoplication was performed at the same time. The other 44 patients were treated medically. Seven of these also underwent one or more dilatations of strictures.

An attempt was made to establish the treatment being taken by the patients three to four years after diagnosis and the overall outcome of therapy at this time. Since many patients had been discharged from outpatient clinic attendance, information in many instances was obtained from the patient's general practitioner. In all, information was obtained in respect of 43 of the original 50 patients (Table 20.4).

Table 20.4 Treatment and outcome of 43 patients with oesophagitis at three to four years after diagnosis.

Therapy 3-4 years after diagnosis	
12 patients	No regular therapy (3 had undergone surgery)
26 patients	Various regimes based on antacids, alginates, metoclopramide, cimetidine or Pyrogastrone, or some combination of these
Outcome 3-4 years after diagnosis	
1 worse ⎫ 2 unchanged ⎬ compared with time 35 better ⎭ of diagnosis	
5 died during follow up period	

Between three and four years after diagnosis, 12 patients were taking no regular medication at all. Three of these had undergone operation. Twenty-six were receiving regular medication, based on various combinations of antacids, alginate–antacid mixtures, metoclopramide, cimetidine and Pyrogastrone. Overall clinical assessments of the patient's condition at three to four years rated 35 better, two unchanged and one worse than at the time of diagnosis. Five patients had died during the period, four from causes unrelated to their oesophageal disease. One patient had died from bronchopneumonia associated with chronic renal failure due to the milk–alkali syndrome.

These findings do not of course prove that the patient's oesophageal mucosa was any less inflamed or ulcerated than it had been at the time of diagnosis, but they do indicate that most patients had either improved symptomatically or had come to tolerate their symptoms. The figures seem entirely compatible with the study of Rex et al (1961), conducted when antacids were the only available medication. They found that 60 per cent of medically treated patients were asymptomatic or improved 10 years after diagnosis. In addition, they noted that only 3 of the 75 deaths recorded during their follow-up period were attributable to oesophageal disease.

The fact that some patients abandon regular medication was also observed by Rex et al (1961) and by Palmer (1968). The latter found that oesophagitis disappeared in about one-third of these patients. Nevertheless it is still not clear whether most patients who abandon medication do so because of diminution in their gastro-oesophageal reflux, a change in their perception of discomfort or simply because their symptoms are a lesser nuisance than their medication. We have no information on the condition of the oesophageal mucosa in our patients who abandoned therapy nor indeed any satisfactory information from follow-up endoscopy in the majority of the group of 43. However, it seems clear that from the patient's point of view, most found their condition acceptable.

HOW SHOULD SEVERE OESOPHAGITIS BE MANAGED?

A study by Behar et al (1976) is reasonably representative of the observations of several authors who attempted to compare medical and surgical treatment of severe oesophagitis before the modern generation of drugs became available. They reported that approximately 20 per cent of patients with severe oesophagitis showed a good symptomatic response to a simple medical regime based on antacid administration, although no improvement was observed in the oesophageal mucosa, in lower sphincter pressures or in the results of objective tests of gastro-oesophageal reflux. However, symptomatic improvement occurred in more than 70 per cent of patients who had undergone surgery, who also exhibited improvement in the objective tests. Nevertheless, it should be noted that a more recent study has indicated that the objective improvement demonstrable eight months after operation is not sustained at five years (Brand et al, 1979).

In our group of 50 patients, 15 were judged to have severe oesophagitis, and follow-up information was obtained for 13. Two had died during follow-up — neither from causes related to their oesophageal disease. Three had undergone operation and all were symptomatically improved compared with the time of diagnosis, but one still required antacids and cimetidine for symptom control. Seven were receiving medical therapy only, of whom six were considered improved and one unchanged. One patient was taking no medication at all and was asymptomatic. Although these numbers are small, they do seem to bear out the belief that the modern drugs, particularly cimetidine, facilitate symptom suppression. This is in accord with the information available from short-term studies (see pp. 153-166). In addition, it is our impression that improvement in the oesophagitis also occurs, though this may be less dramatic than the symptom suppression. Further studies are needed to clarify the point.

A source of major concern is the patient who continues to have severe oesophagitis despite substantial improvement in symptoms. At present there is no satisfactory information from which an optimum policy of management may be deduced. Elderly patients whose symptoms are well controlled cannot be sent for operation simply because it will make their doctors feel better. Similarly, the notion that operation should be undertaken in such patients to prevent the development of stricture or the occurrence of major haemorrhage is highly questionable. Given that strictures are readily managed by dilatation, many elderly patients will understandably prefer to accept symptom control and take their chance on the future. Their eventual death is seldom due to oesophageal disease.

For the present therefore it seems reasonable to pursue medical therapy of most patients with severe oesophagitis for at least one year before considering operation. In addition to general advice, including stopping smoking, weight reduction where necessary, and so on, our current practice is to recommend alginate/antacid preparations (Gastrocote or Gaviscon) and cimetidine, 1 g daily, together with supplementary antacid as required. The addition of metoclopramide can be justified in terms of its actions on the oesophagus (Stanciu and Bennett, 1973; Behar and Biancani, 1976) and also because of the possibility that impaired gastric emptying contributes to the occurrence of reflux (McCallum et al, 1981). With this type of medical therapy, an improvement in symptoms can be anticipated in the majority of patients with severe oesophagitis, perhaps with modest improvement in the condition of the oesophageal mucosa. It remains to be shown whether the long-term results of surgery are any better.

IS STRICTURE DILATATION SUCCESSFUL?

In recent years, the management of oesophageal strictures by dilatation, repeated as required, has gained widespread favour. Disenchantment with the results of stricture resection with direct oesophagogastric anastomosis led to the development of alternative operations such as the Thal procedure (Thal, 1968) but the simplicity of dilatation alone as a means of relieving dysphagia had obvious attractions despite the likelihood of recurrence. In 1974, Price et al described the dilatation of benign oesophageal strictures using Eder–Puestow dilators in conjunction with fibreoptic endoscopy and the technique rapidly gained popularity, particularly among gastroenterologists. There is no doubt that the results are good (Price et al, 1974; McIntyre et al, 1979; Ogilvie et al, 1980). Relief of dysphagia is almost always obtained and although the problem of gastro-oesophageal reflux continues, and restricturing seems likely, most patients find that the benefits of dilatation last many months. For those in whom repeated dilatation is necessary, it is not so frequent as to be unacceptable. Continued medication may be required for the relief of reflux symptoms but appears not to reduce the interval at which repeat dilatations are required (Ferguson et al, 1979).

Eder–Puestow dilatations with fibreoptic endoscopy are now being performed by many endoscopists who have little or no experience of rigid oesophagoscopy and other dilatation procedures. Thus the undoubted popularity of the Eder–Puestow method is not in itself evidence that it gives the best outcome; a reappraisal of more 'old-fashioned' methods may be appropriate.

Table 20.5 shows our results in respect of 34 consecutive patients who underwent dilatation of benign oesophageal strictures by rigid oesophagoscopy and bouginage during the last two and a half years. The group is biased towards the more severe cases, since we have continued to use the Eder–Puestow technique with fibreoptic endoscopy for some patients with mild strictures. All 34 patients suffered dysphagia for solids and in five cases for liquids also. There were 13 men aged between 42 and 83 years and 21 women aged between 32 and 91 years. Ten patients were over 80 years of age. Oesophagoscopy was performed under general anaesthesia using a rigid oesophagoscope and bouginage carried out with gum elastic bougies to 28 English gauge (15 mm). This was followed by hydrostatic dilatation with a Negus bag filled to a 40 ml volume. After stricture dilatation the patients were treated with antacids and, if necessary, cimetidine to control reflux symptoms. Dilatations were repeated if recurrent dysphagia proved troublesome. As shown in Table 20.5, more than half the patients have so far required only a single dilatation and on average have gained acceptable relief of dysphagia for more than a year. In all, 65 dilatations have been performed, producing relief of dysphagia immediately after the procedure in all cases. No complications were encountered. However in five patients, relief of dysphagia has been relatively brief and thus the outcome of the procedure is not particularly satisfactory. In four of these, operative treatment is considered contraindicated on grounds of age or general ill health but it seems likely that one patient will come to surgery in the near future.

Table 20.5 Duration of relief of dysphagia resulting from dilatation of oesophageal stricture. Sixty-five dilatations were performed in 34 patients in 2.5 years.

No. of patients	No. of dilatations	Duration of relief of dysphagia (months)	
		mean	range
18	1	13	7-23
11	2	11	4-19
1	3	6	2-12
1	4	5	2-10
3	6	4	1-10

The advantages of rigid oesophagoscopy with bouginage over the fibreoptic endoscopy/Eder–Puestow method are that it is carried out under direct vision and that a more sustained dilatation of the strictured area can be achieved. Is it significantly more hazardous in expert hands? As far as the oesophagoscopy is concerned, it may be noted that a large American study of the complications of endoscopy carried out before the era of fibreoptic instruments found that serious complications occurred in 0.25 per cent of oesophagoscopies (Palmer and Wirts, 1957). In 1974, when fibreoptic instruments were in general use, a similar American survey found that major complications occurred in 0.23 per cent of oesophagoscopies (Silvis et al, 1976). These figures may or may not reflect the current state of affairs in the United Kingdom but they do suggest that the reduction in morbidity attributable to the advent of fibreoptic instruments may not be so great as is often supposed. As regards stricture dilatation itself, perforation of the oesophagus occurs in approximately one per cent of dilatations carried out with the Eder–Puestow technique (Price et al, 1974; Silvis et al, 1976; Ogilvie et al, 1980). Perforation is allegedly more frequent with gum elastic bouginage carried out through a rigid oesophagoscope — a four per cent perforation rate has been reported (Raptis and Mearns Milne, 1972) — but our experience is more encouraging. Nevertheless, it seems likely that both skill and caution are necessary. It should not be forgotten that the Eder–Puestow dilators were first developed for use with a rigid oesophagoscope and if any difficulty is encountered in passing the smallest gum elastic bougie through an oesophageal stricture, an attempt should be made to introduce the Eder–Puestow guide wire and begin the procedure with the metal olives.

Very occasionally, long oesophageal strictures are encountered which are not suitable for dilatation and in such patients there is probably no alternative to resection. However, these are exceptional. For most patients with oesophageal strictures dilatation is highly successful in relieving dysphagia, whether undertaken by fibreoptic endoscopy and the Eder–Puestow method or by rigid endoscopy and bouginage. Both techniques carry an acceptably low morbidity.

CONCLUSIONS

The facts available on the outcome of management of patients with gastro-oesophageal reflux justify an optimistic view. While medical therapy will not abolish reflux, and complete healing of the oesophageal mucosa is unlikely, symptoms are satisfactorily controlled in a substantial majority of patients. Perhaps inevitably, many clinicians tend to be especially conscious of the difficulties presented by the minority of patients who respond poorly and there is understandable disappointment when symptomatic remission is not matched by improvement in the endoscopic appearances of the oesophageal mucosa. Nevertheless, even for patients with severe oesophagitis, symptom control is usually possible with the aid of a multiple drug regime which will comprise some combination of antacids, antacid/alginate mixtures, metoclopramide and cimetidine. The advantages and disadvantages of indefinite medical treatment in comparison with antireflux surgery remain to be determined.

Despite the persistence of oesophagitis in most medically treated patients, and thus the continuing risk of complications, death is seldom due to oesophageal disease. In competent hands, even the dilatation of strictures is relatively safe as well as successful.

The development of a treatment — medical or surgical — which would abolish reflux and facilitate complete healing of the oesophageal mucosa would, no doubt, be an advance. A more realistic hope perhaps would be a treatment which improved on our present levels of success in these respects. However the limitations of present therapy should not be allowed to obscure the fact that a reasonably acceptable outcome is obtained three to four years after diagnosis in 80 per cent of patients with problems attributable to gastro-oesophageal reflux.

REFERENCES

Behar J, Biancani P 1976 Effect of oral metoclopramide on gastro-oesophageal reflux in the post-cibal state. Gastroenterology 70: 331-335

Behar J, Sheahan D G, Biancani P, Spiro H M, Storer E H 1975 Medical and surgical management of reflux esophagitis. New England Journal of Medicine 293: 263-268

Brand D L, Eastwood I R, Martin D, Carter W B, Pope C E 1979 Esophageal symptoms, manometry and histology before and after antireflux surgery. Gastroenterology 76: 1393-1401

Ferguson R, Dronfield M W, Atkinson M 1979 Cimetidine in treatment of reflux oesophagitis with peptic stricture. British Medical Journal 2: 472-474

McCallum R W, Berkowitz I M, Lerner E 1981 Gastric emptying in patients with gastro esophageal reflux. Gastroenterology 80: 285-291

McIntyre R I E, Lee E G, Kettlewell G W 1979 Conservative treatment alone for benign oesophageal stricture. Gut 20: A917

Ogilvie A L, Ferguson R, Atkinson M 1980 Outlook with conservative treatment of peptic oesophageal stricture. Gut 21: 23-25

Palmer E D 1968 The hiatus hernia - esophagitis - esophageal stricture complex. American Journal of Medicine 44: 566-579

Palmer E D, Wirts C W 1957 Survey of gastroscopic and esophagoscopic accidents. Journal of the American Medical Association 164: 2012-2015

Price J D, Stanciu C, Bennett J R 1974 A safer method for dilating oesophageal strictures. Lancet 1: 1141-1142

Price S, Castell D O 1978 Esophageal mythology. Journal of the American Medical Association 240: 44-46

Raptis S, Mearns Milne D 1972 A review of the management of 100 cases of benign stricture of the oesophagus. Thorax 27: 599-603

Rex J C, Andersen H A, Bartholemew L G, Cain J C 1961 Esophageal hiatal hernia — a 10 year study of medically treated cases. Journal of the American Medical Association 178: 117-130

Silvis S E, Nebel O, Rogers G, Sugawa C, Mandelstam P 1976 Endoscopic complications. Results of the 1974 American Society for Gastrointestinal Endoscopy Survey. Journal of the American Medical Association 235: 928-930

Stanciu C, Bennett J R 1973 Metoclopramide in gastro-oesophageal reflux. Gut 14: 275-279

Thal A P 1968 A unified approach to surgical problems of the esophagogastric junction. Annals of Surgery 168: 542-549

Discussion on Oesophageal Reflux Disease

Chairman: Dr J. R. Bennett

Dr Bennett. Professor Tytgat has described short-term management, and he is very experienced in stricture management. Do Dr Heading's results on long-term management surprise him?

Professor Tytgat. No, they do not surprise me at all. We recently analysed our material and found that 88 per cent of the dilated patients became truly symptom-free, 50 per cent within six months. The follow-up now lasts up to six or seven years, so I am not surprised by Dr Heading's results.

Dr Bennett. Would this more radical form of dilatation produce better results? Your results were obtained with Eder–Puestow dilatation?

Professor Tytgat. Yes, they were all done as outpatients, either with Eder–Puestow dilators or mercury bougies without general anaesthesia. The overall results are about the same. I like to dilate more gradually than is achieved by the one dilatation under anaesthesia.

Dr Bennett. Did Dr Heading draw any conclusions about respiratory disease in the follow-up of the 55 patients?

Dr Heading. No, we did not draw any conclusions and, after Dr Bernstein's paper, we should think again. The difficulty is to balance the fact that respiratory disease is common in patients with reflux against the fact that in our community chronic respiratory disease is common in everybody. Which is the chicken and which is the egg? Indeed, is there any relationship between that particular chicken and that particular egg?

Mr Earlam. I would like to compare today's analysis of the treatment of hiatus hernia with yesterday's on duodenal ulcer. With hiatus hernia it is known that there is little correlation between hiatus hernia, reflux, oesophagitis and symptoms. It is very unfair to expect cimetidine to repair either an anatomical hiatus hernia or a mechanical stricture. That is why we concentrated on the Bernstein test. Are we not becoming slightly worried in duodenal ulcer disease because the treatment is being assessed by looking at the duodenal ulcer itself? We have heard that the duodenal ulcer may be present with or without symptoms: there are all sorts of combinations. Would it not be a good idea to start to analyse the failures of cimetidine, doing a few Bernstein tests, and determining whether many of those failures were in fact due to mechanical problems with emptying and to other symptoms?

Professor Tytgat. I would agree completely with these comments. The failures on routine medical therapy definitely comprise the most interesting group. This may well be a different entity from the ordinary patient with reflux.

Dr Heading. I agree. The problem is similar to that of those who fail to respond to medical therapy for duodenal ulcers. We need to be careful about what we mean by 'failure' to respond to cimetidine. Are we talking about clinical failures of symptomatic control, or about the lesion, that is, failure to suppress oesophagitis. The two do not necessarily go together. 'Failure to respond' needs a subsidiary definition.

Professor Tytgat. Why was the study not repeated a third time, with perfusion of the asthma patients without anaesthesia of the oesophagus, to be absolutely sure there was no bias. To what extent is the treatment of asthma affecting reflux? For example, theophylline can certainly weaken the sphincter, as can several other anti-asthmatic drugs.

Dr Bernstein. In answer to Professor Tytgat's first point, we are doing that now. There are certain ethical limitations to such studies. Asthma patients do not like having a tube put down their nose. Further work is also being done with two pH electrodes in series to determine at what level pH changes — whether low or high in the oesophagus.

With respect to treatment, theophylline derivatives lower oesophageal pressure and create reflux. There is no doubt about that symptomatically. β-blocking drugs have the same effect. We must be aware of the patient who recognises that reflux provokes asthma; that is the patient to look for. The other patients who have reflux and asthma probably fall into the 'chicken and egg' problem.

Dr Stoddard. Professor Tytgat said that his patients with Barrett oesophagus on cimetidine showed an improvement in the histological appearance, yet there was no regression of the columnar epithelium. What does improve?

Dr Heading said that the long-term effects of operation in Seattle were not good. In fact, in that particular paper four different types of operation were reviewed. What does Dr Heading think about the results of any specific type of operation, rather than a mixed group?

Professor Tytgat. In the patients with Barrett oesophagus the ulcers healed and disappeared, and in all of them the oesophagitis at the level of the squamocolumnar junction healed. Healing usually took about two months and this state was maintained on cimetidine therapy.

Dr Heading. It is quite right to say that the Seattle report was a miscellany of operations, but more than two-thirds of them were Nissens. The surgeons that I have talked to suspected what was confirmed in the Seattle report — that patients may do best initially but the longer they go on the more question marks arise. I am not suggesting that surgery is a failure; I am merely suggesting that on a long-term basis its best achievement is symptom control.

Section 4
HAEMORRHAGE

21. Treatment of haemorrhage with cimetidine

J. J. Misiewicz

Department of Gastroenterology, Central Middlesex Hospital,
London

Haemorrhage originating in the upper alimentary tract is a frequent and important cause of emergency admission to hospital and carries an appreciable mortality. In a study of 2149 emergency admissions because of haematemesis and melaena during a 15-year period from 1953 to 1967, Schiller et al (1970) found the mean mortality to be 8.9 per cent. Analysis of mortality figures separately for each quinquennium in the period under study showed little change in the percentage of patients dying.

Allan and Dykes (1976) reported a prospective analysis of 300 consecutive patients admitted because of acute gastrointestinal haemorrhage. They found an overall mortality rate of 9.7 per cent, a figure very similar to the previous study. Examination of percentage mortality rates from acute alimentary bleeding reported in many studies shows little change from the mid-thirties to the present day. It has been pointed out however (Allan and Dykes, 1976) that the constant mortality rate may conceal advances due to improved medical, surgical and anaesthetic techniques. This is because the average age of the population admitted with acute bleeding has progressively risen, and old age carries an increased risk of dying.

Many factors, apart from age, affect the prognosis of an episode of bleeding. Bleeding from oesophageal varices or from gastric erosions in a patient suffering from hepatic cirrhosis complicated by portal hypertension carries an especially high mortality related to the degree of liver failure, coagulopathy and similar factors.

Most patients with acute haemorrhage in this country, however, will be bleeding either from chronic or acute duodenal and gastric ulcers. A minority present with rare conditions, such as the Mallory–Weiss syndrome and the like. The impact of histamine H_2-receptor antagonists on the main diagnostic groups is therefore of particular interest. The outcome of alimentary bleeding is affected by variables such as the age of the patient, the underlying diagnosis, hypotension, gross anaemia, concomitant disease outside the alimentary tract and also perhaps by the enthusiasm for early surgical intervention. In some series the data have been interpreted as showing that more frequent emergency operations should lower the incidence of death (Schiller et al, 1970), but other studies have suggested the opposite (Allan and Dykes, 1978; Dronfield et al, 1979). The value of aggressive surgery in bleeding peptic ulcer is therefore questionable and it would seem proper to test this question in a prospective randomised trial. Nor is it certain whether the availability of early endoscopy, with consequent improvement in the accuracy of diagnosis, will have a significant effect on mortality rates. It can thus be seen that none of the factors discussed so far can be affected by chemotherapy in general and by H_2-receptor blockade in particular.

There is, however, another variable with a bearing on the outcome of alimentary bleeding and theoretically this may be affected by medical treatment — this is the pattern of bleeding after the initial episode. Continuous haemorrhage, or early recurrence of bleeding will adversely affect the outcome and may carry a serious prognosis both in absolute terms and in terms of the risks of subsequent operations. It is, therefore, this aspect of acute gastrointestinal haemorrhage that some controlled studies have examined. Treatment of established bleeding from peptic ulcers or from other causes has to be clearly differentiated from prevention of bleeding by prophylactic pretreatment with cimetidine. This aspect of cimetidine therapy is dealt with in the following contribution.

La Brooy et al (1979) studied 101 patients in a multicentre prospective double-blind controlled trial assessing the effect of oral cimetidine 800 mg on entering the study and then 400 mg six-hourly on the continuance, or recurrence, of upper gastrointestinal haemorrhage. The source of bleeding was identified endoscopically within a median time of 8.2 hours after admission in 92 per cent of the patients, of whom 70 had bled from a peptic ulcer. Patients with carcinoma, renal, or hepatic failure and those bleeding from oesophageal varices, were excluded. Bleeding continued in 11 of 51 (22 per cent) patients on cimetidine and in 12 of 50 (24 per cent) on placebo. Analysis of the effect of cimetidine with respect to age or severity of haemorrhage showed no significant advantage for the drug.

In a similar study (Hoare et al, 1979) cimetidine 200 mg i.v. every 4 hours for 48 hours and then 400 mg orally four times daily for 7 days, or placebo, was given to 66 patients with acute gastrointestinal haemorrhage. Further bleeding within the study period was detected in 8 patients on cimetidine and in 15 on placebo. Cimetidine had no effect on the prognosis of bleeding from duodenal ulcer but only two of 14 patients with gastric ulcer on treatment with cimetidine bled again, compared with 10 of 19 on placebo. This advantage for the drug (at the 0.05 level) was apparent only in those aged 65 years or older.

Galmiche et al (1980) compared the effect of cimetidine 1.6 g/day i.v. for 3 days followed by 1 g orally for 4 days with placebo; all patients were also treated with antacids for the first 48 hours. In addition to the usual exclusions, however, patients with obvious arterial bleeding at endoscopy were not admitted to this study. The results in 96 patients show that the incidence of treatment failure (persistent or recurrent bleeding) was significantly less ($P < 0.05$) in those with gastric ulcer, in those older than 50 years and in those who took anti-inflammatory drugs prior to the bleed.

The results of these last two studies (Galmiche et al, 1980; Hoare et al, 1979) contrast with negative results reported by Eden and Kern (1978) on 51, Pickard et al (1979) on 69, Macklon et al (1978) on 30 and Carstensen et al (1980) on 88 patients. The results of prospective randomised trials of cimetidine in the treatment of upper alimentary bleeding are summarised in Table 21.1.

Table 21.1 Results of controlled trials of cimetidine in acute upper alimentary haemorrhage.

Negative trials	N	Positive trials	N
Eden et al (1978)	51	Hoare et al (1979)	66
Pickard et al (1979)	62	Galmiche et al (1980)	96
Macklon et al (1979)	30		
La Brooy et al (1979)	101		
Carstensen et al (1980)	88		

Comparisons of cimetidine with other drugs in the treatment of bleeding peptic ulcer are few. In one such sequentially designed controlled trial on 20 patients, i.v. cimetidine 200 mg four-hourly for 48 to 120 hours was compared with i.v. somatostatin $250 \mu g$/hour following an initial bolus of $250 \mu g$. In seven of the ten pairs of patients somatostatin was more effective than cimetidine; in two pairs both were ineffective; and in one pair the drugs were equally effective (Kayasseh et al, 1980).

Results of other studies are also of interest. Burland and Parr (1977) reviewed results of treatment with cimetidine of 119 patients with gastrointestinal haemorrhage who were also suffering from other complicating conditions. Bleeding stopped in 67 per cent during treatment with cimetidine intravenously or orally, and there was some control of bleeding in a further 8 per cent.

Treatment of haemorrhagic gastritis with H_2-receptor antagonists deserves special attention. The first report initially concerned patients in an intensive care unit given metiamide, which controlled 17 episodes of bleeding from gastric erosions. Subsequently cimetidine was used successfully in 24 of 27 patients (MacDonald et al, 1978).

Mühe et al (1977) studied 61 patients with massive bleeding from stress ulcers given cimetidine 1.2 g/day i.v. for two days and then continued orally: surgical intervention was needed in only five cases and bleeding stopped within 24 hours in 57 (93.4 per cent) of the patients. Similar results in haemorrhagic gastritis have been reported by, among others, Dunn et al (1978) in 13 and by Schulz and Schiessel (1979) in 40 patients.

Should a patient with acute upper alimentary bleeding be treated with cimetidine? Unfortunately it is not possible to answer this question unequivocally on the evidence presently available. If the haemorrhage originates from a chronic duodenal ulcer, there are no data to support the view that cimetidine will affect the outcome and there is therefore no point in administering the drug to arrest continuing, or to prevent the recurrence of, bleeding. However, the clinician may wish to start healing therapy for the duodenal ulcer without delay and there is no contraindication for doing this immediately after the diagnosis has been established. Full routine clinical observations used for monitoring the progress of patients with bleeding from a peptic ulcer must not be abandoned just because the patient is receiving cimetidine. Available data suggest that the older patient bleeding from a gastric ulcer may benefit from cimetidine therapy and in this group such treatment should not be withheld. It is necessary, in the absence of more definite evidence, to observe the same criteria in the management of these patients as outlined for duodenal ulcer. Haemorrhage from stress ulceration, or erosive gastritis may well respond to cimetidine therapy, but more properly controlled trials are needed before definite guidelines can be established. It is important to remember that in the elderly or in severely ill patients cimetidine may occasionally cause mental confusion.

It is not clear how cimetidine acts to arrest established haemorrhage from the oesophagus, stomach or duodenum. As the predominant pharmacological effect of H_2-receptor blockade is inhibition of acid and pepsin output, it can be hypothesised that reduction in the volume of these components of gastric secretion must play a part: the concomitant decrease in the mucosal blood flow may be important in the case of haemorrhage originating from the gastric mucosa. The lessened availability of hydrogen ions for back-diffusion may also be a factor. There are as yet no data to indicate whether the widespread use of cimetidine has affected the incidence of mortality after acute bleeding from the upper alimentary tract.

REFERENCES

Allan R, Dykes P 1976 A study of the factors influencing mortality rates from gastrointestinal haemorrhage. Quarterly Journal of Medicine 45: 533-550
Burland W L, Parr S N 1977 Experiences with cimetidine in the treatment of seriously ill patients. In: Burland W L, Simkins M (eds). Cimetidine: Proceedings of the Second International Symposium on histamine H_2-receptor antagonists. Excerpta Medica, Amsterdam, p 345-357
Carstensen H E, Bulow S, Hansen O H, Jacobsen B H, Krarup T, Pedersen T, Tahave D, Svendsen L B, Backer O 1980 Cimetidine for severe gastroduodenal haemorrhage: a randomised controlled trial. Scandinavian Journal of Gastroenterology 15: 103-105
Dronfield M W, Atkinson M, Langman M J S 1979 Effect of different operation policies on mortality from bleeding peptic ulcer. Lancet 1: 1126-1128
Dunn D H, Fischer R C, Silvis S E, Onstad G R, Howard R J, Delaney J P 1978 The treatment of haemorrhagic gastritis with cimetidine. Surgery, Gynecology and Obstetrics 147: 737-739
Eden K, Kern F Jr 1978 Current status of cimetidine in upper gastrointestinal bleeding. Gastroenterology 74 (part 2): 466-467
Galmiche P J, Colin R, Veyrac M, Hecketsweiler P, Ouvry D, Tenière P, Ducrotté P 1980 Double blind controlled trial of cimetidine in bleeding peptic ulcer. In: Torsoli A, Lucchelli P E, Brimblecombe R L S (eds) H_2-antagonists: Proceedings of a European Symposium. Excerpta Medica, Amsterdam, p 164-173
Hoare A M, Bradby G V H, Hawkins C F, Kang J Y, Dykes P W 1979 Cimetidine in bleeding peptic ulcer. Lancet 2: 671-673
Kayasseh L, Gyr K, Keller V, Stalder G A, Wall M 1980 Somatostatin and cimetidine in peptic ulcer haemorrhage. Lancet 1: 844-846
La Brooy S J, Misiewicz J J, Edwards J, Smith P M, Haggie S J, Libman L, Sarner M, Wyllie J H, Croker J, Cotton P 1979 Controlled trial of cimetidine in upper gastrointestinal haemorrhage. Gut 20: 892-895
MacDonald A S, Pyne D A, Freeman A N G, Holland S G, Badley D W D 1978 Upper gastrointestinal bleeding in the intensive care unit. Canadian Journal of Surgery 21: 81-84
Macklon A F, Roberts S H, James O 1979 Cimetidine in bleeding peptic ulcer. Lancet 2: 1135-1136

Mühe E, Gentsch H-H, Groitl H, Hager Th 1977 Clinical experience in the treatment of massive stress ulcers with cimetidine. In: Harrengt C, Deschepper P J, Bogaert R, Cremer M, Sharpe P C (eds) Proceedings of the National Symposium on cimetidine. Excerpta Medica, Amsterdam, p 138-143

Pickard R G, Sanderson I, South M, Kirkham J S, Northfield T C 1979 Controlled trial of cimetidine in acute upper gastrointestinal bleeding. British Medical Journal 1: 661-662

Schiller K F R, Truelove S C, Williams G D 1970 Haematemesis and melaena with special reference to factors influencing the outcome. British Medical Journal 1: 7-14

Schulz F, Schiessel R 1979 Cimetidine for treatment of stress-induced ulcer haemorrhage. Deutsche Medizinische Wochenschrift 104: 1845-1848

22. Prevention of bleeding with cimetidine

V. Speranza, N. Basso and M. Bagarani

Clinica Chirurgica VI, University of Rome, Rome, Italy

Stress ulcer syndrome is an extremely important problem, not only because of the lack of certainty surrounding its cause but also because of its high incidence. In fact, about 25 per cent of all upper gastrointestinal bleeding is attributable to stress lesions (Byrne and Guardione, 1973; Byrne et al, 1970; Ivey, 1971).

Acute stress lesions and their most frequent clinical manifestation, haemorrhage, are seen in almost every type of patient in the intensive care unit, including those with burns (Czaja et al, 1976; Rosenthal et al, 1977), respiratory insufficiency (Pariente and Wanstok, 1972; Voisin et al, 1970), uraemia (Fischer and Stremple, 1972; Jungers et al, 1972), head injury, sepsis, multiple trauma, and other conditions, or after operation (Dalgaard, 1959; David and Kelly, 1969; Goodman and Frey, 1968; Kamada et al, 1977; Lewis, 1973; Taylor et al, 1973) (Table 22.1).

Table 22.1 Conditions associated with upper gastrointestinal bleeding from acute gastroduodenal lesions in patients with 'stress'.

Condition	N	Number and percentage bleeding	Number and percentage of deaths from bleeding
Respiratory insufficiency	1 221	90(7.4)	66(73)
Cranial trauma	552	91(16)	25(27)
Renal failure	2 371	435(18)	296(68)
Burns	7 942	657(8.3)	438(67)
Following			
general surgery	243 282	125(0.05)	75(60)
heart surgery	5 000	38(0.8)	9(24)
neurosurgery	1 087	23(2.1)	—
vascular surgery	1 298	16(1.2)	—
Multiple trauma	2 297	69(3)	—
Total	265 050	1 544(0.6)	

Since statistical analysis permits identification of those with the highest risk of developing stress lesions, we have examined data on approximately 2200 patients in intensive care units in Rome between 1974 and 1976. We matched clinical characteristics and the incidence of stress ulcer-related gastrointestinal bleeding in our retrospective study and in a review of the literature (Czaja et al, 1976; Fischer and Stremple, 1972; Kamada et al, 1977; Pariente and Wanstok, 1972) and this provided profiles for high-risk patients (Table 22.2).

Table 22.2 Highly rated risk factors for developing stress lesions.

Condition	Risk factors
Lesions of the central nervous system	Lesions of the midline Cranial trauma with coma
Respiratory insufficiency	Endotracheal intubation $pCO_2 > 50$ mm Hg; $pO_2 < 60$ mm Hg
Acute renal failure	Oliguria: < 500 ml/24 hrs Anuria: (for > 24 hrs) Hyperazotaemia: > 0.8 g/100 ml (> 48 hrs) Creatinaemia: > 2 mg/100 ml (48 hrs)
Hypotension in previously normotensive patients	Fall in arterial systolic pressure of more than 30 to 40 mm Hg below the usual pressure for more than 24 hours
Hypotension in previously hypertensive patients	Fall in arterial systolic pressure to 100 mm Hg or below for 24 hours
Burns	Burns covering more than 20% of the total body surface
Serious infections	Infective foci (peritonitis, pneumonia, subphrenic abscess, pleural empyema) or septicaemia
Multiple trauma	Lesions of two or more systems creating multiple problems
Postoperative complications	Development of any of the indicated risk factors after surgery

For those already critically ill, further damage from gastrointestinal bleeding or from a perforating acute ulcer is associated with a mortality rate that can reach 70 per cent.

Since the treatment of stress ulcer syndrome is often difficult and still associated with a high mortality rate, prophylaxis offers the most rational approach to treatment.

ANTACIDS AND CIMETIDINE IN THE PREVENTION OF ACUTE STRESS LESIONS

At present antacids and cimetidine are the most widely used drugs. Both preparations significantly prevented upper gastrointestinal bleeding (UGIB) from acute stress lesions in controlled trials.

Prophylactic antacids

In three controlled studies (Hastings et al, 1978; McAlhany et al, 1976; MacDougall et al, 1977) (Table 22.3) 7 per cent of 88 patients with prophylactic antacids experienced UGIB; in the control group the percentage of bleeders was significantly higher.

Table 22.3 Prophylactic treatment for stress lesions: antacid versus control.

	Number of patients		Percentage of UGIB	
	Antacid	Control	Antacid	Control
Acute liver				
failure (MacDougall et al, 1977)	13	12	23	50
Burns (McAlhany et al, 1976)	24	24	4	25
ICU (Hastings et al, 1978)	51	49	4	24
Total	88	85	7	28

Prophylactic cimetidine

In two controlled studies (Fischer et al, 1980; Halloran et al, 1980) (Table 22.4) UGIB from stress lesions was present in 12 per cent of patients treated prophylactically with cimetidine. This percentage was significantly lower than

Table 22.4 Prophylactic treatment for stress lesions: cimetidine versus control

	Number of patients		Percentage of UGIB	
	Cimetidine	Control	Cimetidine	Control
Polytrauma (Fisher and Stremple, 1972)	14	14	0	35
Head injury (Halloran et al, 1980)	26	24	19	75
Total	40	38	12	60

that in patients receiving no treatment. Halloran et al (1980) administered cimetidine 300 mg or placebo every 4 hours to 50 brain-injured patients. All patients received conventional neurosurgical treatment in addition to cimetidine. The drug was initially given as an intravenous bolus injection, and patients were switched to oral medication when tube feeding or a diet was started. Patients were closely monitored for bleeding, and gastric analysis and endoscopy were performed serially over the course of the three-week study.

It is clear that antacids and cimetidine are more effective than no treatment in preventing stress lesions.

Antacids compared with cimetidine

Controversy exists as to which of the two drugs is most effective.

In three clinical trials (MacDougall et al, 1977; McElwee et al, 1979; Zumtobel et al, 1979) (Table 22.5) conducted on patients with acute liver failure, polytrauma or burns, the percentage of cimetidine-treated patients presenting

Table 22.5 Prophylactic treatment for stress lesions: cimetidine versus antacid.

	Number of patients		Percentage of UGIB	
	Cimetidine	Antacid	Cimetidine	Antacid
Acute liver				
failure (MacDougall et al, 1977)	26	24	4	54
Polytrauma (McElwee et al, 1979)	146	38	5	24
Burns (Zumtobel et al, 1979)	13	14	0	0
ICU (Priebe et al, 1980)	38	37	18	0
Total	223	113	7	19

with UGIB was 5 per cent (total number of patients: 185), while it was 29 per cent in antacid-treated patients (total number of patients: 76). This difference is statistically significant.

Zumtobel et al (1979) treated 204 intensive care patients prophylactically with either oral antacids (2 litres/day by stomach tube) or 200 mg cimetidine intravenously 8 times a day. All patients had multiple-organ insufficiency, with or without sepsis. In the group without sepsis, bleeding occurred in 12.5 per cent of antacid-treated patients and only 1.6 per cent of cimetidine-treated patients. Patients with sepsis were at greater risk of bleeding, which was noted in 42.9 per cent of those given antacid therapy. The 13.6 per cent incidence of bleeding among cimetidine-treated patients with sepsis was higher than for the cimetidine group without sepsis, but still well below that of the antacid-treated group with sepsis.

McElwee et al (1979) in a study on 40 patients with a greater than 30 per cent surface burn area randomly compared cimetidine 400 mg every 4 hours and antacid or placebo antacid 30 ml every 2 hours. Thirteen patients died from complications of the burns before the study was completed. Of the 27 survivors, 13 received cimetidine and 14 received antacids for at least 10 days. There were no catastrophic gastrointestinal complications (haemorrhage or perforations) in any of the patients during the study period.

On the other hand, in the study of Priebe et al (1980) on high-risk patients, 18 per cent of the cimetidine-treated patients presented with UGIB, while no bleeding occurred in the antacid-treated patients.

A closer analysis of the data in the literature may partly explain some of the contradictory results.

Criticism of cimetidine therapy (Herrmann and Kaminski, 1979; Martin et al, 1979; Priebe et al, 1980) is mainly related to the high incidence of UGIB and of gastroduodenal lesions as seen at routine endoscopy when compared to the low incidence in studies which are not subject to routine endoscopy.

At routine endoscopy (Table 22.6), the incidence of gastroduodenal lesions during prophylactic cimetidine therapy was 64 per cent within 36 hours of the cranial trauma (Halloran et al, 1980) and 20 per cent and 77 per cent within 72 hours of cranial trauma (Silvestri et al, 1980) and burns (McElwee et al, 1979), respectively.

Table 22.6 Cimetidine prophylaxis: endoscopic lesions and UGIB.

	Lesions (percentage)	UGIB (percentage)
Head injury: Halloran et al (1980)	64	19
Head injury: Silvestri et al (1980)	20	
Burns: McElwee et al (1979)	77	0

However, further endoscopy (McElwee et al, 1979; Silvestri et al, 1980) demonstrated that, during cimetidine prophylaxis, the percentage of patients with lesions fell close to zero on the sixth to tenth day, while in the control group (Silvestri et al, 1980) or in the antacid group (McElwee et al, 1979) the percentage rose (Table 22.7).

Table 22.7 Routine endoscopic studies

Type of trauma	Treatment	Days from commencement of treatment		
		0	3	6
Head injury: Silvestri et al (1980)	Cimetidine	0%	20%	0%
	No treatment	0%	50%	70%
		0	3	10
Burns: McElwee et al (1979)	Cimetidine	30%	77%	30%
	Antacid	29%	71%	79%

When considering the occurrence of UGIB during cimetidine prophylactic treatment, in McElwee et al's study the incidence was zero while in Halloran et al's study the incidence was 19 per cent (although lesions were present at endoscopy in 64 per cent of patients), and in Priebe's study, 47 per cent. In the first study, with zero UGIB, only clinically relevant haemorrhages were considered, while in the last two studies the occurrence of haemorrhage was determined by testing the gastric aspirate using the Guaiac or the Hemoccult test. Cimetidine was less effective only when the results to these tests were considered. It should be added, however, that recent studies have demonstrated high false positives to Hemoccult during cimetidine theapy (Norfleet et al, 1980).

The above data may help to explain some of the discrepancies in the different studies. Furthermore, in the various studies the risk categories and the type of prophylactic therapy used were not homogeneous.

For these reasons it was considered necessary to study the prophylaxis of stress lesions, using two criteria: the evaluation of clinical data (clinically relevant haemorrhage) and mandatory endoscopic control. Each group of patients treated was as far as possible homogeneous for risk categories.

We have now completed a clinical study assessing the prophylactic effectiveness of cimetidine compared with antacid treatment and placebo in high-risk patients. Patients at significant risk of stress ulcer syndrome (Table 22.2) were selected (Basso et al, 1981; Speranza and Basso, 1980) from a population of

800 drawn from several intensive care units. Following randomization, the patients were assigned to one of three groups. All patients in whom upper gastrointestinal haemorrhage was suspected or confirmed underwent oesophagogastroduodenoscopy. The maximum duration of treatment in this study was 10 days. Each patient was routinely monitored for: heart rate, arterial blood pressure, urine output, haematocrit, haemoglobin, blood electrolytes, urea and glucose.

Table 22.8 Risk categories (percentages) for each treatment group.

	Cimetidine	Antacid	Control
Respiratory failure	41	48	45
Sepsis	18	18	18
Postop. complications	16	4	16
Acute renal failure	11	14	16
Polytrauma	9	7	—
Hypotension	9	7	12
Neurosurgery	25	25	26
Head injury	7	2	8
Burns	9	9	8
Mean risk factor per patient	1.5	1.4	1.5

Of the 168 patients selected, 137 completed the study (Table 22.8). Reasons for non-completion included death unrelated to stress lesions (16 patients), transfer to other divisions (9 patients), and failure to follow the protocol (6 patients).

The results are summarized in Table 22.9. No gastrointestinal haemorrhages were noted in the group A (cimetidine 200 mg 6-hourly i.v. or p.o.) patients. In group B (antacids: Maalox 10 ml/h via nasogastric tube or p.o.) one haemorrhage occurred. Eight patients in group C (neither treatment) experienced haemorrhage, and this result was significantly different from that achieved with either cimetidine ($P < 0.005$) or antacid ($P < 0.05$).

Table 22.9 Incidence of bleeding in high risk patients with stress ulcers.

	Number of patients	Number bleeding
Cimetidine	44	0
Antacid	44	1 } $P < 0.05$ } $P < 0.005$
Control	49	8

Untreated patients having only one risk factor were found to have a 14 per cent chance of bleeding which increased to 25 per cent when two or more risk factors were present.

All nine patients who had UGIB received cimetidine 200 mg every three hours. In seven patients haemorrhage was controlled. Angiographic embolization was necessary in one patient. One patient died because of myocardial infarction.

None of the 632 low-risk patients presented with bleeding, thus confirming the clinical accuracy of the criteria.

CONCLUSION

In conclusion, prophylaxis is the best therapeutic approach to patients at high risk of UGIB due to stress lesions.

Cimetidine and antacids are equally effective in diminishing the incidence of UGIB in such patients.

However, cimetidine is easier to use, with a higher patient compliance, and can be administered both per os and parenterally.

A number of problems are still unsolved: the low efficacy of prophylactic measures in patients with sepsis, the effectiveness of the second generation H_2-blockers, the possible advantages of combined therapies, etc. In due time all these problems will be solved.

The complete understanding of stress lesions still eludes us. However, because of advances in prophylaxis, stress ulcer syndrome is no longer an inevitable complication of critically ill patients.

REFERENCES

Basso N, Bagarani M, Materia A, Fiorani S, Lunardi P, Speranza V 1981 Cimetidine and antacid prophylaxis of acute upper G.I. bleeding in high risk patients. A controlled, randomized trial. American Journal of Surgery, in press

Byrne J J, Guardione V A 1973 Surgical treatment of stress ulcers. American Journal of Surgery 125: 464-468

Byrne J J, Guardione V A, Williams L F 1970 Massive gastrointestinal haemorrhage. American Journal of Surgery 120: 312-315

Czaja A J, McAlhany J C, Pruitt B A Jr 1976 Gastric acid secretion and acute gastroduodenal disease after burns. Archives of Surgery 111: 243-245

Dalgaard J B 1959 Peptic ulceration complicating cerebral operations: a post-mortem study of 23 cases. Acta Neurochirurgica 7: 1-12

David E, Kelly K A 1969 Acute postoperative peptic ulceration. Surgical Clinics of North America 49: 1111-1121

Fischer M, Lorenz W, Rohde H 1980 The use of cimetidine in preventing clinically manifest stress ulcers in patients with severe polytrauma. In: Dresse A, Barbier F, Harvengt C, Tijtgat G N (eds) Second National Symposium on Cimetidine. Excerpta Medica, Amsterdam, p 45-51

Fischer R P, Stremple, J F 1972 Stress ulcers in post-traumatic renal insufficiency in patients from Vietnam. Surgery, Gynecology and Obstetrics 134: 790-794

Goodman A A, Frey C F 1968 Massive upper gastrointestinal hemorrhage following surgical operations. Annals of Surgery 167: 180-184

Halloran L G, Zfass A M, Gaule W E, Wheeler C B, Miller J D 1980 Prevention of acute gastrointestinal complications after severe head injury: a controlled trial of cimetidine prophylaxis. American Journal of Surgery 139: 44-48

Hastings P R, Skillman J J, Bushnell L S, Silen W 1978 Antacid titration in the prevention of acute gastrointestinal bleeding. New England Journal of Medicine 298: 1041-1045

Herrmann V, Kaminski D L 1979 Evaluation of intragastric pH in acutely ill patients. Archives of Surgery 114: 511-514

Ivey K J 1971 Acute haemorrhagic gastritis: modern concepts based on pathogenesis. Gut 12: 750-752

Jungers P, Kleinknecht D, Barbanel C 1972 Les Hémorragies digestives chez l'insuffisant rénal aigu. Annales de Chirurgie 26: 893-896

Kamada T, Fusamoto H, Kawano S, Noguchi M, Hiramatsu K, Masuzawa M, Abe H, Fujii C, Sugimoto T 1977 Gastrointestinal bleeding following head injury: a clinical study of 433 cases. Journal of Trauma 17: 44-47

Lewis E A 1973 Gastroduodenal ulceration and haemorrhage of neurogenic origin. British Journal of Surgery 60: 279-283

McAlhany J C, Czaja A J, Pruitt B A 1976 Antacid control of complications from acute gastroduodenal disease after burns. Journal of Trauma 16: 645-648

MacDougall B R D, Bailey R J, Williams R 1977 H$_2$-receptor antagonists and antacids in the prevention of acute gastrointestinal haemorrhage in fulminant hepatic failure: two controlled trials. Lancet 1: 617-619

McElwee H P, Sirinek K R, Levine B A 1979 Cimetidine affords protection equal to antacids in prevention of stress ulceration following thermal injury. Surgery 86: 620-626

Martin L F, Staloch D K, Simonowitz D A, Dellinger E P, Max M H 1979 Failure of cimetidine prophylaxis in the critically ill. Archives of Surgery 114: 492-496

Norfleet R G, Rhodes R A, Saviage K 1980 False-positive 'Hemoccult' reaction with cimetidine. New England Journal of Medicine 302: 467

Pariente R, Wanstok E 1972 Les hémorragies digestives au cours des insuffisances respiratoires. Annales de Chirurgie 26: 897-902

Priebe H J, Skillman J J, Bushnell L S, Long P C, Silen W 1980 Antacid versus cimetidine in preventing acute gastrointestinal bleeding. A randomized trial in 75 critically ill patients. New England Journal of Medicine 302: 426-430

Rosenthal A, Czaja A J, Pruitt B A Jr 1977 Gastrin levels and gastric acidity in the pathogenesis of acute gastroduodenal disease after burns. Surgery, Gynecology and Obstetrics 144: 232-235

Silvestri N, Curzio M, Motta U, De Pietri P, Bonacina F, Minoja G 1980 Cimetidine to prevent stress ulcers. Lancet 1: 885

Speranza V, Basso N 1980 Stress ulcer syndrome. A current medical perspective. Smith Kline Corporation

Taylor P C, Loop F D, Hermann R E 1973 Management of acute stress ulcer after cardiac surgery. Annals of Surgery 178: 1-5

Voisin C, Guerrin F, Wattel F, Tonnel A B 1970 Hémorragies et lésions gastro-duodénales en cours de réanimation respiratoire. Lille Médical 15: 1140-1145

Zumtobel V, Teichmann R K, Inthorn D 1979 Prophylaxis and treatment of gastroduodenal stress bleedings in intensive care patients with the histamine H$_2$-receptor antagonist cimetidine. Langenbecks Archiv für Chirurgie, p 247-250

Discussion on Haemorrhage

Chairman: Dr J. R. Bennett

Dr Bennett. How does Dr Misiewicz think cimetidine might affect the outcome of established bleeding from chronic lesions?

Dr Misiewicz. I can think of no mechanism other than the obvious one — that there is less acid and less pepsin, the pH may be higher, and healing and clotting might be more efficient. Grave doubts have been voiced about cimetidine and platelet function, which might have an adverse effect on the outcome of bleeding but I do not think that this effect has ever been demonstrated in the concentrations attained in the patient.

Dr Bardhan. Is there any rational basis for using cimetidine for bleeding from a chronic ulcer? After all, it is surely naive to think that when the ulcer is burrowing away and hits a blood vessel some sort of seal can be put in. Is there not a biological subgroup of people who bleed without being exposed to factors like analgesic drugs and who, having bled once, are likely to bleed again in the future?

In those patients in whom Dr Speranza was able to prevent bleeding was there any correlation with ultimate mortality? Is cimetidine being over-used in the intensive therapy unit?

Dr Speranza. I have no special data on the ultimate results of cimetidine treatment. As regards haemorrhage, only one of the patients died from myocardial infarction. Six out of the seven patients stopped bleeding on cimetidine treatment, and one after embolisation. Our results are better than other people's, but in this case it was therapy with cimetidine — prophylaxis is completely different.

Professor Langman. The problem of gastric bleeding is very similar to that of myocardial infarction where the mortality rate is so low that very large groups of patients have to be studied to come to any satisfactory conclusion. None of the trials presented is large enough to study what really matters, which is whether people die and whether the surgeons can be kept away. It is significant that Dr Misiewicz has presented data only on re-bleeding, which is not very easy to assess in some of our patients. So far we have admitted 300 patients to a controlled trial of cimetidine, placebo and antifibrinolysis, but I have no intention of trying to sort out the results until 600 patients have been put into the trial, and even then, our conclusions must be tentative. At the moment, there are as many patients in our trial as in all the others put together.

Dr Misiewicz. I agree. The other problem, as Dr Bardhan pointed out, is that many of the deaths are inevitable and no form of therapy, drugs or operation, would make any difference to the patient. To determine whether there is any effect on mortality a very large series is needed, possibly as a multicentre, national or international study.

Mr Keighley. With respect to mortality, would Dr Misiewicz like to comment, not just on drug therapy but on management? The one group in the world which has reduced mortality in gastrointestinal bleeding is an Australian group; patients are centralised, carefully monitored and are managed concurrently by physicians and surgeons. I believe that this rather than drug therapy is one of the most important factors in reducing mortality.

Dr Misiewicz. What Mr Keighley is saying is very attractive. Let us all get together, let us put these patients in intensive care, let us get the physician and the surgeon in on it together, let us endoscope the patients from the very beginning, let us get the diagnosis established very early and then let us see what happens. Dr Hansky published the most remarkable improvement in mortality figures in his series. I wonder what happened before he started agitating about the treatment of these patients. If we take a critical look at what happens to the mortality when all these actions have been taken, the answer is not very much. Professor Langman, for example, carried out a study in which the outcome of an episode of gastro-intestinal bleeding was assessed in a random fashion, whether the patient had an endoscopy or a barium meal (which is now perhaps a rather old-fashioned way of diagnosing what is happening, and which gives lower diagnostic accuracy). The outcome of the haemorrhage was still the same. Therefore, although in theory Mr Keighley is right, in practice I doubt whether a great deal of impact can be made on the mortality of these patients.

Dr Speranza. I agree that the ideal is a high-standard centre for each hospital to which all the bleeding patients may be referred, but this is only an ideal. What is important is to know which patients are at high risk. The easiest way to manage these high-risk patients is prophylaxis with antacids or cimetidine, and this can be done in every kind of hospital and in every kind of situation. That is a real improvement in management — much more than building beautiful centres.

Section 5
CIMETIDINE AND OTHER CONDITIONS

23. Cimetidine in the treatment of acute pancreatitis — report of an ongoing multicentre study

G. Bommelaer[1]

Service des Maladies de l'Appareil Digestif, CHU Rangueil, Toulouse, France

Three primary objectives have been proposed for the medical treatment of acute pancreatitis:

1. To limit the severity of pancreatic inflammation itself.

2. To decrease the incidence of complications by interrupting their pathogenesis.

3. To support the patient and treat complications as they arise.

Non-specific measures, including respiratory support, nutritional support and electrolyte replacement, are commonly employed in order to achieve the third goal, and their usefulness will not be discussed any further.

Various specific measures have been proposed in order to limit the severity of pancreatitis or to interrupt the pathogenesis of its complications. They include nasogastric suction, inhibition of pancreatic secretion by glucagon, anticholinergics, hyperthermia, inhibition of pancreatic enzymes, and prevention of complications by antibiotics, heparin, vasopressin and dextran. None of these specific measures has been proved unequivocally to be useful, particularly in view of controlled clinical studies; see complete references in Di Magno (1979) and Ranson (1979).

The basis for assessing the clinical usefulness of cimetidine in acute pancreatitis is essentially theoretical. By decreasing gastric acid secretion, cimetidine would suppress secretin release and thereby diminish pancreatic secretion. As a matter of fact it has been shown that cimetidine did decrease pancreatic enzyme secretion during acute pancreatitis (Regan et al, 1980). By raising the gastric pH, cimetidine could prevent gastric haemorrhage — a possible complication of acute pancreatitis (Lawson et al, 1980). So far, available data from clinical trials have shown:

1. Either an improvement (Perez Oteyza et al, 1980) or no benefit from cimetidine on the clinical outcome of patients (Alcala Santaella et al, 1980; Meshkinpour et al, 1979).

[1]Members of the working party were: Pr Fekete (Clichy), Pr Gaucher (Nancy), Pr Gauthier (Marseille), Pr Gillet (Besançon), Pr Grenier (Strasbourg), Pr Launois (Rennes), Pr Ribet (Toulouse).

2. Either an increase (Meshkinpour et al, 1979) or a decrease in hyperamylasaemia (Damman and Augustin, 1978) following cimetidine therapy so that no definite conclusion on the usefulness of this treatment can be drawn.

Our study was undertaken in order to re-evaluate the effect of cimetidine on the clinical outcome and biological evolution of acute pancreatitis.

PATIENTS AND METHODS

Patients
Selected for inclusion in the study were patients, both male and female over 18 years old, suffering for less than 48 hours from upper abdominal pain and tenderness and having one or more of the following:

serum amylase more than 200 Somogyi units or amylase versus creatinine clearance ratio over 3 per cent

hyperamylasaemia

serum glucose over 1.2 g/l;

serum calcium under 80 mg/l;

segmental small bowel ileus or a sentinel loop;

evidence obtained by laparotomy or ultrasonography for acute pancreatitis.

Pregnant women, patients suffering from renal insufficiency with a serum creatinine over 212 μmol/l, and subjects admitted after 48 hours following the initial symptoms were excluded.

Treatment
Treatment consisted of cimetidine (or placebo) i.v. 1.6 g/24 hours until oral feeding was resumed and then cimetidine (or placebo) per os 1.6 g/24 hours for a maximum of one month. Anticholinergics, enzyme inhibitors, glucagon and oral anticoagulants were excluded, but treatment could include nasogastric suction (if vomiting), parenteral feeding, antibiotics, electrolyte replacement, and pentazocine as sole analgesic when needed. Patients were randomly assigned to a schedule prepared from a table of random numbers and given either cimetidine or placebo tablets which were identical with respect to colour and taste. Resumption of oral feeding took place when the patient was pain-free and the serum amylase level had returned to normal.

Statistical analysis
Student's t-test for independent samples and the Chi square test were used for comparison between the cimetidine and placebo group.

RESULTS

Thirty-three patients have been placed on the protocol. One was withdrawn from the trial because of granulocytopenia and excluded from the analysis; code-breaking revealed that this patient was actually on placebo treatment but he died a few days later.

Finally 15 patients received cimetidine and 17 placebo. Both groups were comparable for age, duration of pain before inclusion in the study, presumed aetiology of the pancreatitis and admission values for serum amylase (Table 23.1).

Table 23.1 Comparison of cimetidine and placebo groups.

	Cimetidine	Placebo
Number of patients	15	17
Sex: male	10	13
female	5	4
Age (years)	48.8 ± 16.8^1	50.4 ± 14.8^1
Time between onset of symptoms and treatment (hours)	16.9 ± 10.5^1	21.7 ± 11.3^1
Admission serum amylase		
$<$Normal $\times$ 3	10	11
$>$Normal $\times$ 3	5	6
Presumed aetiology		
cholelithiasis	3	7
alcohol	7	9
other	0	1

^{1} mean $\pm$ SD.

There were no differences in inclusion criteria between the two groups (results not shown).

The mean durations of symptoms, signs, elevated serum amylase values and treatment, as well as the number of patients who required surgery during the trial, are summarized in Table 23.2.

Table 23.2 Clinical observations and serum amylase values studied in 32 cases of acute pancreatitis.

	Cimetidine (N = 15) (mean $\pm$ SD)	Placebo (N = 17) (mean $\pm$ SD)	P
Days of:			
Abdominal pain	3 ± 1.2	3.4 ± 1.8	NS
Nausea	2 ± 1.3	2 ± 0.9	NS
Vomiting	1.5 ± 0.7	1.5 ± 0.5	NS
Raised serum amylase	3.9 ± 2.5	2.9 ± 1.4	NS
Treatment: total	19.3 ± 9.8	20.3 ± 10.7	NS
i.v.	6.6 ± 2.44	6.2 ± 4.4	NS
oral	12.6 ± 10.4	14 ± 9.65	NS
Number of patients operated	8	9	NS

There was no statistically significant difference between the treatment and control groups in any of the results despite a trend towards a higher mean duration for a raised serum amylase in the cimetidine group. Mean values for serum amylase were compared between the two groups every day from inclusion until the fifth day of the study and again no statistically significant difference appeared.

Results for the outcome of the patients and incidence of complications are listed in Table 23.3.

Table 23.3 Outcome of patients and complications in 32 cases of acute pancreatitis.

Parameters	Cimetidine (N = 15)	Placebo (N = 17)	P
Death	4	0	NS
Hyperthermia	2	1	NS
Haemorrhage	2	1	NS
Pseudocysts or abscess	2	1	NS
Septicaemia	2	0	NS
Renal failure	1	0	NS
Fistula	0	1	NS
Pneumopathy	0	1	NS

Various complications were observed in both groups and their incidence seemed to be higher in the cimetidine group, although never reaching a statistically significant level. The striking difference between the two groups, although not statistically significant, is related to the death rate since four subjects died in the cimetidine group and none in the placebo group. Two deaths occurred respectively in the 4th and 25th day after the end of the cimetidine treatment and were related in one case to a coma of unknown origin, and in the other case to a pancreatic abscess with septicaemia and renal failure. The two other deaths occurred while under treatment and were attributed to cholangitis in one case and in the other to a haemorrhage following surgical pancreatectomy.

DISCUSSION

Our results suggest:

1. Cimetidine seems to be no more effective than placebo in the clinical and biological evolution of acute pancreatitis.

2. Cimetidine treatment could be hazardous in the management of acute pancreatitis.

Several explanations may be advanced to account for this. First, the two treatment groups may have been too dissimilar to permit a valid comparison. This is unlikely since we are unable to find any difference between the two groups in the pretreatment clinical and laboratory assessments. Second, inhibition of gastric acid secretion, as induced by cimetidine, may not be of great importance in the management of acute pancreatitis. In support of this is the fact that reducing gastric secretion by nasogastric suction has not proved helpful (Levant et al, 1974). Third, since so far no statistically significant level has been reached, the apparent increase in death rate in the cimetidine group could be due to a random distribution. If this is not the case, and contrary to previous results (Meshkinpour et al, 1979; Perez Oteyza et al, 1980), cimetidine would appear to be dangerous when given to acute pancreatitis patients.

The mechanism by which cimetidine could worsen the outcome of acute pancreatitis is unknown. Results concerning a possible harmful effect of cimetidine in experimental pancreatitis induced in animals are conflicting (Hadas et al, 1978; Lawson et al, 1980) and do not offer any explanation regarding the possible mechanism of action of cimetidine. Hypotheses concerning a direct effect of cimetidine on pancreatic acinar cells are purely speculative. However, in view of the published data and our own experience it does not seem that at present cimetidine can be recommended in the treatment of acute pancreatitis.

REFERENCES

Alcala-Santealla R, Robles J, Cos E 1979 Therapeutic study in acute pancreatitis. In: Dresse A, Barbier F, Harvengt C, Tijtgat G N (eds) Proceedings of the Second National Symposium on cimetidine. Excerpta Medica, Amsterdam, p 10-26
Damman H G, Augustin H J 1978 Cimetidine and acute pancreatitis. Lancet 1: 666
Di Magno E P 1979 What is appropriate non-operative treatment of acute pancreatitis. Digestive Diseases and Sciences 24: 337-338
Hadas J, Wapnick S, Grosberg S J 1978 Cimetidine in pancreatitis (letter). New England Journal of Medicine 299: 487
Lawson M J, Alp M H, Van Deth A, Leong A, Read Tr 1980 The progression of experimental pancreatitis with cimetidine I.R.C.S. Medical Science 8: 449
Levant J A, Secrist D M, Resin H, Sturdevant R A L, Guth Ph 1974 Nasogastric suction in the treatment of alcoholic pancreatitis. Journal of the American Medical Association 229: 51-52
Meshkinpour H, Molinari L G, Berk J E, Hoehler F K 1979 Cimetidine in the treatment of acute alcoholic pancreatitis. Gastroenterology 77: 687-690
Perez Oteyza C, Rebollar J, Ballarin M, Chantres M T, Garcia Calvo M I, Gilsanz V 1980 Treatment of acute pancreatitis with cimetidine. Double blind controlled trial. Hepatogastroenterology Suppl., XI International Congress of Gastroenterology, 366
Ranson J H 1979 Acute pancreatitis. In: Ravitch M (ed) Current problems in surgery. Yearbook Medical Publishers, Chicago
Regan P T, Malagelada J R, Go W L N, Wolf A M, Di Magno E P 1980 The effect of cimetidine and glucagon in pancreatitis and gastric secretion and outcome in human acute pancreatitis. Gastroenterology 78: 1242

24. Treatment of pancreatic and ileectomy steatorrhoea

Timothy C. Northfield, Patrick L. Zentler-Munro, William J. Fitzpatrick, David R. Fine

Department of Medicine, St George's Hospital Medical School, London

Pancreatic exocrine insufficiency and ileal resection can both give rise to severe steatorrhoea. Apart from reflecting malabsorption of fat and fat-soluble vitamins, steatorrhoea can itself be a very troublesome symptom to the patient and resistant to treatment. This contribution will attempt to answer the following six questions:

1. What is the mechanism of the steatorrhoea in these conditions?
2. How effective is conventional treatment?
3. Why use cimetidine?
4. Does cimetidine improve fat digestion and solubilisation?
5. Does it improve steatorrhoea?
6. What is the optimum current treatment?

WHAT IS THE MECHANISM OF STEATORRHOEA?

According to the micellar theory of fat absorption, dietary fat requires both pancreatic lipolysis and micellar solubilisation before it can be absorbed. Dietary fat is largely triglyceride, which is hydrolysed by pancreatic lipase to form fatty acids and monoglyceride, which can then undergo micellar solubilisation by bile acids. If postprandial jejunal content is ultracentrifuged, it separates into three phases: an upper oil phase, an intermediate aqueous phase and a precipitate. Physically, the oil phase contains droplets of emulsified fat, whilst the aqueous phase contains fat dissolved in micelles. Micelles are capable of crossing the 'unstirred layer' next to the small intestinal mucosa very much more rapidly than the emulsion droplets, and hence facilitate fat absorption. Chemically, the oil phase consists of triglyceride and unionised fatty acid. The aqueous phase consists of monoglyceride, ionised fatty acid and bile acids. Triglyceride, being a hydrophobic lipid, is unable to enter the aqueous phase, whereas ionised fatty acids and monoglyceride, being hydrophilic lipids, are capable of entering it, so long as there is an adequate concentration of bile acids for their micellar solubilisation. Thus, lipolysis of dietary triglyceride is regarded as a prerequisite for aqueous solubilisation by bile acids. The products of lipolysis — fatty acids and monoglyceride — can be regarded as the solute for the aqueous phase and bile acid as the solvent.

Solute deficiency results from reduced lipolysis due to pancreatic insufficiency. The pancreas has considerable reserve function, and it has been shown that lipase secretion must be reduced by more than 90 per cent before steatorrhoea ensues (Di Magno et al, 1973). Solvent deficiency results from a reduced jejunal bile acid concentration, and the most important cause of this is interruption of the enterohepatic circulation of bile acids due to removal of the ileum — the site of active bile acid reabsorption. Again, there is considerable reserve function, since the liver can compensate by increasing bile acid synthesis so as to maintain jejunal bile acid concentration. In practice, steatorrhoea usually results if more than 100 cm of ileum has been resected (Hofmann and Poley, 1969); smaller resections result in diarrhoea alone, due to the cathartic effect of unabsorbed bile acids on the colon.

HOW EFFECTIVE IS CONVENTIONAL TREATMENT?

Pancreatic steatorrhoea
Pancreatic enzyme supplements are available in the form of pancreatin tablets, powder and capsules. Tablets have the disadvantage of being slow to dissolve. Powder sprinkled over the food is effective, but makes the food taste unpleasant. Capsules are probably the best preparation, because they rapidly dissolve to release powder in the stomach. Steatorrhoea usually continues despite large doses of pancreatin, because 90 per cent of the enzyme activity is destroyed by acid in the stomach (Di Magno et al, 1977). Many patients need 10 capsules with each meal, and we have experience of one patient regularly taking 100 capsules a day without complete control of steatorrhoea. High doses lead to hyperuricosuria, because the pancreas has a high purine content.

Enteric-coated pancreatin tablets are designed not to dissolve till the pH rises above 6, thus protecting the pancreatin from gastric inactivation. Since they do not dissolve in gastric acid, however, these tablets may be retained in the stomach after the meal has emptied. To circumvent this, enteric-coated microspheres have been developed in the USA, but are not yet available in the UK. These preparations are clinically satisfactory in many patients. In some, however, steatorrhoea is little changed. In these patients jejunal pH may rarely rise above 6, so that disintegration is unlikely to occur even in the jejunum. This problem is discussed in more detail below.

Acid-stable enzymes intended to resist gastric inactivation have been developed, but have not been convincingly demonstrated to be better than pancreatin. Bromelain is a proteolytic enzyme derived from the pineapple, which is active at intragastric pH. Acid-stable cellulases have also been developed, but no acid-stable lipase preparation has been marketed. The important theoretical advantage of acid-stable animal tongue and pharyngeal lipases has not yet been exploited commercially.

Ileectomy steatorrhoea

The most effective conventional treatment consists of non-specific restriction of dietary fat (Andersson et al, 1974) together with the use of isotonic drinks to avoid osmotic diarrhoea. Cholestyramine is of value for diarrhoea, because it binds bile acids and thus prevents their cathartic action on the colon (Hofmann and Poley, 1969). It is contraindicated, however, in steatorrhoea because it aggravates it by further reducing jejunal bile acid concentration. Although medium-chain triglyceride can be absorbed without lipolysis or bile acids, its use as a dietary supplement is of doubtful benefit. Reports of a reduction in faecal fat excretion are probably artefactual, because the conventional method of estimating faecal fat does not measure medium-chain triglyceride.

WHY USE CIMETIDINE?

There are several theoretical reasons why cimetidine is likely to be of benefit:

1. Pancreatic enzymes are sensitive to acid, and are 50 per cent inactivated if the pH falls to 5. As a result, 90 per cent of orally administered enzyme is destroyed before it leaves the stomach (Di Magno et al, 1977).

2. Glycine-conjugated bile acids precipitate in vitro if the pH falls below 5. This could have a critical effect on aqueous solubilisation of fat if total bile acid concentration is reduced, as in ileectomy steatorrhoea, or if jejunal pH is reduced to an abnormal extent due to hyposecretion of bicarbonate in patients with pancreatic insufficiency. We have found from jejunal intubation studies that about 40 per cent of a meal enters the jejunum at pH less than 5 in pancreatic steatorrhoea due to adult cystic fibrosis, compared with 15 per cent in healthy controls (Zentler-Munro et al, 1979). At pH less than 5, approximately 50 per cent of the bile acids precipitate in vivo compared with about 20 per cent at pH more than 6.

3. In vitro we have shown that binding of bile acids to dietary protein is also increased at pH less than 5, thus further decreasing aqueous phase bile acid concentration.

4. The partitioning of unionised fatty acid into the oil phase increases if pH falls below 6.

Thus, there are four ways in which acid interferes with intraluminal digestion and solubilisation of lipid. These pH-dependent effects were demonstrated in our intubation studies, where there was a significant reduction in aqueous phase lipid and fatty acid concentration at pH less than 5. All these effects are potentially correctable by cimetidine.

DOES CIMETIDINE IMPROVE FAT DIGESTION AND SOLUBILISATION?

We have examined this question in eight patients with pancreatic steatorrhoea due to adult cystic fibrosis (Zentler-Munro et al, 1981). We compared jejunal aspirate on three different regimens in random order: pancreatin alone, cimetidine alone, and pancreatin plus cimetidine. Results were compared with those on no treatment from the study described above. On pancreatin alone, there was a significant increase in mean lipase activity from 4 to 15 μ/l and in lipolysis from 9 to 12 per cent. This improvement in lipolysis was not accompanied by an improvement in aqueous phase lipid concentration, because bile acid precipitation remained unchanged. On cimetidine alone, all the meal entered the jejunum at a pH above 6. Mean bile acid precipitation was reduced from 31 to 18 per cent, and aqueous phase lipid increased from 6 to 9 mmol/l, despite minimal lipase activity and lipolysis.

The combination of pancreatin plus cimetidine was significantly better than either pancreatin or cimetidine alone for lipase (40 μ/l), lipolysis (20 per cent) and bile acid precipitation, which fell to 4 per cent. This further decrease in bile acid precipitation on addition of pancreatin to cimetidine is attributable to a reduction both in pH-dependent precipitation, and in protein-binding due to improved digestion of protein. As a result, there was a marked improvement in aqueous phase lipid concentration to 19 mmol/l on the combined regimen. We conclude that for optimal therapy of pancreatic steatorrhoea, bile acid precipitation and binding must be prevented, in addition to prevention of pancreatin inactivation.

Another study has shown a similar improvement in lipid solubilisation on addition of cimetidine to pancreatin (Regan et al, 1979). Since cimetidine alone was not studied, it failed to demonstrate whether this was due to prevention of gastric inactivation of pancreatin, or intrajejunal precipitation of bile acids. The distinction is important because, while enteric-coating or acid-stable enzymes may avoid the former, only cimetidine can prevent the latter.

In ileectomy steatorrhoea also, we found that treatment with cimetidine caused a significant reduction in bile acid precipitation. This resulted in a significant increase in overall micellar lipid concentration from 9 to 16 mmol/l (Fitzpatrick et al, 1979).

DOES CIMETIDINE IMPROVE STEATORRHOEA?

Several studies have shown that cimetidine improves the efficacy of pancreatin therapy in pancreatic steatorrhoea. In the best of these (Regan et al, 1977), five different treatment regimens were given in random order to patients on a carefully controlled fat intake (Figure 24.1). Viokase, an American preparation of pancreatin in tablet form, failed to control steatorrhoea, reducing mean faecal fat excretion from 60 to 30 g/day. An enteric-coated preparation and combinations of Viokase with two different antacid preparations (sodium

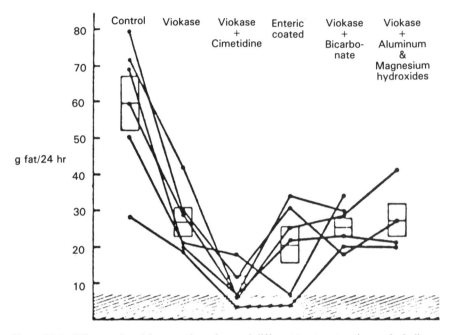

Figure 24.1   Effect on faecal fat excretion of several different treatment regimens, including pancreatic enzyme supplement (Viokase) plus cimetidine (from Regan et al, 1977, with kind permission of the Editor of *New England Journal of Medicine*). The double boxes represent mean ± SEM.

bicarbonate 2.5 g/meal and a magnesium/aluminium hydroxide combination — Maalox — 30 ml/meal) performed no better. Only Viokase plus cimetidine produced a significantly greater reduction in faecal fat excretion to 10 g/day. Thus, cimetidine does improve steatorrhoea in patients receiving pancreatin, and its effect is greater than enteric-coating or simultaneous administration of antacids.

Figure 24.2 shows our results for faecal fat excretion in 10 patients with ileectomy steatorrhoea. Patients were admitted to hospital for two weeks and put on a 100 g/day fat diet. Cimetidine 400 mg 30 minutes before meals, and a matching placebo, were given in random order for one week each. On both regimens, a two-day equilibration period preceded a five-day faecal fat collection. Faecal fat excretion (mean ± SEM) was 44.5 ± 10.0 mmol/24 hours on placebo, compared with 27.6 ± 4.7 mmol/24 hours on cimetidine; median values were 29.1 and 24.3 mmol/24 h ($P < 0.05$) by Wilcoxon matched pairs signed rank test. This represents a 40 per cent reduction in faecal fat excretion on cimetidine. The reduction was greatest in the three patients with the most severe steatorrhoea. We did not find any reduction in mean faecal wet weight (1957 g/24 h on placebo and 1958 g/24 h on cimetidine) but another group has reported a significant reduction in faecal volume and sodium in ten patients with diarrhoea due to extensive small bowel resection (Ali et al, 1980).

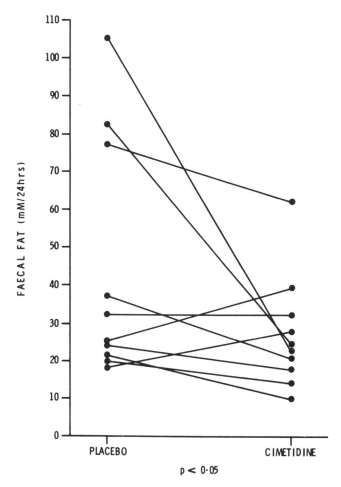

Figure 24.2   Effect of cimetidine on faecal fat excretion in 10 patients with ileectomy steatorrhoea.

WHAT IS OPTIMUM CURRENT TREATMENT?

For pancreatic steatorrhoea, enteric-coated pancreatin offers a satisfactory treatment for many patients. If this fails, optimum treatment can be achieved by pancreatin capsules taken with meals, plus cimetidine 200–400 mg taken 40 minutes before meals. For ileectomy steatorrhoea, the mainstay of treatment remains dietary fat restriction. In patients with severe ileectomy steatorrhoea that does not respond satisfactorily to this dietary regimen, a further improvement in steatorrhoea can be obtained by taking cimetidine 200–400 mg 40 minutes before meals.

REFERENCES

Ali A, Barany F, Kollberg B, Monsen U, Wisen O, Johansson C 1980 Effect of an H_2-receptor blocking agent on diarrhoea after extensive small bowel resection in Crohn's disease. Acta Medica Scandinavica 207: 119-122

Andersson H, Isaksson B, Sjogren B 1974 Fat-reduced diet in the symptomatic treatment of small bowel disease. Gut 15: 351-359

Di Magno E P, Go V L W, Summerskill W H J 1973 Relations between pancreatic enzyme outputs and malabsorption in severe pancreatic insufficiency. New England Journal of Medicine 288: 813-815

Di Magno E P, Malagelada J R, Go V L W, Moertel C G 1977 Fate of orally ingested enzymes in pancreatic insufficiency. New England Journal of Medicine 296: 1318-1322

Fitzpatrick W J F, Zentler-Munro P, Bird R, Northfield T C 1979 Acid mediated bile acid precipitation in ileal resection patients. Gut 20: A941

Hofmann A F, Poley J R 1969 Cholestyramine treatment of diarrhoea associated with ileal resection. New England Journal of Medicine 281: 397-402

Regan P T, Malagelada J R, Di Magno E P, Galnzman S L, Go V L W 1977 Comparative effects of antacids, cimetidine and enteric coating on the therapeutic response to oral enzymes in severe pancreatic insufficiency. New England Journal of Medicine 297: 854-858

Regan R T, Malagelada J R, Di Magno E P, Go V L W 1979 Reduced intraluminal bile acid concentrations and fat maldigestion in pancreatic insufficiency: correction by treatment. Gastroenterology: 77, 285-289

Zentler-Munro P L, Fitzpatrick W J F, Bird R, Northfield T C 1979 Acid-mediated bile acid precipitation in pancreatic insufficiency due to cystic fibrosis. Gut 20: A920

Zentler-Munro P L, Fine D R, Gannon M, Northfield T C 1981 Effect of cimetidine on intraduodenal bile acid precipitation, pancreatin inactivation and lipid solubilisation in pancreatic steatorrhoea. Gut, in press

25. Cimetidine in anaesthetic practice

J. Moore, J. P. Howe, J. W. Dundee, J. R. Johnston, W. McCaughey
Department of Anaesthetics, The Queen's University of Belfast, Northern Ireland

Acid pulmonary aspiration is a well recognised complication of anaesthesia and occurs most commonly in those patients with a large gastric residue of pH less than 2.5. The obstetric patient requiring general anaesthesia is particularly at risk during labour because gastric emptying is prolonged, especially if narcotic analgesics have been given (Nimmo et al, 1977). Mendelson (1946) drew attention to this anaesthetic hazard in obstetrics, and the condition resulting from inhaled gastric contents is frequently called Mendelson's syndrome. As its severity is related to the acidity of the aspirate, routine antacid therapy is now considered essential prior to general anaesthesia (Moir, 1980).

The most commonly used antacid is magnesium trisilicate mixture BPC given in 25 to 30 ml doses at two-hourly intervals throughout labour. Recently, however, the efficacy of such treatment has been questioned. In the report on Confidential Enquiries into Maternal Deaths for England and Wales, 1973-75 (DHSS, 1979) nine deaths were attributed to acid aspiration pneumonitis, and the assessor considered that in eight of these antacid treatment had been adequate. Indeed animal studies have shown that inhalation of emulsion alkalis either per se or mixed with gastric contents can induce a pneumonitis which is no less severe than that due to acid (Gibbs et al, 1979).

A different approach to the problem of reducing intragastric acidity seemed worthy of investigation and a series of studies using H_2 receptor blockade by cimetidine have been carried out at the Department of Anaesthetics, The Queen's University of Belfast. All of these were approved by the local Ethical Committee.

INTRAVENOUS INVESTIGATION

A preliminary study, in which cimetidine 200 mg was given intravenously to 20 women in active labour, revealed no harmful effects on uterine contractility, fetal heart rate or newborn wellbeing (McGowan, 1979). A similar intravenous dose was given at predetermined time intervals (30, 60, 90 and 120 minutes) before elective Caesarean section. The gastric samples were obtained by aspirating the total stomach contents through a double lumen Salem sump tube following the establishment of endotracheal anaesthesia. The volume was measured using a graduated cylinder and pH determined by a Corning 133 pH meter. Cimetidine significantly reduced gastric acidity but the gastric pH was maintained above 2.5 perioperatively only when the drug was administered at 60 minutes prior to anaesthesia (Figure 25.1) (Howe et al, 1980). Cimetidine had no significant effect on gastric volume when comparison was made with untreated patients.

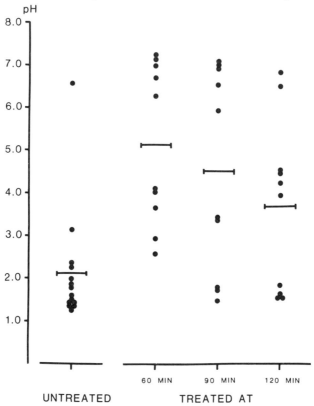

Figure 25.1   pH of gastric contents at 60, 90 and 120 minutes after i.v. cimetidine 200 mg.

ORAL TREATMENT

To be widely accepted in clinical practice cimetidine had to be shown to be effective when given orally. Twenty patients scheduled for elective Caesarean delivery were given two doses of cimetidine 400 mg by mouth, one the evening before and the other between one and three hours before induction of anaesthesia. The pH of the gastric aspirates, obtained as in the intravenous study, were all above the critical value of 2.5 only when obtained between 90 and 150 minutes after ingestion of cimetidine (Figure 25.2) (Johnston et al, 1982a).

The effects of a single oral dose of 400 mg given to 44 patients undergoing similar surgery showed that those anaesthetised within the above times had an acceptable reduction in gastric acidity. The volumes of the aspirates from these women were significantly less than those of a similar group given 20 ml magnesium trisilicate mixture BPC within one hour of surgery. It was apparent

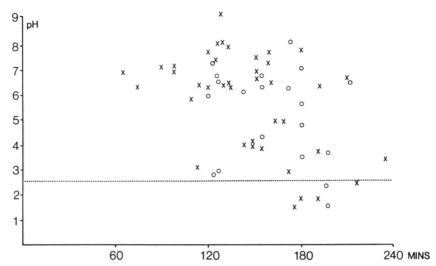

Figure 25.2   pH of gastric contents after oral cimetidine 400 mg (×, single dose; o, two doses).

that while cimetidine effectively reduced intragastric acidity this remained satisfactory only for a relatively short time. To be continuously effective throughout labour repetitive dosage at fixed time intervals was needed.

FIELD TRIAL

A field trial was then undertaken in which oral cimetidine was used as the sole antacid treatment throughout labour (Johnston et al, 1982b). Following an initial dose of 400 mg, a further dose of 200 mg was given at two-hourly intervals to a maximum of six doses, giving a total intake of 1.6 g. The limitation of total dosage was considered necessary because of the possible cumulative effects on mother and infant. Of the 1323 women included, 128 required a general anaesthetic for Caesarean section. This was electively carried out in 44, and the findings for this group have already been presented in the oral treatment section. The remaining 84 had been in active labour for varying lengths of time. Gastric samples were obtained from 54 of these, no attempt being made to aspirate the stomach in the remaining 30 for a variety of reasons. Their pH values together with those for samples obtained from 16 patients anaesthetised for forceps delivery or manual removal of placenta are shown in Figure 25.3.

Examination of Figure 25.3 shows that after the first 90 minutes there is a gradual rise in pH above 2.5 to a plateau level at about 6 to 7. Some patients, on post-delivery questioning, were found not to have adhered to the prescribed treatment schedule and these are indicated by crosses on the graph. Five of the nine aspirates obtained within 90 minutes of the initial dose had low pH values and the blood cimetidine concentration of four of these was below 0.5 μmol/ml, a level considered necessary for a therapeutic effect (Burland et al, 1975).

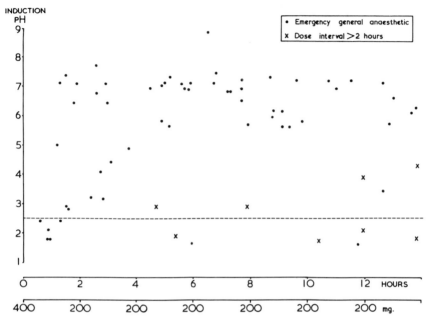

Figure 25.3 pH of gastric contents from patients in field trial of oral cimetidine.

The results for the volumes of gastric aspirate are shown in Table 25.1 and are compared with those obtained from a similar group given magnesium trisilicate mixture BPC 20 ml, 2-hourly. Whilst the mean volume for the cimetidine series was less than that of the oral alkali treated group the difference was not statistically significant. The effect of narcotic analgesics in delaying gastric emptying is also evident and occurred irrespective of the type of treatment.

Table 25.1 Effect of narcotic analgesia on the average and range of the volume of gastric contents from 28 women receiving magnesium trisilicate mixture BPC and 70 receiving cimetidine as their antacid during labour. Figures inside brackets indicate numbers of women.

Antacid regime	Magnesium trisilicate mixture BPC		Cimetidine	
Volume of gastric contents at induction	Average	Range	Average	Range
with narcotic analgesia	104.5 (13)	4-350	70.3 (54)	0-325
without narcotic analgesia	54.7 (15)	1-238	34.9 (16)	1-163
Total	77.8 (28)	1-350	62.2 (70)	0-325

Maternal side-effects specifically related to the use of cimetidine were not observed or complained of in any of these studies. In the field trial vomiting occurred in 14.8 per cent of the 1323 patients and only five refused treatment. Uterine contractility was not affected and blood loss or the incidence of placental retention was not increased by the repetitive use of oral cimetidine.

PLACENTAL TRANSFER

With any new treatment in obstetrics the wellbeing of the infant is of prime concern. During our intravenous studies the placental transfer of cimetidine 200 mg was investigated in 16 patients in normal labour and 40 patients undergoing elective Caesarean section (Howe et al, 1981). Cimetidine crossed the placental barrier, blood levels in mothers and infants being lower with increasing time from injection (Figure 25.4).

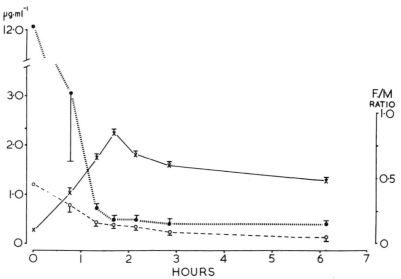

Figure 25.4 Cimetidine concentrations in maternal venous (●) and mixed umbilical cord blood (o) following an i.v. dose of 200 mg to the mother. The fetal/maternal ratio (×) is also shown.

Umbilical cord blood levels were markedly lower than those of the mother during the first hour following administration but thereafter levels were similar. The mean fetal–maternal ratio at delivery was highest (0.84) at one and a half to two hours. Post-delivery infant and maternal blood samples showed that cimetidine could not be detected in most cases at 19 hours after treatment.

Detailed assessment of infant status at birth and during the post-delivery period was carried out in all studies. No untoward effects were found in the newborn which could be related to maternal cimetidine treatment. The pH of the gastric juice of the neonate was high at birth but fell two hours after delivery indicating that gastric acid was being secreted.

COMMENTS

The ideal antacid should act rapidly to raise the gastric pH to above 2.5, not increase the volume of stomach contents, be non-irritant if inhaled alone or mixed with gastric juice and not harm the mother or her infant. Cimetidine is not rapidly effective even if given intravenously so it is of no value in the untreated emergency patient. Following oral treatment some 90 minutes must elapse before safe conditions are present. The delay is due in part to the presence of existing acid as well as the latent period associated with the absorption and onset of effect of cimetidine. Nevertheless beyond this time it proved to be an acceptable antacid having the major advantage that it did not increase the volume of gastric contents. Patient acceptability is high and its use is associated with a negligible incidence of maternal side-effects. Newborn wellbeing is not jeopardised but the placental transfer and infant eliminations of cimetidine following repetitive treatment remains to be investigated.

A single oral dose of 400 mg given 120 ± 30 minutes before an elective anaesthetic will consistently reduce intragastric acidity to safe levels without adding to the volume of stomach contents. If cimetidine is to be used as the sole antacid throughout labour it is important that dose times are strictly adhered to. Some of the problems associated with cimetidine treatment for the parturient may be overcome by combining its administration with a single dose of a saline antacid immediately before induction of anaesthesia.

REFERENCES

Burland W L, Duncan W A M, Hesselbo T, Mills J G, Sharpe P C 1975 Pharmacological evaluation of cimetidine. A new histamine H_2-receptor antagonist in healthy man. British Journal of Clinical Pharmacology 2: 481-486
Department of Health and Social Security 1979 Report on Confidential Enquiries into Maternal Deaths in England and Wales, 1973-75. HMSO, London.
Gibbs C P, Schwartz D J, Wynne J W, Hood I C, Kuck E I 1979 Antacid pulmonary aspiration in the dog. Anesthesiology 51: 380-385
Howe J P, Moore J, McCaughey W, Dundee J W 1980 Effect of cimetidine in reducing intragastric acidity in patients undergoing elective Caesarean Section. In: Torsoli A, Luchelli P E, Brimblecombe R W (ed) H_2 receptor antagonists in peptic ulcer disease and progress in histamine research. Excerpta Medica, Amsterdam, p 174-184
Howe J P, McGowan W A W, Moore J, McCaughey W, Dundee J W 1981 The placental transfer of cimetidine. Anaesthesia 36: 371-375
Johnston J R, McCaughey W, Moore J, Dundee J W 1982a Cimetidine as an oral antacid before elective caesarean section. Anaesthesia 37, in press
Johnston J R, McCaughey W, Moore J, Dundee J W 1982b A field trial of cimetidine as the oral antacid in obstetric anaesthesia. Anaesthesia 37, in press
McGowan W A W 1979 Safety of cimetidine in obstetric patients. Proceedings of the Royal Society of Medicine 72: 902-907
Mendelson C L 1946 The aspiration of stomach contents into the lungs during obstetric anaesthesia. American Journal of Obstetrics and Gynecology 52: 191-204
Moir D D 1980 Obstetric anaesthesia and analgesia, 2nd ed, Balliere Tindall, London, p 147
Nimmo W S, Wilson J, Prescott L F 1977 Gastric emptying. Further studies of gastric emptying during labour. Anaesthesia 32: 100-101

Discussion on Cimetidine and Other Conditions

Chairman: J. Alexander-Williams

QUESTIONS ON DR BOMMELAER'S PAPER

Mr Alexander-Williams. Dr Bommelaer, do you intend to continue the trial?

Dr Bommelaer. The trial will be continued until a statistically significant level is reached, and it will be stopped if we reach that.

Mr Alexander-Williams. Has anyone else done a study on the effects of cimetidine in pancreatitis? How many people have used cimetidine as part of their treatment for acute pancreatitis?

Dr Bommelaer. Some controlled studies have been done, especially one Spanish study which has shown that cimetidine improves the clinical outcome. So far, there is no reason for not using it.

Dr Baron. There were no deaths in Dr Bommelaer's 17 placebo patients. Is this low mortality usual in France, or does it reflect his special units? If so, the nil mortality means that no additional drugs are required beyond the basic conservative medical supportive care; any additional drugs could only increase the mortality — which is what happened!

Dr Bommelaer. That is the reason for continuing the study. Mortality for non-postsurgical acute pancreatitis in France is the same as everywhere else — about 15 per cent; for postsurgical pancreatitis the mortality is much higher — about 45 per cent. The low mortality rate in the placebo group is probably due to random distribution and, by continuing the study, there will probably be a higher mortality rate in that group.

Dr Pounder. If I heard correctly, one of the deaths in the cimetidine-treated group was a patient with coma of unknown origin. I suggest that perhaps that was a cimetidine-induced problem because changes in mental status have been detected in gravely ill patients.

Dr Bommelaer. I do not know about this particular patient.

QUESTIONS ON DR NORTHFIELD'S PAPER

Dr Russell. Has Dr Northfield any data on the composition of faecal fat before and after cimetidine and, in particular, of hydroxystearic acid?

221

Dr Northfield. We did not measure it, and I do not know of anyone who has done so.

Dr Wormsley. The problem of steatorrhoea in chronic pancreatitis and its theoretical treatment is delightful and exciting. In practice it is extremely disappointing for several reasons: first, because most pancreatic extracts do not contain much lipase and, second, most of them contain no co-lipase. However, it is the bile acid problem that presents most difficulties. This is because cimetidine alone does not suppress acid secretion satisfactorily. The upper small intestinal contents still remain acid in many patients with chronic pancreatitis. The acid can be buffered with antacids, but which antacids should we use — they all bind or precipitate bile salts? It is a problem I have found insuperable.

Dr Northfield. In our studies in the patients with pancreatic steatorrhoea all the jejunal samples that were aspirated had a pH greater than 6, instead of finding 40 per cent of them less than pH 5.

Professor Tytgat. Has Dr Northfield studied patients with mild or moderate pancreatic steatorrhoea of, say, 20 to 30 g, giving them only cimetidine? Does it make any difference whether the cimetidine is given 30 minutes before meals or with meals?

Dr Northfield. I know of no evidence that cimetidine given by itself improves faecal fat excretion. We have not tried giving cimetidine with a meal — but because there is a time lag of onset of gastric acid inhibition, it seems logical to give the drug 30 or 40 mins before a meal.

QUESTIONS ON DR MOORE'S PAPER

Mr Alexander-Williams. What about the use of cimetidine in anaesthesia other than obstetric anaesthesia? Does it have a theoretical value in emergency surgery for intestinal obstruction, for example?

Dr Moore. No, I would not give cimetidine intravenously in that specific situation, nor do I use it in emergency anaesthesia other than in obstetric situations. I believe, however, that in the United States there is increasing use of antacids, and in some cases of cimetidine, for non-obstetric patients coming for elective surgery.

Mr Keighley. Are there theoretical dangers if cimetidine were to be used more frequently in this country for elective surgical procedures? Dr Moore has already shown — and we all know — that cimetidine has a rapid effect on gastric pH. If an operation is being performed on the stomach that rise in gastric pH is invariably associated with colonisation of the stomach with pathogenic organisms and in our experience, there is a risk from infection.

Dr Moore. I cannot comment on the problem of possibly introducing enteritis into the adult patient, but we have studied this particular problem in the newborn infant. In the amount transferred from mother to infant cimetidine does not alter the pattern of gastric acidity in the newborn. This hazard may well occur with the adult patient given cimetidine.

Another point to make is that we are talking in this meeting of doing gastroscopies in patients. Regurgitation of gastric contents into the pharynx is a not uncommon complication of gastroscopy, particularly in a heavily sedated patient. Such patients are at risk of an aspiration pneumonitis, the severity of which may, as with the obstetric patient, be related to the acidity of the aspirate.

Section 6
SAFETY OF CIMETIDINE IN TREATMENT

26. Cimetidine and the cardiovascular system

Malcolm J. Boyce

Smith Kline and French Research Ltd, Welwyn Garden City, Hertfordshire, England

The various cardiovascular responses to histamine in laboratory animals are mediated via two classes of histamine receptor, designated H_1 and H_2 (Owen, 1977). Knowledge of the existence of cardiovascular H_2-receptors in animals naturally led to speculation that cimetidine, an H_2-receptor antagonist, might adversely affect cardiovascular function in patients treated with this novel drug. A number of in vitro and in vivo pharmacological studies have now been done to characterise human cardiovascular histamine receptors and to assess the effect of cimetidine on cardiovascular function in healthy subjects and patients. The purpose of this paper is to review these pharmacological studies and to interpret those adverse cardiovascular effects reported in association with cimetidine therapy in routine clinical practice.

CARDIOVASCULAR HISTAMINE RECEPTORS

Peripheral blood vessels

In healthy subjects, exogenous histamine causes dose-dependent flushing of the skin, increases in forearm blood flow and falls in systolic and diastolic blood pressure. Classical antihistamines, e.g. chlorpheniramine, mepyramine, which selectively inhibit histamine H_1-receptors, can completely prevent the responses to a small dose of histamine (Duff and Whelan, 1954). However, a combination of an H_1 and an H_2-antagonist is more effective than either antagonist alone in preventing the increase in forearm blood flow (Chipman and Glover, 1976), skin flushing and the falls in blood pressure (Boyce and Wareham, 1980; Boyce et al, 1980b; Figure 26.1) caused by a large dose of histamine.

Thus, human peripheral blood vessels contain both H_1- and H_2-receptors. Each class of receptor can contribute to the vasodilator responses to exogenous histamine.

Heart

Histamine causes increases in the rate (positive chronotropic response), contractility (positive inotropic response) and cyclic AMP content of the human myocardium in vitro (Wolleman and Papp, 1979; Gristwood et al, 1980;

227

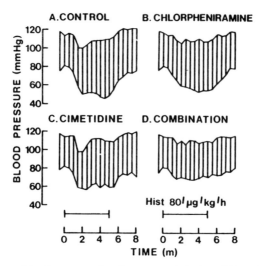

Figure 26.1 Effects on blood pressure of an intravenous infusion of histamine (80 μg/kg/hour for 5 min) (A) alone and in the presence of (B) chlorpheniramine 10 mg i.v., (C) cimetidine 200 mg i.v. and (D) chlorpheniramine plus cimetidine. Mean values, n = 6 healthy subjects (Boyce and Wareham, 1980).

Ginsburg et al, 1980). These responses are mimicked by specific H_2-receptor agonists, antagonised by cimetidine, but not propranolol or mepyramine, and are therefore mediated via H_2-receptors (Figure 26.2).

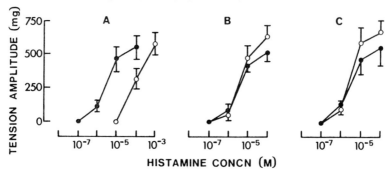

Figure 26.2 Effects of histamine on human right atrial contractility alone (●) and (n = 5) in the presence of (A) cimetidine 10^{-5} M (o), (B) propranolol 10^{-6} M (n = 4) or (C) mepyramine 10^{-7} M (n = 3). Mean ± s.e., n indicates sample numbers. (Redrawn with permission from Gristwood et al, 1980).

Exogenous histamine also causes positive chronotropic (Boyce and Wareham, 1980) and inotropic (Dargie et al, 1980) responses in healthy subjects. However, exogenous histamine can stimulate the heart in vivo both *directly,* at myocardial H_2-receptors, and *indirectly,* by reducing blood pressure and thereby activating the baroreceptor reflex or releasing adrenaline from the adrenal medullae (Boyce, Clancy, Dalton and Toseland, unpublished observations). H_1-receptors play a major role in these indirect effects.

Impromidine, a highly specific histamine H_2-receptor agonist, recently developed for use in man (Durant et al, 1978), is a pharmacological tool with which to identify cardiovascular H_2-receptors, particularly those in the myocardium. Healthy subjects have been studied by non-invasive methods, including impedance cardiography to assess left ventricular function. Impromidine causes dose-dependent skin flushing, falls in diastolic blood pressure and peripheral resistance and increases in cardiac rate, contractility and output. Systolic pressure is unaffected. Cimetidine antagonises the various responses to impromidine (Boyce and Wareham, 1980; Boyce et al, 1980a; Boyce et al, 1981; Figure 26.3).

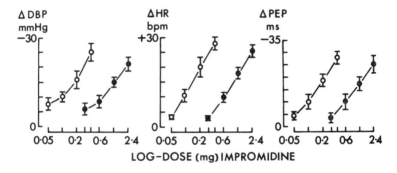

LOG–DOSE (mg) IMPROMIDINE

Figure 26.3 Effects of impromidine on diastolic blood pressure (DBP), heart rate (HR) and pre-ejection period (PEP) in the presence of (o) placebo and (●) cimetidine, 400 mg q.d.s. by mouth for one week. Mean ± sem; n = 6 healthy subjects. Shortening of PEP reflects a positive inotropic response. Cimetidine antagonises the response to impromidine displacing the placebo dose-response curves to the right. However, cardiovascular function, assessed at rest and during exercise prior to administration of impromidine, was unaffected by cimetidine (Boyce et al, 1981).

These results, which are similar to those obtained in laboratory animals, are consistent with the presence of H_2-receptors in the peripheral blood vessels and myocardium of man. Stimulation of H_2-receptors in the peripheral vasculature causes vasodilatation. Stimulation of cardiac H_2-receptors causes positive chronotropic and inotropic responses. Cimetidine is a competitive antagonist at cardiovascular H_2-receptor sites. The distribution and effects of stimulation of cardiovascular histamine receptors in man are summarised in Table 26.1.

Table 26.1. Stimulation of cardiovascular histamine receptors in man.

	Effect	Receptor
Peripheral blood vessels	vasodilatation	H_1 and H_2
Heart:		
sinus rate	increase	H_2
contractility	increase	H_2
cyclic AMP	increase	H_2

CIMETIDINE AND CARDIOVASCULAR FUNCTION — PHARMACOLOGICAL STUDIES

Various pharmacological studies have been carried out in healthy subjects and patients to assess whether cimetidine, oral or intravenous, can intrinsically affect cardiovascular function.

Oral cimetidine

In placebo-controlled studies in healthy subjects, cimetidine 1.6 g/day for one week did not affect supine blood pressure, the electrocardiogram or left ventricular function, assessed non-invasively by systolic time intervals, apex cardiography or impedance cardiography (Barbat and Warrington, 1981; Boyce et al, 1981). Barbat and Warrington (1981) reported that supine heart rate was slightly (3.3 beats/min) but significantly lower during cimetidine treatment whereas others found no differences between cimetidine and placebo for heart rates at rest, supine or standing (Boyce et al, 1981), and during or recovery from, exercise (Warburton et al, 1979; Boyce et al, 1981). The increase in systolic blood pressure, which normally occurs with exercise, was also unaffected by cimetidine.

In a placebo-controlled study of 19 out-patients in symptomatic remission from peptic ulcer disease, some of whom had pre-existing cardiovascular disease, cimetidine 1.6 g/day for one month did not affect blood pressure, at rest or during exercise, or left ventricular function, assessed by echocardiography. Neither did cimetidine affect heart rate at rest, during exercise nor during 24 hour monitoring of the ambulatory electrocardiogram (Saltissi et al, 1981; Figures 26.4-26.6).

In general, these studies show that oral cimetidine, at doses of up to 1.6 g/day and capable of antagonising basal and stimulated gastric acid secretion, lacks effect on cardiovascular function at rest and during exercise. Such a dose of cimetidine, however, substantially antagonised the cardiovascular responses to impromidine (Boyce et al, 1981; Figure 26.3), which would suggest that histamine H_2-receptors in the cardiovascular system, unlike those in the stomach, do not have a major physiological role.

Intravenous cimetidine

The cardiovascular effects of single intravenous doses of cimetidine have been assessed by non-invasive methods in healthy subjects, at doses varying from 200 to 800 mg, and by invasive methods in patients at doses of up to 400 mg. The results have been variable and dependent on the dose of cimetidine, its rate of administration and the state of health of the subject.

Healthy subjects. 200 mg cimetidine, the conventional intravenous dose in clinical practice, had no effect on blood pressure, heart rate or left ventricular function in healthy subjects (Gianrossi et al, 1979; Barbat and Warrington, 1981). The rate of administration of cimetidine in the first study was not reported; cimetidine was infused over five minutes in the latter study.

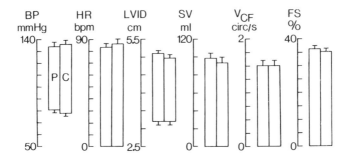

Figure 26.4 Cimetidine (C), 400 mg q.d.s. by mouth for 4 weeks did not significantly affect blood pressure (BP), heart rate (HR) and left ventricular function at rest. Left ventricular internal dimensions (LVID), stroke volume (SV), circumferential fibre shortening (V_{CF}) and fractional shortening (FS) were measured by echocardiography. Means, sem; n = 19 patients. P = placebo (drawn from data of Saltissi et al, 1981).

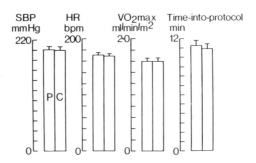

Figure 26.5 Maximal treadmill-exercise test variables (means, sem; n = 19 patients) after oral cimetidine (C) 400 mg q.d.s. or placebo (P) for four weeks. There were no significant differences between treatments for systolic blood pressure (SBP), heart rate (HR), maximal oxygen uptake (VO_2 max) and time-into-exercise protocol (drawn from data of Saltissi et al, 1981).

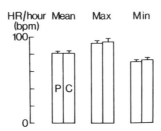

Figure 26.6 Lack of effect of oral cimetidine (C) 400 mg q.d.s. for four weeks on minimum, maximum and mean hourly ambulatory heart rates. Mean values, sem; n = 19 patients. P = placebo (drawn from data of Saltissi et al, 1981).

When healthy subjects (mean weight 70 kg) were given a large dose (800 mg) of intravenous cimetidine over one minute, there were increases in heart rate and left ventricular ejection time, corrected for heart rate, and shortening of the pre-ejection period, derived from the externally recorded systolic time intervals. Blood pressure was unaffected. The responses to cimetidine were acute in onset and of 15–20 minutes duration (Boyce, 1981; Figure 26.7).

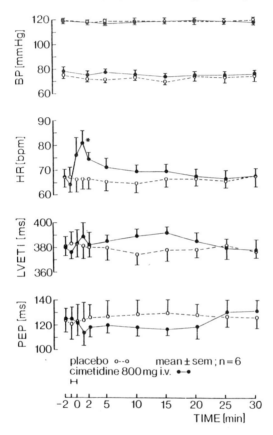

Figure 26.7   Effects of a large dose (800 mg) of intravenous cimetidine on blood pressure (BP), heart rate (HR), left ventricular ejection time (LVET), corrected for HR, and pre-ejection period (PEP). Means, ± sem; n = six healthy subjects. *p = < 0.05; analysis of variance. PEP and LVET were derived from external recordings of the carotid pulse, second heart sound and the ECG (Boyce, 1981).

200 and 400 mg cimetidine given in a similar manner to the same group of subjects showed that the changes in heart rate and systolic time intervals observed in the first study were dose-dependent (Boyce, 1981). Responses to 200 mg cimetidine were very slight and of few minutes duration. Neither the 200 nor 400 mg dose affected blood pressure. In the two studies, changes in heart rate with dose were linear with an increase of approximately 4 beats/minute/200 mg cimetidine.

These transient heart rate and systolic time interval responses, which are not consistent with H_2-receptor blockade, can be interpreted with the aid of data from animal studies. Intravenous bolus injections of cimetidine (doses 2.52, 8.32 and 25.20 mg/kg) caused transient, dose-dependent falls in blood pressure and increases in blood flow in anaesthetised animals (Brimblecombe and Duncan, 1977; Figure 26.8).

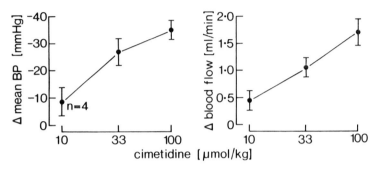

Figure 26.8   Intravenous bolus injections of cimetidine cause dose-dependent falls in blood pressure and increases in blood flow in anaesthetised rats (drawn from data of Brimblecombe and Duncan, 1977).

Thus, vasodilatation occurred in animals with doses of cimetidine equivalent on a mg/kg basis to those given to the healthy subjects. Blood pressure was maintained in healthy man probably as a consequence of activation of the baroreceptor reflex, which would be impaired in anaesthetised animals. The increase in heart rate and minor changes in the systolic time intervals in healthy subjects probably represent indirect myocardial stimulation. Adrenaline released from the adrenal medullae, may contribute to the cardiovascular responses to the large dose (800 mg) of cimetidine (Boyce, Dalton and Toseland, unpublished observations).

Large doses of cimetidine when given slowly by intravenous infusion do not affect cardiovascular function in anaesthetised animals (Brimblecombe and Duncan, 1977). Similarly, in healthy subjects the responses to a very rapid intravenous injection of 400 mg cimetidine were avoided by infusion over ten minutes (Boyce, 1981).

Patients. Heart rate, sinus node function and atrioventricular conduction were assessed in ten patients, three with sick sinus syndrome, before and 30 minutes after intravenous infusion of 300 mg cimetidine. There were no significant differences (Engel and Luck, 1979).

Samuel and Dundee (1979) assessed the cardiovascular effects of a rapid, atrial injection of 400 mg cimetidine in ten patients requiring intermittent positive pressure ventilation on an intensive care unit. Heart rate, mean blood pressure and cardiac output were measured before and from five minutes after dosing. There were essentially no differences between control and post dosing values in nine patients. In one patient, however, there were falls in blood pressure and cardiac output of approximately 20 and 30 per cent, respectively, after cimetidine compared with control values. Heart rate was unaffected.

Lee et al (1981) reported acute but transient (less than ten minutes) falls in systemic and pulmonary arterial pressure in systole and diastole, systemic vascular resistance and total pulmonary resistance in patients given 400 mg cimetidine as a rapid intravenous injection. Falls were greater in a group of patients with chronic obstructive airways disease and pulmonary hypertension than in a group with normal lung function. Falls in pressure were accompanied by increases in heart rate. This study and that of Samuel and Dundee (1979) will be discussed in the next section.

CIMETIDINE AND CARDIOVASCULAR FUNCTION IN ROUTINE CLINICAL PRACTICE

Data from various sources (Gifford et al, 1980; Davis et al, 1980; Register of Adverse Reactions, U.K. Committee of Safety of Medicines (CSM), September, 1980) show the reported incidence of adverse cardiovascular events in association with cimetidine therapy in routine clinical practice to be low, approximately 0.1–1.0 per 10 000 patients treated. Spontaneous reports of adverse events do not appear to follow any clearly discernible pattern (Rowley-Jones et al, 1980). Isolated case reports of disturbances of heart rate and rhythm or hypotension in association with cimetidine therapy in a small number of patients have been published. In general, these published reports appear to represent two groups of patients.

In the first group, bradycardia occurred hours to weeks after dosing with either oral or intravenous cimetidine, usually oral, and was slow to recover on cimetidine withdrawal (Reding et al, 1977; Bournerias et al, 1978; Jefferys and Vale, 1978; Luciano et al, 1978; Stimmesse et al, 1978). All but one had suffered gastro-intestinal haemorrhage or had pre-existing disease, e.g. renal failure, cirrhosis. Subsequent rechallenge of one patient with cimetidine was associated with a recurrence of bradycardia (Jefferys and Vale, 1978), a finding which is consistent with an adverse drug-related effect. In other instances, however, assessment of specific culpability is more difficult. For instance when cimetidine was restarted at a lower dose after haemodialysis of a patient with renal failure, heart rate remained normal (Stimmesse et al, 1978); in the patient with bradycardia reported by Ligumsky et al (1978), cimetidine was associated with reversal of a tachyarrhythmia. A total of nine patients with bradycardia in association with cimetidine therapy were reported to the CSM between Nov. 1976 and Sept. 1980. The authors of published reports of bradycardia have postulated that bradycardia was a consequence of myocardial H_2-receptor blockade by cimetidine. Even if in some of these patients cimetidine were responsible for bradycardia, its rarity and the general lack of experimental evidence that myocardial H_2-receptors serve a major physiological role do not favour such a hypothesis.

In the second group, hypotension or more serious arrhythmias followed administration of intravenous cimetidine, usually at high dose and/or by bolus injection to ill patients (Mahon and Kolton, 1978; Cohen et al, 1979; Shaw et al, 1980).

Two patients on an intensive care unit became abruptly hypotensive on several occasions following a large dose (600 mg) of cimetidine given intravenously over 4-5 minutes (Mahon and Kolton, 1978). Hypotension lasted 5-25 minutes. Cimetidine 300 mg was associated with falls in blood pressure which were smaller in magnitude and of shorter duration. Heart rate did not change during episodes of hypotension. Cimetidine did not induce hypotension in 50-60 other patients requiring intensive care. Mahon and Kolton (1978) were of the opinion that hypotension could be avoided in intensive care patients by giving cimetidine by infusion rather than by injection.

Cohen et al (1979) reported two patients with asystole following 400 mg of intravenous cimetidine. One had been hypotensive following a previous dose of intravenous cimetidine. Autopsy of this patient showed polyarteritis nodosa involving the heart as well as other organs. The other patient was anuric and septicaemic, from which he eventually died, and had been resuscitated from asystole prior to the start of cimetidine therapy. A further three patients with cardiac arrest following intravenous cimetidine, given over 1-2 minutes in the post-operative period, have recently been reported (Shaw et al, 1980). Asystole occurred in one of these patients after 150 mg of a 200 mg dose. She was known to suffer from ischaemic heart disease, hypertension and episodes of supraventricular tachycardia. The interval between administration of cimetidine and asystole in the other two patients was ten minutes and one hour, respectively.

There is good circumstantial evidence in some but not all of this second group of case reports to implicate cimetidine as the cause of the adverse event. Most patients were ill, had pre-existing cardiovascular malfunction or severe renal impairment and were given intravenous cimetidine at high dosage and/or by bolus injection. The acute hypotensive episodes in these patients and those of Samuel and Dundee (1979) and Lee et al (1981) are consistent with the intrinsic vasodilator activity of intravenous cimetidine discussed previously. Unlike healthy subjects, ill patients and those with cardiovascular malfunction may not be able to maintain blood pressure following a bolus injection of cimetidine. Asystole could be a consequence of acute hypotension in the ill patient who has already received a number of other drugs.

Four years of clinical experience with cimetidine and the pharmacological studies in healthy subjects indicate that 200 mg cimetidine, the conventional intravenous dose, is unlikely to cause adverse cardiovascular effects if given by bolus injection to patients with normal cardiovascular function. In patients with cardiovascular malfunction or if high dosage is considered essential, intravenous cimetidine should be given more slowly, e.g. 200-400 mg over 5-10 minutes or ideally by continuous infusion. Dosage must be reduced in patients with renal failure since the kidney is the principal route of excretion of cimetidine.

CONCLUSIONS

Although pharmacological studies in man show that the peripheral blood vessels and heart possess histamine H_2-receptors, to date there is no real evidence that these receptors serve a physiological role. The estimated incidence of untoward cardiovascular events in association with the use of cimetidine in routine clinical practice is low. Oral cimetidine has been associated rarely with bradycardia but a causal role on the available evidence remains unproven. Intravenous cimetidine has the potential to reduce blood pressure if given rapidly, particularly at high dosage to ill patients or those with cardiovascular malfunction. Depressor activity of intravenous cimetidine, which is unlikely to be a consequence of H_2-receptor blockade, can be avoided by attention to dose and its rate of administration.

REFERENCES

Barbat J, Warrington S J 1981 Effects of cimetidine and ranitidine on some non-invasive indices of cardiac function. British Journal of Clinical Pharmacology 72(1): 131P
Bournerias F, Ganeval D, Danan G 1978 Trouble du rythme cardiaque mortel au cours d'un traitement par la cimetidine. Nouvelle Presse Médicale 7: 2069
Boyce M J 1981 Cardiovascular effects of intravenous cimetidine. British Journal of Clinical Pharmacology (in press)
Boyce M J, Wareham K 1980 Histamine H_1 and H_2-receptors in the cardiovascular system of man. In: Torsoli A, Lucchelli P E, Brimblecombe R W (ed) H_2-antagonists. Excerpta Medica, Amsterdam, p 280-293
Boyce M J, Balasubramanian V, Wareham K 1980a Cardiovascular effects in man of impromidine, a novel and specific histamine H_2-receptor agonist. British Journal of Pharmacology 70: 157-158P
Boyce M J, Owen D A A, Wareham K 1980b Modification of cardiovascular effects of histamine infusions in man by chlorpheniramine and cimetidine. British Journal of Pharmacology 70: 110P
Boyce M J, Wareham K, Balasubramanian V 1981 Oral cimetidine antagonises cardio-vascular histamine H_2-receptors but does not affect normal cardiovascular function. Clinical Science 60: 28P
Brimblecombe R W, Duncan W A M 1977 The relevance to man of pre-clinical data for cimetidine. In: Burland W L, Simkins M A (ed) Cimetidine. Excerpta Medica, Amsterdam, p 54-65
Chipman P, Glover W E 1976 Histamine H_2-receptors in the human peripheral circulation. British Journal of Pharmacology 56: 494-496
Cohen J, Weetman A P, Dargie H J, Krikler D M 1979 Life-threatening arrhythmias and intravenous cimetidine. British Medical Journal 2: 768
Dargie H J, Watkins J, Dollery C T, Brown M, Krikler D M 1980 Myocardial histamine type 2 receptors. British Heart Journal 43: 113-114
Davis T G, Pickett D L, Schlosser J H 1980 Evaluation of a worldwide spontaneous reporting system with cimetidine. Journal of the American Medical Association 243: 1912-1914
Duff F, Whelan R F 1954 The effects of antihistamine substances on the response to histamine on the blood vessels of the human forearm. British Journal of Pharmacology 9: 413-418
Durant G J, Duncan W A, Ganellin C R, Parsons M E, Blakemore R C, Rasmussen A C 1978 Impromidine (SK&F 92676) is a very potent and specific agonist for histamine H_2-receptors. Nature (London) 276: 403-404
Engel T R, Luck J C 1979 Histamine H_2-receptor antagonism by cimetidine and sinus node function. New England Journal of Medicine 301: 591-592
Gianrossi R, Azzolini A, Livi S, Nizzo M C 1979 Effects of cimetidine on systolic time intervals. Clinical Pharmacology and Therapeutics 7: 55
Gifford L M, Aeugle M E, Myerson R M, Tannenbaum P J 1980 Cimetidine postmarket outpatient surveillance program. Journal of the American Medical Association 243: 1532-1533

Ginsburg R, Bristow M R, Stinson E B, Harrison D C 1980 Histamine receptors in the human heart. Life Sciences 26: 2245-2249

Gristwood R W, Lincoln J C R, Owen D A A 1980 Effects of histamine on human isolated heart muscle: Comparison with effects of noradrenaline. Journal of Pharmacy and Pharmacology 32: 145

Jefferys D B, Vale J A 1978 Cimetidine and bradycardia. Lancet 1: 828

Lee P K, Lai C L, Lok A S F, Tse T F, Lai K N, Chow S F, Lam K C 1981 Haemodynamic responses to intravenous cimetidine in subjects with normal lung function and in subjects with chronic airway obstruction. British Journal of Clinical Pharmacology 11: 339-343

Ligumsky M, Schochina M, Rachmilewitz D 1978 Cimetidine and arrhythmia suppression. Annals of Internal Medicine 89: 1008

Luciano J J, Theodorou-Touchais A M, Souteyrand P 1978 Cimetidine: trouble du rythme cardiaque au cours d'un traitement. Nouvelle Presse Médicale 7: 4049

Mahon W A, Kolton M 1978 Hypotension after intravenous cimetidine. Lancet 1: 828

Owen D A A 1977 Histamine receptors in the cardiovascular system. General Pharmacology 8: 141-156

Reding P, Devroede C, Barbier P 1977 Bradycardia after cimetidine. Lancet 2: 1227

Rowley-Jones D, Flind A C, Backhouse J N 1980 The safety of cimetidine: a continuing assessment. In: Dresse A, Barbier F, Harvengt C, Tijtgat G N (eds) Cimetidine. Excerpta Medica, Amsterdam, p 78-88

Saltissi S, Crowther A, Byrne C, Coltart D J 1981 The effects of chronic oral cimetidine therapy on the cardiovascular system in man. British Journal of Clinical Pharmacology 11: 497-503

Samuel I O, Dundee J W 1979 Influence of cimetidine on cardiovascular parameters in man. Journal of the Royal Society of Medicine 72: 889-901

Shaw R G, Mashford M L, Desmond P V 1980 Cardiac arrest after intravenous injection of cimetidine. Medical Journal of Australia 2: 629-630

Stimmesse B, Daoudal P, Neidhardt A 1978 Bradycardie au cours d'un traitement par cimetidine. Nouvelle Presse Médicale 7: 4233

Warburton S, Opie L H, Kennelly B M, Müller F O 1979 Does cimetidine alter the cardiac response to exercise and propranolol? South African Medical Journal 55: 1125-1127

Wolleman M, Papp J G 1979 Blockade by cimetidine of the effects of histamine on adenylate cyclase activity, spontaneous rate and contractility in developing pre-natal heart. Agents Actions 9: 29-30

27. Cimetidine and the immune system

Margaret R. Vickers

Smith Kline and French Research Ltd, Welwyn Garden City, Hertfordshire, England

Histamine is traditionally regarded as a mediator of inflammation and immediate hypersensitivity. These effects are mediated via H_1-receptor stimulation. Recently, interest has focused on the ability of histamine to modulate, usually via an inhibitory action, the functions of leucocytes involved in immune responses. Many of the inhibitory actions of histamine can be partially reversed by burimamide, metiamide and cimetidine, suggesting that H_2-receptors are involved. If endogenous histamine suppresses immune responses in vivo then H_2-antagonists, by blocking this effect, may stimulate immune responses. Cimetidine might then be potentially harmful for hypersensitive patients, those with transplants and those predisposed to auto-immune diseases. In contrast, cimetidine might prove beneficial for patients with depressed immune responses.

In this chapter the effects of histamine and cimetidine, alone and in combination, on some in vitro assays of lymphocyte and granulocyte function are described and the evidence for the involvement of H_2-receptors is examined. The problems of showing a modulatory role for histamine or cimetidine in in vivo models are discussed and the clinical reports of the influence of cimetidine on immunological reactivity in man are reviewed.

CELL FUNCTION IN VITRO

Lymphocyte proliferation

Histamine, in high concentrations (10^{-5}M to 10^{-3}M), inhibits T lymphocyte proliferation induced by antigens and mitogens. In lower concentrations (10^{-9}M to 10^{-6}M), histamine can also enhance the response to sub-optimal mitogenic stimulation. It was initially claimed that the H_2-antagonists, burimamide and metiamide, could reverse the inhibitory effects of histamine (Artis and Jones, 1975) but more recent work shows that the H_2-antagonists *alone* affect proliferation (Brostoff et al, 1980). We find that H_2-antagonists, in concentrations from 10^{-5}M to 10^{-3}M, inhibit proliferation of human lymphocytes induced by phytohaemagglutinin (PHA). These concentrations are far in excess of the blood levels achieved in man during a normal course of cimetidine and this observation may therefore have no clinical relevance. It does, however, indicate

238

that H_2-antagonism reduces rather than stimulates proliferation in vitro. Since the lymphocyte preparation used is contaminated with basophils, and since antigens and mitogens release histamine, the H_2-antagonists may be blocking a stimulation of proliferation induced by endogenous histamine. In contrast to the inhibitory effects of H_2-antagonists in general, cimetidine and structurally related compounds, irrespective of their H_2-antagonist potency, also enhance lymphocyte proliferation. Enhancement of a sub-optimal PHA response is obtained with 10^{-7}M to 10^{-5}M cimetidine, concentrations which would be reached in the blood during cimetidine therapy. The degree of enhancement varies considerably from experiment to experiment, but, in some experiments, increases of more than 250 per cent have been observed. Thus, it appears that cimetidine has immunostimulatory activity unrelated to its H_2-antagonist activity and this may explain the apparent reversal of some of the inhibitory actions of histamine in poorly controlled experiments. It also implies that immunological changes induced by cimetidine would not necessarily be seen with other H_2-antagonists.

Lymphokine production

Histamine, added to in vitro cultures, suppresses the production of macrophage migration inhibitory factor (MIF) by guinea pig lymph node cells (Rocklin, 1976) and of leucocyte migration inhibitory factor (LIF) by human peripheral blood mononuclear cells (PBMC) (Rigal et al, 1979). These effects are partially blocked by burimamide and metiamide but there is no evidence to support interaction at an H_2-receptor. (To claim competitive antagonism at an H_2-receptor, parallel, dose-related displacements of a histamine dose-response curve by H_2-antagonists must be shown.) No independent action of cimetidine on lymphokine production has been demonstrated.

T cell mediated cytolysis

Histamine inhibits the effector function of cytolytic T lymphocytes obtained from alloimmunised mice (Plaut et al, 1975). The inhibition appears to be via H_2-receptor stimulation; H_2-agonists but not H_1-agonists inhibit cytolysis and the effect of histamine can be reversed by H_2-antagonists in a manner suggesting competitive inhibition. If the cytolytic T lymphocytes are generated in vitro, however, the induction, but not the effector function, of the cells is inhibited by histamine (Schwartz et al, 1980). The receptor specificity of this effect has not been clearly defined. There is some evidence that cimetidine enhances murine cell-mediated cytotoxicity in vitro (Gifford et al, 1980) but the cells affected and the involvement of H_2-receptors require further study.

Antibody production

Histamine does not affect the proliferation of B lymphocytes but is thought to inhibit their production of antibody. Fallah et al report that histamine reduces the number of mouse spleen cells producing antibody to sheep erythrocytes in vitro.

However the effect is not dose related and is also observed in background control cultures not stimulated by antigen, suggesting some non-specific action of histamine. Two studies describe the effect of histamine on IgG antibody synthesis by human PBMC stimulated by pokeweed mitogen (PWM). In one report, histamine reduces IgG synthesis (Rocklin and Lima, 1980), but another shows that an H_1-agonist, but not histamine or an H_2-agonist, decreases IgG synthesis (Lai et al, 1980). In our experiments histamine does not inhibit antibody production to SRBC by mouse spleen cells or to PWM by human PBMC. At high concentrations, 10^{-4}M to 10^{-3}M, histamine enhances the PWM response in some individuals. Cimetidine is without effect on the production of antibody to SRBC by mouse spleen cells.

Mediator release from granulocytes
The release of inflammatory mediators from basophils, mast cells and neutrophils is inhibited by histamine. Antigen-induced, IgE-mediated, release of histamine from sensitised human basophils is reduced by histamine and this effect is blocked by burimamide and metiamide in a manner consistent with competitive inhibition at an H_2-receptor (Lichtenstein and Gillespie, 1975). Histamine release from sensitised guinea-pig mast cells, challenged in vitro with antigen, is increased by cimetidine (Dulabh and Vickers, 1978). This is thought to reflect blockade of a histamine, H_2-receptor mediated, feedback inhibition of histamine release. In this system, however, effects on the metabolism or uptake of histamine could also account for the observed increase in extracellular histamine. Lysosomal enzyme release from neutrophils is inhibited by histamine (Busse and Sosman, 1976). The effect of histamine is reversed by metiamide and cimetidine but H_2-receptor antagonism has not been demonstrated.

IMMUNE RESPONSES IN VIVO

Histamine releasing cells participate in most immunological reactions and large amounts of histamine are released by antigen, complement products and lymphocyte derived factors. However, there are few reports describing the effects of histamine on in vivo immune responses in animals. This may reflect the difficulty of analysing the influence of histamine on complex systems where opposing effects could occur. For example, histamine might mediate inflammatory activity via H_1-receptor stimulation and suppressive activity via H_2-receptor stimulation. If so, this may be revealed by treatment with specific histamine antagonists. It is, however, difficult to demonstrate competitive inhibition in vivo and we should therefore be cautious in attributing an in vivo effect of cimetidine to a blockage of the action of histamine.

Delayed hypersensitivity
The expression of delayed hypersensitivity responses is inhibited to a small extent by histamine in the guinea pig (Rocklin, 1976) and the mouse (Schwartz and

Gershon 1978). This may result from an inhibition of lymphokine production or from effects on the vascular system. H_2-antagonists block the inhibition induced by histamine more effectively than do H_1-antagonists. However, H_2-antagonists alone do not enhance either the induction or expression of delayed hypersensitivity responses in the guinea-pig, and in the mouse there is one report that metiamide inhibits the expression of delayed hypersensitivity (Schwartz et al, 1977). These data suggest that endogenous histamine is not an important modulator of delayed hypersensitivity. Further, there is no evidence that cimetidine stimulates delayed hypersensitivity by a mechanism which does not involve H_2-receptors.

Graft survival
Basophils accumulate during allograft rejection and an increase in tissue histamine levels is reported prior to rejection of kidney grafts in man (Moore et al, 1971). Some studies describe an increase in graft survival after treatment with H_1-antagonists (Conway et al, 1953; Boyd and Smith 1960) while others report no effect (Woodruff and Boswell, 1955; Barnes, 1963). Cimetidine does not affect skin allograft survival in the mouse (Festen et al, 1980) but is reported to decrease the survival time of kidney transplants in the dog (Zamitt and Toledo-Pereyra, 1979). Goodwin reports that cimetidine increases the proportion of male skin isografts surviving on female A/J mice. However, in C3H mice, in which male to female grafts normally survive indefinitely, metiamide and cimetidine increase the number of grafts rejected. It is possible that cimetidine promotes rejection only if there is a fine balance between cell-mediated and humoral responses or if the antigenic disparity between host and graft is minimal.

Antibody production
Histamine has no consistent effect on antibody production to SRBC in the mouse in vivo. In our experiments, with doses greater than 100 μmol/kg, small inhibitory effects are observed but in less than one in four experiments. Cimetidine has no effect on antibody production in this system.

Immediate hypersensitivity
Histamine, released from sensitised mast cells and basophils, is an important mediator of immediate hypersensitivity. Stimulation of H_1-receptors produces contraction of respiratory smooth muscle, increases in vascular permeability and dilation of arterioles. However H_2-receptors have also been identified on respiratory smooth muscle and these generally mediate relaxation (Chakrin and Krell, 1980). This finding, combined with the in vitro evidence for an H_2-receptor mediated negative feedback of histamine release, indicates that H_2-antagonists might exacerbate immediate hypersensitivity responses. However, in vivo, in the monkey and the dog, H_2-antagonists do not potentiate an anaphylactic reaction and in the guinea-pig bronchoconstriction is exacerbated only by doses of cimetidine far in excess of those used therapeutically (Chakrin and Krell, 1980).

MODULATION OF REGULATORY CELL FUNCTION

The immune system is controlled by a series of regulatory loops with well defined sub-populations of T lymphocytes helping or suppressing the ability of other cells to respond to antigen. In some situations regulatory signals may be mediated via soluble factors released from lymphocytes. Cells which suppress various immune responses bind to conjugates of histamine and rabbit serum albumin (Shearer et al, 1974; Tartakovsky et al, 1979) and thus it is suggested that histamine might influence the function of T suppressor cells. Depending on the system used, histamine appears to activate, inhibit, or fail to affect T suppressor cell activity. Histamine activates guinea-pig and human suppressor lymphocytes, causing the release of a soluble suppressor factor (Rocklin et al, 1979, 1980). This factor suppresses T lymphocyte proliferation and the production of lymphokines. There is also one report (Hébert et al, 1980) which suggests that histamine activates suppressor T cells in man which suppress T cell proliferation in the absence of a soluble factor. However, other workers are unable to confirm the latter observation (Gerosa et al, 1980). In systems where histamine does appear to induce suppressor cell activity there is no sound evidence regarding the receptor specificity of the effect. Nevertheless, it is generally accepted that H_2-receptors are involved and the possibility that cimetidine might block suppressor cell activity is currently receiving much attention. Osband et al (1979) claim that T suppressor cell activity induced by Concanavalin A (Con A) is blocked by cimetidine. They postulate that Con A does not have a direct effect but causes the release of histamine from basophils which then activates T suppressor cells. Cimetidine would then compete with histamine for H_2-receptors on T suppressor cells. In contrast, Stranegaard reports that histamine inhibits the activation of T suppressor cells induced by Con A. The reason for this discrepancy is not clear. Until further studies are performed, however, the claim that antigen-induced T suppressor cell activation in vivo is mediated via histamine, and is reversible by cimetidine, must be regarded with extreme caution.

EXPERIMENTAL DATA — SUMMARY AND CONCLUSIONS

There is evidence that histamine inhibits some immune cell functions in vitro in man, mouse and guinea-pig. The mechanisms of inhibition are not clear and the receptor specificity of the effects is not well defined. Further, in some systems histamine can also enhance immunological reactivity. There is, therefore, little to suggest that H_2-receptor antagonism would enhance immune responses. In general the data from in vivo studies support this conclusion. It may be important, however, to distinguish between situations where all the components of the immune system are functioning correctly and those where there is some abnormality in cell function, particularly in regulatory cell function. If histamine does influence T suppressor cell activity, and if this effect is H_2-receptor mediated, then cimetidine may cause changes in immune function in some disease states. It is also possible that cimetidine has some immunostimulatory properties unrelated to its H_2-antagonist activity.

CLINICAL STUDIES

In the United Kingdom alone over one million people have now received cimetidine and few reports of adverse effects associated with the immune system have been received. In view of the presumed effects of cimetidine on suppressor cell function it is appropriate to consider three groups of patients: those whose immune system is functioning normally, those in whom immunostimulation might be harmful and those in whom immunostimulation might be beneficial.

In several controlled studies, immunological functions have been examined, in patients with gastro-intestinal disorders and in healthy volunteers, before, during and after a course of cimetidine.

Table 27.1 Immunological studies after cimetidine therapy

	Condition of patients	n	Dose cimetidine g/day	Responses measured	Observations
McGregor et al, 1977	Dyspepsia Healthy	12 5	1 (1 month)	Lymphocyte migration Auto AB, Serum Ig	No alteration
de Pauw et al, 1977	ZE syndrome	1	2 (16 months)	Lymphocyte counts Lymphocyte transformation	No immunological abnormalities detected
		1	0.8 (12 months)	Cutaneous DTH Auto AB, Serum Ig	
André et al, 1978	Duodenal ulcer	10	1 (1 month)	Serum Ig	Small decrease (N.S.) in IgA, IgM, IgG, in some patients
Festen et al, 1980	Peptic ulcer	9	1.6 (37 days)	Lymphocyte counts Lymphocyte transformation	No change due to cimetidine
	Healthy	11		Cutaneous DTH AB levels	
Avella et al, 1978	Duodenal ulcer Healthy	8 8	1.2 (6 weeks)	Cutaneous DTH	Augmentation

N.S. — non-significant

Four of the five reports show no changes in immune responsiveness attributable to cimetidine in 'immunologically normal' subjects. In contrast, the observations of Avella et al (1978) suggest that cimetidine augments delayed cutaneous reactions. Their findings are frequently cited as evidence that histamine activates T suppressor cells in vivo via H_2-receptors, while the other studies are rarely quoted. The main difference between the Avella work and that of other groups is the timing of the tests for immune function. In the Avella study the 'before treatment' skin test was read on day 1 and day 2 of cimetidine treatment and the 'on treatment' tests were made after cimetidine had been discontinued. In these circumstances, the increased cutaneous delayed hypersensitivity responses are more likely to reflect a transient state of hypersensitivity to histamine following withdrawal of cimetidine than an effect on T suppressor cell function. Hence in healthy subjects there is no reason to expect that cimetidine will stimulate immunological reactivity.

Immunostimulation should be avoided in patients receiving transplants, in hypersensitive subjects and in those predisposed to auto-immune diseases. Renal transplant patients are often given cimetidine to prevent upper gastro-intestinal haemorrhage. Primack (1978) reports two irreversible rejection episodes which he attributes to cimetidine. However, controlled studies (Jones et al, 1978) show that cimetidine does not influence the function of the graft or increase the number or severity of rejection episodes. This finding is not surprising in view of the heavy immuno-suppressive therapy also prescribed for these patients. However, in atopics, not receiving any suppressive drugs, cimetidine does not exacerbate hypersensitivity responses (Wolfe et al, 1979), and in some asthmatics may even augment the beneficial effects of H_1-antagonists (Eiser et al, 1978). In extremely rare cases the onset of arthritis or arthralgia appears to be associated with cimetidine therapy (Khong and Rooney, 1980). Other reports suggest that patients with arthritis improve while taking cimetidine (Wallach et al, 1979), a finding consistent with the effect of cimetidine in animal models of arthritis (Al-Haboubi and Zeitlin, 1979). It may, however, be advisable to use cimetidine with caution in patients with a family history of autoimmune disease.

The only consistent clinical effects of cimetidine on immune responses are in immunodepressed patients. Cimetidine may help to restore immunocompetence and appears to act preferentially on cell-mediated responses. This would be consistent with the observations made in animal models. Two reports describe a reversal of tolerance to dinitrochlorobenzene after treatment with cimetidine (Daman and Rosenberg, 1977; Breuillard and Szapiro, 1978). In patients with chronic mucocutaneous candidiasis (Jorizzo et al, 1980) or Crohn's disease (Bicks and Rosenberg, 1980), skin reactivity to common antigens improves after cimetidine therapy. Lymphokine production also increases in the candidiasis patients but there is no significant change in proliferative responses. Perhaps the most interesting observation is the dramatic remission of symptoms in patients with herpes virus infections treated with cimetidine (Van der Spuy et al, 1980). Susceptibility to herpes zoster and herpes simplex infections correlates closely with depressed cell mediated responses to the viruses and it is suggested that cimetidine causes remission by stimulating cellular immunity. Further studies are required to substantiate this claim. Finally, Calvo (1980) reports that lymphocytes from tumour patients, incubated in vitro with cimetidine, have a much greater capacity to mount a cell-mediated response.

CONCLUSIONS

Cimetidine does not stimulate immunological responsiveness in normal subjects, has no adverse effects on transplants and does not exacerbate hypersensitivity responses. In patients with disease states associated with immunodepression, however, cimetidine stimulates cell-mediated responses. It remains to be seen whether this will produce clinical benefit.

REFERENCES

Al-Haboubi H A, Zeitlin I J 1979 The actions of cimetidine, mepyramine, indomethacin and aprotinin (Trasylol) on the inflammatory response in adjuvant rats. British Journal of Pharmacology 67: 446-447

André F, Druguet M, André C 1978 Traitement par la cimetidine et immunite humorale. Gastroenterologie Clinique et Biologique 2: 8-9

Artis W M, Jones H E 1975 Histamine inhibition of human lymphocyte transformation. Federation Proceedings 34, No. 1002

Avella J, Binder H J, Madsen J E, Askenase P W 1978 Effect of histamine H_2-receptor antagonist on delayed hypersensitivity. Lancet 1: 624-626

Barnes A D 1963 Some observation on the effects of histamine, 48/80 and five anti-histaminic drugs on the survival time of orthotopic skin homografts. Transplantation 1: 181-186

Bicks R O, Rosenberg E W 1980 Reversal of anergy in Crohn's disease by cimetidine. Lancet 1: 552-553

Boyd J F, Smith A N 1960 The effect of compound 48/80 on autograft and homograft reaction. British Journal of Experimental Pathology 41: 259-268

Breuillard F, Szapiro E 1978 Cimetidine in acquired tolerance to dinitrochlorobenzene. Lancet 1: 726

Brostoff J, Pack S, Lydyard P M 1980 Histamine suppression of lymphocyte activation. Clinical and Experimental Immunology 39: 739-745

Busse W W, Sosman 1976 Histamine inhibition of neutrophil lysosomal enzyme release: an H_2-histamine receptor response. Science 194: 737-738

Calvo D B, Mavligit G M, Hersh E M, Patt Y Z, Wong W L 1980 Immunorestoration and/or immunoaugmentation of local xenogeneic graft versus host reaction with cimetidine. Proceedings of an Annual Meeting of the American Association for Cancer Research 21: 210, abstract 841

Chakrin L W, Krell R D 1980 Histamine receptors in the respiratory system: a review of current evidence. In: Torsoli A, Lucchelli P E, Brimblecombe R W (eds) H_2-receptor antagonists in peptic ulcer disease and progress in histamine research. Excerpta Medica, Amsterdam, 338-346

Conway H, Jerome A, Stark R B 1953 Observations on the development of circulation in skin grafts VII. Effect of anti-histamine (Benadryl) on homologous skin grafts. Plastic and Reconstructive Surgery 12: 99-101

Daman L A, Rosenberg E W 1977 Acquired tolerance to dinitrochlorobenzene reversed by cimetidine. Lancet 2: 1087

De Pauw B E, Lamers C B H N, Wagener D J Th, Festen H P M 1977 Immunological studies after long-term H_2-receptor antagonist therapy. Lancet 2: 616

Dulabh R, Vickers M R 1978 The effect of H_2-receptor antagonists on anaphylaxis in the guinea-pig. Agents Actions 8: 559-565

Eiser N M, Guz A, Mills J, Snashall P D 1978 Effect of H_1- and H_2-receptor antagonists on antigen bronchial challenge. Thorax 33: 534

Fallah H A, Maillard J L, Voisin G A 1975 Regulatory mast cells I. Suppressive action of their products on an in vitro primary immune reaction. Annals of Immunology (Inst. Pasteur.) 126C: 669-682

Festen H P M, Berden J H M, de Pauw B E 1980 Immunological studies in patients treated with cimetidine, and the influence of cimetidine on skin-graft survival in mice. In: Torsoli A, Lucchelli P E, Brimblecombe R W (eds) H_2-receptor antagonists in peptic ulcer disease and progress in histamine research. Excerpta Medica, Amsterdam, 327-334

Gerosa F, Pezzini A, Pizzighella S, Riviera A P, Tridente G 1980 Role of agonists and antagonists of histamine lymphocyte receptors or functional expression of the immune system. British Journal of Pharmacology 72: 187P-188P

Gifford R R M, Gamble C E, Schmidtke J R, Ferguson R M 1980 Cimetidine augmentation of in vitro generated cell mediated cytotoxicity. Surgical Forum 31: 379-382

Goodwin J S, Goldberg E H, Williams R C 1979 Prevention of skin graft reaction in mice treated with cimetidine. Clinical Research 27: 232A

Hébert J, Beaudoin R, Aubin M, Fontaine M 1980 The regulatory effect of histamine on the immune response: characterization of the cells involved. Cellular Immunology 54: 49-57

Jones R H, Rudge C J, Bewick M, Parsons V, Weston M J 1978 Cimetidine: prophylaxis against upper gastrointestinal haemorrhage after renal transplantation. British Medical Journal 1: 398-400

Jorizzo J L, Sams W M, Jegasothy B V, Olansky A J 1980 Cimetidine as an immuno modulator: chronic mucocutaneous candidiasis as a model. Annals of Internal Medicine 92: 192-195

Khong T K, Rooney P J 1980 Arthritis associated with cimetidine. Lancet 11: 1380

Lai D Y C, Tingle A J, Ford D K, Singh V K 1980 The role of histamine, H_1-and H_2-receptor agonists in the modulation of immune responses in vitro in individuals with respiratory allergies. International Journal of Immunopharmacology 2: 237

Lichtenstein L M, Gillispie E 1975 The effect of H_1- and H_2-antihistamines on 'allergic' histamine release and its inhibition by histamine. Journal of Pharmacology and Experimental Therapeutics 192: 441-450

McGregor C G A, Ogg L J, Smith I S, Cochran A J, Gray G R, Gillespie G, Forrester J 1977. Immunological and other laboratory studies of patients receiving short-term cimetidine therapy. Lancet 1: 122-123

Moore T C, Thompson D P, Glassock R J 1971 Elevation in urinary and blood histamine following clinical renal transplantation. Annals of Surgery 173: 381-388

Osband M, Gallison D T, Miller B, McCaffrey 1979 Concanavalin A activation of suppressor cells is blocked by cimetidine. Blood 54: 89A

Plaut M, Lichtentein L M, Henney C S 1975 Properties of a subpopulation of T cells bearing histamine receptors. Journal of Clinical Investigation 55: 856-874

Primack W A 1978 Cimetidine and renal-allograft rejection. Lancet 1: 284

Rigal D, Monier J C, Souweine G 1979 The effect of histamine on the leucocyte migration test in man. I. Demonstration of a LIF production inhibitor (LIF-P1). Cellular Immunology 46: 360-372

Rocklin R W 1976 Modulation of cellular immune responses in vivo and in vitro by histamine receptor-bearing lymphocytes. Journal of Clinical Investigation 57: 1051-1058

Rocklin R E, Lima M 1980 Effect of histamine on human IgG production in vitro. Clinical Research 28: 508A

Rocklin R E, Beard J, Gupta S, Good R A, Melmon 1980 Characterization of the human blood lymphocytes that produce a histamine-induced suppressor factor (HSF). Cellular Immunology 51: 226-237

Rocklin R E, Greinder D K, Melmon K L 1979 Histamine-induced suppressor factor (HSF): further studies on the nature of the stimulus and the cell which produces it. Cellular Immunology 44: 404-415

Schwartz A, Gershon R K 1978 Activation of regulatory T cells by histamine. Federation Proceedings 27: 1353

Schwartz A, Askenase P W, Gershon R K 1977 The effect of locally-injected vasoamines on the elicitation of delayed type hypersensitivity. Journal of Immunology 118: 159-165

Schwartz A, Askenase P W, Gershon R K 1980 Histamine inhibition of the in vitro induction of cytotoxic T cell response. Immunopharmacology 2: 179-190

Shearer G M, Weinstein Y, Melmon K L 1974 Enhancement of immune response potential of mouse lymphoid cells fractionated over insolubilised conjugated histamine columns. Journal of Immunology 113: 597-607

Stranegaard O, 1979, Spring Meeting, British Society for Immunology

Tartakovsky B, Segal S, Shani A, Hellerstein S, Weinstein Y, Bentwich Z 1979 Segregation of human peripheral blood lymphocytes according to their affinity for insolubilised histamine. Principal differences between males and females. Clinical and Experimental Immunology 38: 166-174

Van der Spuy S, Levy D W, Levin W 1980 Cimetidine in the treatment of Herpes virus infection. South African Medical Journal 58: 112-116

Wallach D, Decazes J M, Cottenot F 1979 Psoriasis sévère améliorè de facon spectaculaire au cours d'un traitement par cimetidine. Nouvelle Presse Médicale 8: 2981

Wolfe J D, Plaut M, Norman P S, Lichtenstein L M 1979 The effect of an H_2-receptor antagonist on immediate and delayed skin test reactivity in man. Journal of Allergy and Clinical Immunology 63: 208A

Woodruff M F A, Boswell T 1955 The effect of phenergan (Promethazine hydrochloride) on homografts of skin and thyroid in the guinea pig. British Journal of Plastic Surgery 7: 211-216

Zamitt M, Toledo-Pereyra L H 1979 Increased rejection after cimetidine treatment in kidney transplants. Transplantation 27: 358-359

28. Review of endocrine studies of cimetidine

Roger J. Crossley, Patricia W. Evers

Smith Kline & French Laboratories, Philadelphia, USA

The first indication that cimetidine might have some effect within the endocrine system came from the pathology/toxicology studies. In rats treated with 950 mg per kg and in dogs treated with 500 mg per kg for three months or more decreased weights of the seminal vesicles and the prostates were noted. No effect on testes weight occurred, and no histopathology in the secondary sex organs was seen. In further studies there was no evidence of changes in serum or pituitary levels of luteinizing hormone or testosterone, and the mating performance and reproductive outcome of mating in rats dosed up to these levels for 70 days was unaffected.

In special studies for 28 days in mature male rats, castrated controls had prostate weights in the region of 10 per cent of intact controls. The upper doses of cimetidine reduced prostate weights to only about 50 per cent of intact controls. Recovery was prompt (within two weeks) after stopping the drug.

Winters et al (1979) studied the effect of cimetidine and metiamide on binding of labelled DHT to DHT binding sites. There was a clear competitive inhibition by both cimetidine and metiamide, indicating that the drugs were antiandrogenic. The doses required to produce this effect, however, were quite high, showing that the effect was weak.

As clinical studies progressed gynaecomastia was reported in one or two subjects in the early days of our experience among those patients with ZE syndrome who were treated for long periods of time and, in some cases, required high doses.

Data on patients with breast changes comes from a number of sources. In cases treated openly because of special circumstances in the USA 10 of 329 patients reported breast tenderness. However seven of these were from the ZE patients (8.5 per cent), while only three out of 247 (1.2 per cent) were non-ZE cases. Interestingly, seven of these 10 cases improved even when the drug was continued and, while endocrine studies on these patients are sparse, no abnormalities were seen. The higher incidence in ZE syndrome might possibly be explained as refeeding gynaecomastia since weight gain was common. It should also be noted that some of them were on other medications known to cause gynaecomastia.

From the maintenance study coordinated in the USA 2.9 per cent (seven of 244) of the cimetidine patients treated with doses ranging from 400 to 600 mg per day showed gynaecomastia, while two of the 53 (3.7 per cent) placebo patients reported the same effect and there was no statistical difference. However, in a similar study coordinated in the UK, five of 460 cimetidine patients (1.1 per cent) reported gynaecomastia, while none of the 447 patients on placebo reported this.

In a post-marketing study done in the USA (Gifford et al, 1980) out of 9907 patients, 18 reported gynaecomastia: an overall incidence of 0.18 per cent. Our experience with gynaecomastia suggests that (1) it definitely occurs as a result of cimetidine; (2) it is probably of a lower order than that suggested by the original special cases studies and (3) it can, and often does, regress with continued therapy.

Questions have been raised as to whether or not altered libido or potency occurs with cimetidine. In the same special cases protocol three of 329 reported problems in this area, although these were to a great extent quite sick patients and it is therefore difficult to interpret this incidence.

In the USA maintenance study three of 244 (or 1.2 per cent) of cimetidine patients reported libido changes while none of 53 placebo patients reported this. However, a one per cent incidence would not necessarily be observed in a placebo population of this size.

In the study coordinated in the UK, four of 460 patients on cimetidine and two of 447 on placebo reported altered libido and this difference is not significant.

In the post-marketing study in the USA three of the 9907 patients reported altered libido: an incidence of 0.03 per cent. Because of the lack of difference between placebo and cimetidine groups and very low incidence in the post-marketing surveillance where patients were specifically studied by their physicians for adverse events, we believe that it is unlikely that altered libido is due to the drug, and other causes must account for the few isolated anecdotal cases.

While the antiandrogenic effect could be used to explain the observed gynaecomastia in a few patients by inhibiting testosterone at the organ site, the question was raised as to whether there might be an effect on prolactin secretion.

A review of the literature shows that there is a consistent rise in prolactin after bolus i.v. doses of cimetidine, but changes in other hormones have not been consistently reported. Interestingly, Delitala et al (1979) gave cimetidine as a constant i.v. infusion rather than as a bolus and did not observe any prolactin increase.

Carlson and Ippoliti (1977) studied a number of hormones in eight normal males given cimetidine 300 mg and diphenhydramine 50 mg as i.v. bolus doses. There was a sharp rise in prolactin immediately following the bolus followed by a rapid fall in blood levels. The pattern is one of bolus release as opposed to sustained release in that the half-life of the prolactin accounts for the shape of the curve.

Carlson et al (in press) demonstrated that an oral dose of cimetidine 300 mg had no effect while a subsequent i.v. dose had an effect similar to that previously observed. It was suggested, therefore, that a rise above a threshold blood level in the immediate post-bolus situation might be high enough to cause a release of prolactin. On the other hand, with oral dosing, or once blood levels had settled down after bolus dosing, this threshold would not be exceeded. To test this

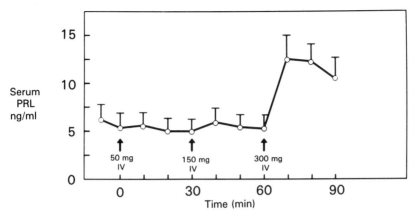

Figure 28.1 Dose-response study: serum prolactin following IV cimetidine (mean ± SE shown)
n = 7

hypothesis they showed that no increase was obtained with 50 mg i.v. nor with 150 mg i.v. but was observed after 300 mg i.v. (Figure 28.1).

This tends to support though not prove that hypothesis. In this study Carlson and co-workers also measured FSH, LH, TSH, GH, serum testosterone and serum cortisol and found no changes whatsoever with any bolus dose of cimetidine.

A review of the literature (Table 28.1) reveals that apart from a single report of prolactin rises in females with oral dosing no rise was seen with oral cimetidine in any of the studies. Also there are sporadic reports for other hormone changes following oral administration which are not substantiated by several other studies.

Carlson et al (in press) studied this question concomitantly with a duodenal ulcer study in patients receiving double-blind randomised medication of either cimetidine 300 mg q.i.d. or Mylanta II 30 ml given seven times a day. There was no effect on serum prolactin throughout the course of this study and similarly

Table 28.1 Effect of chronic oral dosing with cimetidine on serum hormone concentration (dosing with 1.0-1.6 g/day for 3-12 weeks)

Author	Basal					Stimulated						
	PRL	TSH	LH	FSH	Testosterone	LH	FSH	TSH	PRL	GH	Cortisol	T_4
Bohnet (1978)												
males	0		0		0							
females	↑		0		*							
Barber (1979)	0				0	0	0	0				
White (1979)				↑	0	0	0	0	0	0	0	
Valk (1979)	0	0	0	0						**		
May (1979)	0	↑	0	0	0			↑	0	0	0	
Van thiel (1979)			0		↑	↓	0	0	0	0		0

*Oestradiol level unchanged
**Valk et al. (1979) reported ↓ nocturnal GH

measurement of LH showed no changes. However there was a slight rise in testosterone. This was not substantial and occurred equally in both groups.

Van Thiel et al (1979) reported that in seven male subjects, presumed fertile, with a mean age of 39 years, treated with cimetidine 300 mg q.i.d., sperm counts in all subjects fell at the end of nine weeks compared with pre-therapy counts.

The reduction in mean sperm count was from 134 million/mm^3 to 94 million/mm^3, i.e. a 30 per cent decrease. In addition they reported that while basal levels of LH were unchanged and testosterone mildly increased, there was a diminution of LH response to LRF stimulation.

To put some of this in perspective it is necessary to point out that, while the minimum sperm concentration necessary for fertility is variously cited, it is now conventionally accepted at about 20 million per ml. The problem with sperm concentration is that it is highly variable over time and is affected by a number of other issues, in particular febrile illness. Without a control group it is therefore difficult to assess whether other factors influenced the patients in the Van Thiel study.

In general sperm count is not a good predictor of fertility and more recent advances suggest that an in vitro fertilisation test is more accurate (Rogers et al, 1979). In this test the hamster ovum is denuded of its zona pellucida at which point sperm from other species (in this case, man) can penetrate and the initial stages of fertilization take place. This can be evaluated by a standardised technique. Although it requires more widespread experience in the hands of a number of investigators, this test would appear to offer a much better estimation of fertility than any other test.

In order to evaluate the question of spermatogenesis a study was carried out by Paulsen and colleagues (Enzmann et al, 1981). In this study 30 normal male subjects were randomised to three regimens in double-blind fashion: 300 mg q.i.d. cimetidine, 400 mg h.s. cimetidine and placebo. A double-dummy technique was used to maintain the blindness of the regimens. Although subjects were randomised on entry to the trial, the first few months of the trial were carried out without any medication, following which the coded medication was given for six months. In a post-dosing period of three months delayed changes, if any, could be assessed.

Spermatogenesis was evaluated by looking at sperm concentration, ejaculate volume and germ cell morphology every two weeks throughout the 12 months of the study. The sperm penetration assay previously described was performed three times — before, during, and after the drug dosing period.

Table 28.2 shows the mean sperm concentration in the study for the control period and first and second three month periods for each treatment regimen. As can be seen, there was no significant drug effect, although some fall in count was observed in both the 1.2 g a day and placebo groups. Not even a small decrease was seen in the 400 mg h.s. group.

There was no effect of any treatment on germ cell morphology both in the number of oval shapes and in the number of immature germ cell forms. Finally in

Table 28.2 Sperm count data — "raw" counts

Group (n subjects)	Control X S.D.	Drug exposure 1 – 3 months X S.D.	4 – 6 months X S.D.
Placebo (10)	82.8 ± 48.5	85.5 ± 42.9	68.8 ± 22
0.4 g/day (9)	96.2 ± 47.9	103.8 ± 63.9	97.4 ± 60.3
1.2 g/day (9)	92.7 ± 51.3	81.9 ± 49.8	70.4 ± 34.6

the sperm cell penetration assay there was no effect. In fact the most deviant values occurred in the placebo group.

In addition to the spermatogenesis evaluation we also repeated serum hormone levels both before and in the sixth month of the dosing period. There was no effect on serum prolactin levels in this study or on FSH, LH, testosterone or dihydrotestosterone.

Clomiphene stimulation was also done both before dosing and after two months of dosing, the same time at which Van Thiel reported an effect. There was no change in response with any of the three regimens employed.

In summary, therefore, it seems that the effects reported by Van Thiel were due to some factors other than cimetidine — such factors which were not unearthed because of the absence of a control group. We have found no evidence that spermatogenesis is affected by cimetidine. In addition there is consistent evidence that oral cimetidine has no effect on any of the common hormones and it appears that the gynaecomastia is in fact due to an antiandrogen effect, that it is mild and sometimes reversible while on therapy and that no other abnormal endocrine sequelae can be anticipated from the use of cimetidine in chronic therapy.

REFERENCES

Barber S G 1979 Male sexual dysfunction and cimetidine. British Medical Journal 1: 1147
Bohnet H G, Greiwe M, Hanker J P, Aragona C, Schneider H P 1978 Effects of cimetidine on prolactin, LH and sex steroid secretion in male and female volunteers. Acta Endocrinologia 88: 428-434
Carlson H E, Ippoliti A F 1977 Cimetidine, an H_2-antihistamine, stimulates prolactin secretion in man. Journal of Clinical Endocrinology and Metabolism 45: 367-370
Carlson H E, Ippoliti A F, Swerdloff R S 1981 Endocrine effects of acute and chronic cimetidine administration. Digestive Diseases and Sciences (in press)
Delitala G, Stubbs W, Wass J, William S, Besser G 1979 Effects of the H_2 receptor antagonist cimetidine on pituitary hormones in man. Clinical Endocrinology 11: 161-167
Enzmann G D, Leonard J M, Paulsen C A, Rogers J 1981 Effect of cimetidine on reproductive function in men. Clinical Research 29: 26A
Gifford L M, Aeugle M E, Myerson R M, Tannenbaum P J 1980 Cimetidine post-market outpatient surveillance program: Interim report on Phase I. Journal of the American Medical Association 243: 1532-1535
May P, Schneider G, Ayub M, Chandiok S, Ertel N, Giglio W 1979 Evidence for a thyrotropin inhibitory effect of histamine in man. Journal of Clinical Endocrinology and Metabolism 49: 638-641
Rogers B J, van Campen H, Ueno M, Lambert H, Bronson R, Hale R 1979 Analysis of human spermatozoal fertilizing ability using zona-free ova. Fertility and Sterility 32: 664-670

Valk T W, England B, Marshall J 1979 Pituitary function on oral cimetidine therapy —
suppression of growth hormone secretion. Clinical Research 27: 681A (Abstract)
Van Thiel D H, Gavaler J S, Smith W I, Paul G 1979 Hypothalamic-pituitary-gonadal
dysfunction in men using cimetidine. New England Journal of Medicine 300: 1012-1015
White M C, Gore M, Jewell D 1979 Letter to the editor. New England Journal of Medicine 301:
502
Winters S J, Banks J L, Loriaux D L 1979 Cimetidine is an antiandrogen in the rat.
Gastroenterology 76: 504-508

29. Cimetidine and the possible formation of N-nitroso compounds

Roger W. Brimblecombe

Smith Kline & French Research Ltd, Welwyn Garden City, Hertfordshire, England

Nitrosamines, or more properly N-nitroso derivatives, are a class of chemical compounds formed following the attack of nitrosating agents on nitrogen-containing compounds. This leads to the introduction of a nitroso group into the molecule. The resulting compounds (see Figure 29.1) include nitrosamines and nitrosamides.

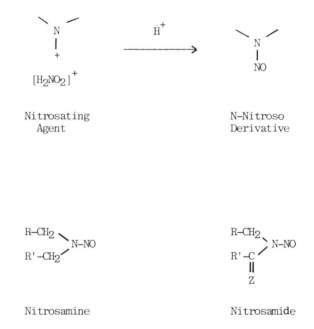

Figure 29.1 Formation of N-nitroso derivatives.

It has been suggested that the acidic conditions in the stomach could form a suitable environment for nitrosation to occur. Thus, dietary nitrite or nitrate could react with nitrogen-containing compounds in foodstuffs.

The potential significance of this suggestion relates to the fact that many nitrosamines and nitrosamides have been shown to be carcinogenic to many species of animals in feeding studies (Magee et al, 1976) although none has been shown to be carcinogenic to man.

Although N-nitroso compounds, or more commonly 'nitrosamines', are often referred to collectively, it is important, as stated above, to distinguish between nitrosamines and nitrosamides chemically but, equally importantly, in relation to their biological properties. Thus, nitrosamides can be directly (or locally) acting carcinogens, for example in the stomach, by chemical generation of an alkylating species. Nitrosamines, on the other hand, require metabolic activation, probably involving the enzyme-catalyzed formation of an alkylating species, before they can act as carcinogens. Thus, they are indirect carcinogens, their carcinogenicity resulting in tumours in organs and tissues remote from their site of entry or formation in the body.

A related point is that in studies where levels of N-nitroso compounds are being measured in, for example, biological fluids, it is essential to be aware of the capabilities of the method employed. As will be indicated later some of the apparently contradictory results in the literature may well be attributable to differences in methodology.

EVIDENCE RELATING TO CIMETIDINE

There have now been a few reports in the literature (for example, Elder et al, 1979) of patients developing gastric carcinoma after treatment with cimetidine. The total number of patients is very small taken in the context of the total use of the drug and the interval between first exposure to cimetidine and diagnosis of cancer is short (in most cases less than six months). Thus, the most probable explanation in most if not all of these cases is that an undiagnosed carcinoma was present prior to the commencement of treatment with cimetidine.

However, on theoretical grounds two possibilities exist: that following the administration of cimetidine it may itself be nitrosated in the stomach to an N-nitroso derivative and/or that there may be an elevation in the levels of total N-nitroso compounds in the stomach. While these two theoretical possibilities exist it is essential that they be examined using all available techniques so that the risk, if any, of gastric carcinoma developing be assessed, put into context and weighed against the benefits of the drug.

On current evidence both possibilities — the formation of nitrosocimetidine and the elevation of total levels of gastric N-nitroso compounds — are hypothetical rather than proven but work is in progress in our own and other laboratories to obtain definitive evidence to enable more informed opinions to be formed as to the actual, rather than the hypothetical, situation.

This article will summarise the present state of knowledge relating to each hypothesis. The field is an active one, however, and clearly the summary can only relate to that which is known to the author at the time of writing (end of February 1981).

Hypothesis A

The first hypothesis, designated 'A', is concerned with the possible formation of the nitrosated derivative of cimetidine in the stomach. For this to occur and for it to constitute a hazard the sequence of events shown in Figure 29.2 would have to occur in the stomach.

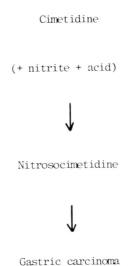

Cimetidine

(+ nitrite + acid)

Nitrosocimetidine

Gastric carcinoma

Figure 29.2   Sequence of events postulated in hypothesis A.

The questions which arise are:

(i) Can cimetidine be nitrosated?
(ii) Is nitrosocimetidine a carcinogen?
(iii) Is nitrosocimetidine formed in the stomach?

The answer to (i) is that in vitro cimetidine reacts with excess nitrite under strongly acidic conditions to form the mono N-nitroso derivative known as N-nitrosocimetidine (Bavin et al, 1980; Foster et al, 1980). The reaction is shown in Figure 29.3 which also illustrates the structure of N-methyl-N'-nitroso-nitroguanidine (MMNG). This is a gastric carcinogen in animals (Sugimura et al, 1966) and attention has been drawn to the fact that the N-nitroso-cyanoguanidino group in nitrosocimetidine bears some chemical resemblance to MNNG.

The kinetics of formation of nitrosocimetidine have been described by Bavin et al (1980). Importantly, the initial rate of nitrosation is directly proportional to hydrogen ion concentration, dropping by a factor of about 10 for each pH unit rise. The rate of formation of nitrosocimetidine is unexceptional when compared with rates of nitrosation of other drugs or chemicals.

The second question as to whether nitrosocimetidine is a carcinogen is still unresolved. Feeding studies in animals with the compound are in progress but results have not been published. All evidence so far available concerning the possible carcinogenicity of nitrosocimetidine is, therefore, indirect.

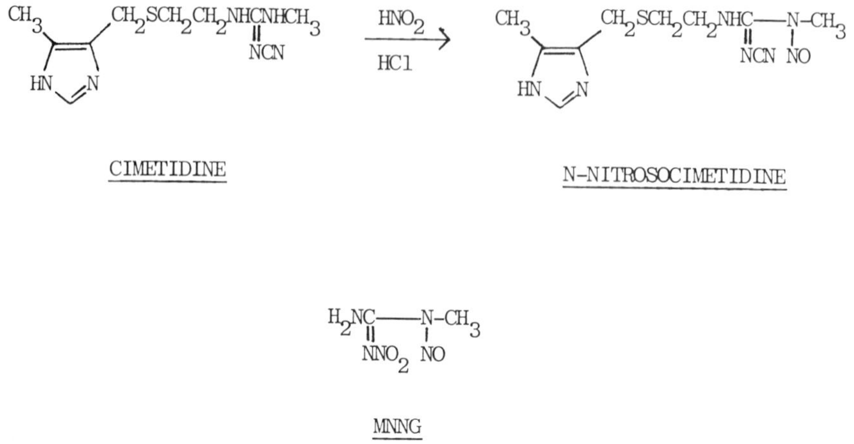

Figure 29.3 Nitrosation of cimetidine

Our own work has indicated that in the Ames test for bacterial mutagenicity nitrosocimetidine is positive in strains TA 100 and TA 1535 at 100 μg per plate with or without microsomal activation. Cimetidine itself is negative at 5000 μg per plate in these and the other three bacterial strains studied.

Similar results have been reported by Pool et al (1979) who have also shown that nitrosocimetidine induces DNA damage in repair-deficient *E. coli* strains at 100 μg per plate. It causes a concentration-dependent increase in damage to DNA in transformed epithelial cell lines in vitro (Schwarz et al, 1980). Again, in these studies cimetidine itself showed no activity and MNNG was considerably more potent than nitroso-cimetidine.

Jensen and Magee (1981) studied the in vitro reaction of MNNG and nitrosocimetidine with DNA and concluded that in the presence of cysteine as an activating nucleophile both compounds methylated DNA with comparable effectiveness. In the absence of cysteine, however, nitrosocimetidine caused no modification of DNA in contrast to MNNG which did. Cimetidine itself was devoid of activity in the absence or the presence of cysteine. In a more recent in vivo study Gombar et al (1981) from Magee's laboratory have administered ^{14}C-labelled cimetidine, nitrosocimetidine or MNNG orally to rats. Following sacrifice 12 hours later DNA was isolated from various tissues. No methylation of DNA was detected in cimetidine-treated rats whereas methylation of DNA from most tissues was observed following MNNG or nitrosocimetidine administration. In all cases MNNG produced a higher level of alkylation than nitrosocimetidine (3 to 50 times higher depending on the tissue). Interestingly MNNG alkylated stomach DNA to the greatest extent whereas the highest level of alkylation with nitrosocimetidine was seen in DNA from the small intestine.

To summarise these findings some of the properties of nitrosocimetidine are similar to those of MNNG but in most respects it is less potent than the latter. A definitive result regarding the carcinogenicity of nitrosocimetidine will presumably be obtained only when the results of current long-term feeding studies become available.

Discussion of the possible hazard associated with nitrosocimetidine becomes relevant only if the compound is formed in vivo (question (iii) above). To date this has not been demonstrated. A method was developed in our laboratories capable of detecting nitrosocimetidine at a concentration of 50 ng/ml in water or gastric juice. Sixteen samples taken from cimetidine treated subjects were examined using this procedure but no nitrosocimetidine was detected. However, this method appears not to be entirely satisfactory for use in gastric juice samples contaminated with food. Currently efforts are being made to improve the specificity and sensitivity of the method.

So hypothesis A remains unproven but is still under investigation.

Hypothesis B

The second hypothesis relates to the possibility that reduction in gastric acidity could allow colonization of the stomach by bacteria not normally present there. If the organisms include those capable of reduction of nitrate to nitrite then elevated levels of gastric nitrite could lead to a faster nitrosation of amines from food stuffs and hence to increased levels of total N-nitroso compounds, some of which could be carcinogenic.

As with hypothesis A a sequence of events must occur if hypothesis B is to be considered proven.

Clearly cimetidine leads to a reduction in gastric acidity but normal therapeutic doses do not produce achlorhydria; the pH fluctuates over the 24 hour period. In individuals on normal regimens of food it rarely falls outside the range pH 1.5 to 5.5. In other hypochlorhydric states caused, for example, by disease (as in

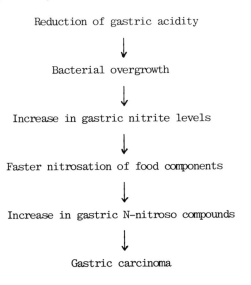

Reduction of gastric acidity

↓

Bacterial overgrowth

↓

Increase in gastric nitrite levels

↓

Faster nitrosation of food components

↓

Increase in gastric N-nitroso compounds

↓

Gastric carcinoma

Figure 29.4 Sequence of events postulated in hypothesis B.

pernicious anaemia) or by surgery (e.g. gastrectomy or vagotomy) the hypochlorhydria is sustained.

Evidence is somewhat conflicting over whether bacterial overgrowth, or perhaps more accurately bacterial colonization, occurs in individuals taking cimetidine. That this occurs in fasting subjects seems to have been established beyond doubt. For example, there are studies by Ruddell et al (1980) and Deane et al (1980) in which patients fasted for 9 to 12 hours overnight, were then given 200 mg cimetidine and remained in a fasting state for a further 2 to 4 hours before samples of gastric juice were taken. Bacterial colonization was present.

However the protocol used in these studies does not reflect the normal habits of subjects routinely treated with cimetidine. More recently Muscroft et al (1981) have studied normal subjects taking full dose or maintenance cimetidine and eating normally. Nocturnal hypochlorhydria was found only rarely, i.e. the intragastric pH seldom exceeded 4. The incidence of bacterial colonization was also low and levels of nitrite in gastric juice were rarely elevated.

This leads on to the next stage in hypothesis B — the question of whether gastric nitrite levels are elevated. Again there is a discrepancy between results of studies in which fasting subjects have been investigated and the results of the study by Muscroft et al (1981) in which fed subjects were used. Elevated levels of nitrite have been found in gastric juice from fasting subjects dosed with cimetidine. This is probably a consequence of the fact that in these subjects the pH of the gastric juice was higher than in fed subjects.

The same kind of considerations apply to levels of N-nitroso compounds. Reed et al (1980), again using subjects fasted overnight, reported a near linear relationship between pH and nitrosamine levels. The mean gastric nitrosamine concentration in all cimetidine-treated patients in this study was 890 nmol/l compared with 540 nmol/l in untreated patients. Although methodological details are not given in this abstract it seems probable that the method used measured stable nitrosamines rather than total N-nitroso compounds.

So evidence relating to hypothesis B is conflicting. Most of the studies so far reported have been carried out in the unusual circumstance of prolonged fasting. This has resulted in greater reduction in the acidity of the gastric juice than cimetidine produces in normally fed subjects — consequently bacterial colonization, nitrite and nitrosamine levels have apparently been affected more than may be the case in more normal circumstances.

As with hypothesis A work is in progress to elucidate hypothesis B more completely.

Results of animal studies

Since the results of the studies reviewed above are inconclusive and conflicting the potential hazard from cimetidine remains a hypothetical one and current views must take account of the results of carcinogenicity studies in animals. These results are unequivocal and have shown no gastric cancer.

Thus, two 2-year carcinogenicity studies in rats using dose levels of up to 950 mg/kg/day cimetidine (about 60 times the human daily dose) have been completed; one has been published (Brimblecombe et al, 1978) and the other is being prepared for publication (Leslie et al, 1981). No gastric carcinoma was detected in either study.

In an ongoing dog study oral daily doses of 144 mg/kg have been given for nearly five years. Regular gastroscopy and multiple biopsy have revealed no evidence of ulceration, dysplasia, cellular atypia or neoplasia of the gastric mucosa (Crean et al, 1979; 1981). Thus in all these studies the administration of large doses of cimetidine for long periods has not resulted in gastric carcinoma.

SUMMARY AND CONCLUSIONS

Concern about a causal relationship between cimetidine administration is based, at the moment, on anecdotes and hypothetical considerations. The hypotheses are being tested.

Evidence currently available suggests that the nitrosated derivative of cimetidine shares some of the properties of known carcinogens but is, in practically all test systems, less active than the carcinogen MNNG. Cimetidine itself is negative in all systems used. There is no direct evidence for carcinogenicity of nitrosocimetidine, neither has nitrosocimetidine been shown to be formed in patients in vivo although some studies are still in progress.

The suggestion that cimetidine, by reducing gastric acidity, could lead to bacterial overgrowth and hence to increase in nitrite and thus total nitrosamine levels in the stomach may be valid in fasted subjects but apparently not in normally fed individuals. Further work is required, particularly in patients with peptic ulcer as opposed to normal subjects. Whatever the result of further work this possible phenomenon of bacterial overgrowth is not specific to H_2-receptor antagonists since it will presumably occur in other situations where gastric acidity is reduced as in surgery (gastrectomy or vagotomy) for peptic ulcer disease.

The most definitive evidence available at present is from long-term studies in rats and dogs where daily administration of high doses of cimetidine have not produced gastric carcinoma.

ACKNOWLEDGEMENTS

Much of the work described here has been carried out by, or discussed with, my colleagues in the Research Institute of Smith Kline and French Research Limited. In particular, I acknowledge the contributions of Dr P. M. G. Bavin, Mr D. W. Darkin, Dr G. J. Durant, Dr A. D. Gribble and Mr G. B. Leslie.

REFERENCES

Bavin P M G, Durant G J, Miles P D, Mitchell R C, Pepper E S 1980 Nitrosation of cimetidine. Journal of Chemical Research (S): 212-213
Brimblecombe R W, Duncan W A M, Durant G J, Emett J C, Ganellin C R, Leslie G B, Parsons M E 1978 Characterization and development of cimetidine as a histamine H_2-receptor antagonist. Gastroenterology 74: 339-347

Crean G P, Leslie G B, Roe F J C 1979 Cimetidine and gastric cancer: negative studies in dogs. Lancet ii: 797-798

Crean G P, Morson B, Leslie G B, Roe F J C 1981 Cimetidine: further evidence of non-carcinogenicity in dogs. New England Journal of Medicine 304: 672

Deane S A, Youngs D J, Poxon V A, Keighley M R B, Alexander-Williams J, Burdon D W 1980 Cimetidine and gastric microflora. British Journal of Surgery 67: 371

Elder J B, Ganguli P C, Gillespie I E 1979 Cimetidine and gastric cancer. Lancet i: 1005-1006

Foster A B, Jarman M, Manson D, Schulten H R 1980 Structure and reactivity of nitrosocimetidine. Cancer Letters 9: 47-52

Gombar C T, Jensen D E, Magee P N 1981 To be read at the 1981 Meeting of the American Association for Cancer Research

Jensen D E, Magee P N 1981 Methylation of DNA by nitrosocimetidine in vitro. Cancer Research 41: 230-236

Leslie G B, Noakes D N, Pollitt F D, Roe F J C, Walker T F 1981 Toxicology and Applied Pharmacology (in press)

Magee P N, Montesano R, Preussman R 1976 In: Searle C (ed) Chemical carcinogens, ACS Monograph 173: 491-625

Muscroft T J, Youngs D J, Burdon D W, Keighley M R B 1981 Cimetidine is unlikely to increase formation of intragastric N-nitroso-compounds in patients taking a normal diet. Lancet i: 408-410

Pool B L, Eisenbrand G, Schmähl D 1979 Biological activity of nitrosated cimetidine. Toxicology 15: 69-72

Reed P I, Smith P L R, Walters C L 1980 The influence of cimetidine treatment on gastric pH and nitrosamine concentration. Hepatogastroenterology Suppl., XI International Congress of Gastroenterology, p 58, Abstract E8.3

Ruddell W S J, Axon A T R, Findlay J M, Bartholomew B A, Hill M J 1980 Effect of cimetidine on the gastric bacterial flora. Lancet i: 672-674

Schwarz M, Hummel J, Eisenbrand G 1980 Induction of DNA strand breaks by nitrosocimetidine. Cancer Letters 10: 223-228

Sugimura T, Nagao M, Okada Y 1966 Carcinogenic action of N-methyl-N'-nitro-N-nitrosoguanidine. Nature (London) 210: 962-963

30. Continuing evaluation of the safety of cimetidine

D. Rowley-Jones, A. C. Flind

Medical Department, Smith Kline & French Laboratories Ltd.
Welwyn Garden City, Hertfordshire

In this review we report on clinical problems concerning which either new evidence has emerged or there has been further discussion of the role of cimetidine since we last reviewed the overall safety profile of the drug (Flind et al, 1980). Conclusions regarding gynaecomastia, mental confusion, interstitial nephritis and the absence of rebound hypersecretion of acid when cimetidine treatment is stopped have not materially altered since our last report and will not be further discussed. Attention will be directed, therefore, to topics of safety which are not dealt with elsewhere in this volume, namely, acute pancreatitis, white blood cell disorders and drug interactions.

METHOD

Pharmacological activity is always associated with unwanted effects as well as clinical benefits. It is important, therefore, that the risks of treatment are accurately defined, so that the effect of treatment can be quantified not only in terms of the expected therapeutic benefit but also in terms of potential harm. We have already described in some detail the sources from which data can be obtained and evaluated so that the safety profile of a drug can be established (Flind et al, 1980). Some advantages and disadvantages of these sources are set out in Table 30.1.

Both post-marketing surveillance studies involving cimetidine, in the United Kingdom and the United States respectively, are progressing. An interim report on the former can be found in this publication (see p. 270). The US study involves around 10 000 patients, as in the UK, although a different protocol is followed and there is no control population. Gifford et al (1980) have published their interim findings on all subjects in the study. To date, results available from both studies have not indicated any adverse reactions to cimetidine not already raised from other sources.

Data obtained from voluntarily reported adverse events to Smith Kline & French (SK&F) remain probably the most valuable single source of information in the continuing evaluation of the safety profile of cimetidine. The number of adverse events reported to SK&F (UK) occurring in association with cimetidine

Table 30.1 Sources of data

	Advantages	Disadvantages
Clinical trials	Controlled	Small population
	Carefully monitored	
Published reports	Wide audience	Anecdotal
	Stimulates further reports	
Spontaneous reports	Large population	Uncontrolled
		Underestimate
Post marketing surveillance	Controlled	Relatively small population
	Monitored	

per quarter since the drug was first marketed in November 1976 has remained relatively constant, running at about 50–70. The implications of this are probably two-fold; first, the medical profession is in no way complacent about the safety of cimetidine and, second, large amounts of data are still being provided, upon which assessment of safety can be based.

RESULTS

Between November 1976 and the end of 1980 SK&F (UK) had received a total of 1039 reports of unpublished adverse events associated with cimetidine. During the period November 1976 to September 1980 the Committee on Safety of Medicines (CSM) had received 2370 such reports. All reports received by SK&F (UK) are passed to the CSM and are included in this figure. To date it is estimated that well over a million patients in the UK have been treated with cimetidine. Even allowing for a considerable degree of under-reporting, inherent in any voluntary system, the incidence of adverse events associated with cimetidine treatment, therefore, is low.

ACUTE PANCREATITIS

The usual treatment for this condition consists largely of analgesia, fluid replacement and an attempt to reduce pancreatic secretion. This latter aspect is usually by means of nasogastric suction on the basis that the reduction in acid gastric juice entering the duodenum will lessen pancreatic output. In theory the same effect could be achieved by administering cimetidine.

In a double-blind study of cimetidine 1.2 g/day and placebo in the treatment of established acute alcoholic pancreatitis, Meshkinpour and his colleagues (1979) found no significant difference between the two treatments. They found, however, that in the group receiving cimetidine the mean serum amylase concentration, although falling to normal after 5 days — the same as in the placebo group, was always higher than in the control population. For the first 48 hours of treatment the difference reached statistical significance, but in spite of this biochemical difference the cimetidine-treated patients did not fare any worse than those on placebo. There appear to be two possibilities to account for their finding. Either cimetidine interfered with renal mechanisms for the excretion of amylase or it produced pancreatic damage.

To March 1981 SK&F have received seven UK reports of patients in whom acute pancreatitis has occurred de novo in patients treated with cimetidine, three of which have been published (Arnold et al, 1978; Wilkinson et al, 1981). In Wilkinson and colleagues' two patients the development of acute pancreatitis can probably be attributed to cimetidine as both are without evidence of alcoholism or recent biliary disease and pancreatitis recurred on rechallenge. Each patient developed pancreatitis about two weeks after first starting cimetidine, there being a recurrence within 24 hours following reintroduction of the drug. On each occasion the pancreatitis resolved rapidly with conventional treatment when cimetidine was discontinued. Of the remaining four unpublished reports, one is unrelated to cimetidine, having occurred in a patient with disseminated intravascular coagulation, whilst details of the other three are not known.

It appears, therefore, that cimetidine, on rare occasions, can produce acute pancreatitis and a statement to this effect has recently been included in the Data Sheet. Although Joffe and Lee (1978) and Hadas et al (1978) considered that, under certain conditions, pancreatitis in the rat could be a direct toxic effect of cimetidine, the time scale of events in the two clinical cases described above is more consistent with a hypersensitivity phenomenon.

WHITE BLOOD CELL DISORDERS

The relationship of a fall in white cell count to cimetidine treatment has become clearer since we last reported. In animal toxicological studies there was no evidence of marrow toxicity nor is cimetidine concentrated in the bone marrow (Cross, 1977). There is, however, evidence that H_2-receptors exist on marrow stem cells (Byron, 1977), so that any effect of cimetidine may be the result of H_2-receptor antagonism and not due to toxicity of the cimetidine molecule itself.

Up to the end of 1980 there had been 29 UK reports of a fall in white cell count of which four have been published (Craven and Whittington, 1977; Johnson et al, 1977; Corbett and Holdsworth, 1978; James and Prout, 1978). Of the 25 unpublished reports all except five are unlikely to be related to cimetidine treatment, or have incomplete data. The five were all thought to have a possible relationship to drug administration in that a fall in white count had occurred with a temporal relationship to cimetidine. On each occasion, however, other factors, which could in themselves have adversely affected the marrow, were present.

It is estimated that more than 11 million patients worldwide have received cimetidine to date. Up to February 1981 there were 192 worldwide reports (including the UK figures) of a fall in white count associated with the drug. Of these, laboratory data were available from 150 and 84 had a total white cell count of $2000/mm^3$ or less or a neutrophil count of $1000/mm^3$ or less. In only two were there no other factors such as other drugs or serious concomitant illness present and details of these two have been published (Carloss et al, 1980; Chang and Morrison, 1979). One was a 66-year-old male who developed aplastic anaemia and died, whilst the other was a 67-year-old man with reversible granulocytopenia. The latter patient had previously been treated with methotrexate for four years, although he had not received this drug for 4-5 months before cimetidine was first started.

It is likely, therefore, that cimetidine per se has no effect on bone marrow. It is in those patients whose marrow may be 'under stress' for other reasons, e.g. drugs, serious illness, irradiation, that H_2-receptor antagonism may have a marrow suppressive potential.

In a recent survey carried out at the Renal Unit, King's College Hospital, London (Rudge, unpublished report) data were collected from 59 consecutive patients, who received cimetidine prophylactically for 6-8 weeks following renal transplantation. They were operated upon between June 1978 and December 1979 and all routinely received azathioprine, anti-lymphocytic globulin and methylprednisolone post-operatively, so would therefore qualify as having a 'stressed' marrow. Virtually complete data were obtained from 42 patients. Of the other 17, three died within 48 hours of surgery, a further eight died during the assessment period, but in none was the death related to a bone marrow problem. Six rejected their kidneys and returned to dialysis. The starting dose of cimetidine was 200 mg b.d. and this was increased according to renal function to 1 g/day, usually over a two-week period. The mean white cell counts during the period of cimetidine administration are shown in Figure 30.1. There was clearly no adverse effect of cimetidine and the mean platelet counts behaved in the same way.

In summary, therefore, the possibility that administration of cimetidine to a patient with an already compromised bone marrow could produce an adverse effect should be borne in mind. Even in these circumstances, however, the complication is unlikely.

DRUG INTERACTIONS

It is essential to assess drug interactions, whether potential or actual, in terms of their clinical importance. Thus, despite its effect in reducing intragastric acidity, cimetidine has been shown, in general, not to interfere with the absorption of drugs where this factor could be important, e.g., benzylpenicillin (Fairfax et al, 1978), enteric-coated prednisolone (Morrison et al, 1980), ampicillin (Rogers et

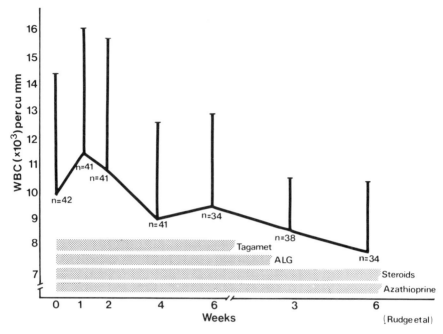

Figure 30.1 Mean white cell counts during cimetidine administration following renal transplantation in patients with 'stressed' marrow.

al, 1980), co-trimoxazole (Rogers et al, 1980) and tetracycline (Garty and Hurwitz, 1980; Fisher et al, 1980).

Puurunen and Pelkonen (1979) showed in the rat that cimetidine inhibited microsomal drug metabolism. They demonstrated that the hexobarbital sleeping time was significantly prolonged in cimetidine-treated rats and suggested that this was due to an effect on the cytochrome P-450 linked mono-oxygenase enzyme system. Subsequently Grygiel and his colleagues (1980) have confirmed these animal data and have suggested that the action of cimetidine may exhibit some specificity to enzymes induced by the polycyclic hydrocarbon 3-methylcholanthrene.

In man, cimetidine can interfere with the elimination of drugs in which oxidation is a significant part of the metabolic pathway. This has been illustrated by Patwardhan et al (1980) who showed that the metabolism of oxazepam and lorazepam, which are eliminated by glucuronidation, was unaffected by cimetidine in contrast to other benzodiazepines, diazepam and chlordiazepoxide, which are eliminated by an oxidative process. Some other pharmacological interactions in man resulting in decreased elimination of drugs in use in the UK have subsequently been identified (Table 30.2) of which possibly the best known is the prolongation of prothrombin time by cimetidine in patients on oral anticoagulants.

In terms of clinical importance, the effect of cimetidine in patients on warfarin is potentially serious and a caution is included in the Data Sheet. Klotz and

Table 30.2

Drug	Author
Warfarin	Desmond et al
	Klotz et al
	Serlin et al
Diazepam, chlordiazepoxide (*not* lorazepam, oxazepam)	Patwardhan et al
Phenytoin	Neuvonen et al
Theophylline	Jackson et al
	Miners et al
	Wood et al
Propranolol	Donovan et al
	Feely et al
Chlormethiazole	Shaw et al
Caffeine	Broughton and Rogers

Reimann (1980) found that the elimination half-life of diazepam and its metabolite desmethyldiazepam were significantly prolonged in subjects receiving cimetidine. They suggested that steady state blood concentrations could be expected to increase by about a third in patients given cimetidine. Up to the end of February 1981, adverse events had been reported to SK&F (UK) in a total of 25 patients who coincidentally were receiving benzodiazepines. In only three of these, however, was a drug interaction a reasonable hypothesis, even retrospectively, to account for the reported event. The possibility, therefore, that a significant interaction could occur has been noted in the Data Sheet, although experience suggests it is unlikely to be of great clinical significance.

Neuvonen and his colleagues (1980) showed that in nine patients receiving phenytoin who were given cimetidine 1 g/day for three weeks the mean serum phenytoin concentration ($\pm$ SE) increased from a steady state level of 5.7 $\pm$ 1.3 mg/l to 9.1 $\pm$ 1.4 mg/l and fell to 5.8 $\pm$ 1.2 mg/l two weeks after cimetidine had been discontinued. This represents a 63 per cent increase in blood concentration and, for a drug with a narrow therapeutic index such as phenytoin, could be of clinical consequence. This may also be true for theophylline, although the effect of cimetidine on theophylline clearance, which is in any case slow, appears to be a reduction of about one-third. One study has shown the changes in smokers only (Miners et al, 1980).

Donovan et al (1981) reported in the *Lancet* one patient in whom the bioavailability of propranolol increased by 340 per cent whilst he was receiving cimetidine. These data have now been extended to six subjects and an average increase in bioavailability of a single dose of propranolol 80 mg of 62 per cent has been found (data to be published). The data are consistent with an effect on first pass metabolism. Feely et al (1980) showed that in volunteers the pulse rate was significantly reduced following a single dose of propranolol 80 mg when they were concomitantly receiving cimetidine. On the other hand, Warburton and her colleagues (1979) in healthy volunteers found no increased effect of a combination of cimetidine and propranolol on pulse rate, blood pressure or response to exercise compared with propranolol alone. This was in spite of the mean steady state propranolol blood concentration ($\pm$ SE) increasing from 38.1 $\pm$ 7.8 mg/l to 48.6 $\pm$ 7.8 mg/l when cimetidine was co-administered. It would seem, therefore, that this interaction is unlikely to be of any clinical significance, other than in patients unusually sensitive to the effect of β -blockade, who are also already on cimetidine and who are given propranolol for the first time.

The interaction between cimetidine and chlormethiazole, where clearance of a very rapidly cleared drug is reduced by about a third, and between cimetidine and caffeine is unlikely to be clinically important.

Up to the end of 1980 there had been 67 reports of events classified as potential drug interactions involving cimetidine, to SK&F (UK). Of these, 25 concerned anticoagulants of which about 80 per cent suggested a potentiation of effect. Of the remaining 42 reports, none of these was probably related to cimetidine administration, 9 were possibly related, 6 were unlikely to be or were not related to drug therapy, whilst in 27 insufficient information was available to make an attribution.

So far, these data tend to confirm that with the exception of patients on warfarin, where dosage reduction may be required, and possibly those on phenytoin, concomitant administration of cimetidine with drugs metabolised by oxidation in the liver, is unlikely to produce changes which are of clinical significance.

CONCLUSION

Extensive and increasing experience continues to indicate that, for the vast majority of patients who need cimetidine, the benefits of treatment far outweigh the risks. As expected for any clinically useful drug, knowledge of cimetidine continues, even after over four years of widespread use, to increase steadily with progressively better understanding of its safety profile. Further progress depends greatly on continued reporting by vigilant doctors of all adverse experience, whether or not apparently drug-related, to SK&F and the CSM.

REFERENCES

Arnold F, Doyle P J, Bell G 1978 Acute pancreatitis in a patient treated with cimetidine. Lancet i: 382-383
Broughton L J, Rogers H J Decreased clearance of caffeine due to cimetidine. Unpublished data
Byron J W 1977 Mechanism for histamine H_2-receptor induced cell-cycle changes in the bone marrow stem cell. Agents & Actions 7: 209
Carloss H W, Tavassoli M, McMillan R 1980 Cimetidine-induced granulocytopenia. Annals of Internal Medicine 93: 57-58
Chang H K, Morrison S L 1979 Bone marrow suppression associated with cimetidine. Annals of Internal Medicine 91: 580
Corbett C L, Holdsworth C D 1978 Fever, abdominal pain, and leucopenia during treatment with cimetidine. British Medical Journal 1: 753-4
Craven E R, Whittington J M 1977 Agranulocytosis four months after cimetidine therapy. Lancet ii: 294-5
Cross S A M 1977 The localisation of histamine H_2-receptor antagonists. Acta Pharmacologica et Toxicologica 41(Suppl 1): 116-117

Desmond P V, Patwardhan R V, Schenker S, Speeg K V 1980 Cimetidine impairs elimination of chlordiazepoxide (Librium) in man. Annals of Internal Medicine 93: 266-268

Donovan M A, Heagerty A M, Patel L, Castleden M, Pohl J E F 1981 Cimetidine and bioavailability of propranolol. Lancet i: 164

Fairfax A J, Adam J, Pagan F S 1978 Effect of cimetidine on absorption of oral benzylpenicillin. British Medical Journal 1: 820

Feely J, Wilkinson G R, Wood A J J 1980 Cimetidine administration results in increased effects of propranolol and higher propranolol blood levels. Circulation 62: Suppl 3: 257

Fisher P, House F, Inns P, Morrison P J, Rogers H J, Bradbrook I D 1980 Effect of cimetidine on the absorption of orally administered tetracycline. British Journal of Clinical Pharmacology 9: 153-158

Flind A C, Rowley-Jones D, Backhouse J N 1980 The safety of cimetidine — a continuing assessment. In: Torsoli A, Lucchelli P E, Brimblecombe R W (eds). H$_2$-receptor antagonists in peptic ulcer disease and progress in histamine research. Excerpta Medica, Amsterdam, p 209-217

Garty M, Hurwitz A 1980 Effect of cimetidine and antacids on gastrointestinal absorption of tetracycline. Clinical Pharmacology and Therapeutics 28: 203-207

Gifford L M, Aeugle M E, Myerson R M, Tannenbaum P J 1980 Cimetidine postmarket outpatient surveillance program. Journal of the American Medical Association 243: 1532-1535

Grygiel J J, Drew R, Miners J O, Rowell J, Willoughby J O, Birkett D J 1980 The effects of cimetidine on the theophylline clearance in rat. 14th Annual Meeting Australasian Society of Clinical and Experimental Pharmacology: Abstract 58

Hadas N, Wapnick S, Grosberg S J 1978 Cimetidine in pancreatitis. New England Journal of Medicine 299: 487

Jackson J E, Powell J R, Wandell M, Bentley J, Dorr R 1980 Cimetidine–theophylline interaction. Pharmacologist 22: 231: Abstract 396

James C, Prout B J 1978 Marrow suppression and intravenous cimetidine. Lancet i: 987

Joffe S N, Lee F D 1978 Acute pancreatitis after cimetidine administration in experimental duodenal ulcers. Lancet i: 383

Johnson N McI, Black A E, Hughes A S B, Clarke S W 1977 Leucopenia with cimetidine. Lancet ii: 1226

Klotz U, Reimann I 1980 Delayed clearance of diazepam due to cimetidine. New England Journal of Medicine 302: 1012-1014

Meshkinpour H, Molinari M D, Gardner L, Berk J E, Hoehler F K 1979 Cimetidine in the treatment of acute alcoholic pancreatitis. Gastroenterology 77: 687-690

Miners J O, Grygiel J J, Drew R, Birkett D J 1980 Interaction between cimetidine and theophylline in smokers and non-smokers. 14th Annual Meeting Australasian Society of Clinical and Experimental Pharmacology: Abstract 61

Morrison P J, Rogers H J, Bradbrook I D, Parsons C 1980 Concurrent administration of cimetidine and enteric-coated prednisolone; effect on plasma levels of prednisolone. British Journal of Clinical Pharmacology 10: 87-89

Neuvonen P J, Tokola R A, Kaste M 1980 Cimetidine–phenytoin interaction: effect on serum phenytoin interaction: effect on serum phenytoin concentration and antipyrine test in man. Naunyn Schmiedebergs Archives of Pharmacology 313 (Suppl): Abstract 239

Patwardhan R V, Yarborough G W, Desmond P V, Johnson R F, Schenker S, Speeg K V 1980 Cimetidine spares the glucuronidation of lorazepam and oxazepam. Gastroenterology 79: 912-916

Puurunen J, Pelkonen O 1979 Cimetidine inhibits microsomal drug metabolism in the rat. European Journal of Pharmacology 55: 335-336

Rogers H J, James C A, Morrison P J, Bradbrook I D 1980 Effect of cimetidine on oral absorption of ampicillin and cotrimoxazole. Journal of Antimicrobial Chemotherapy 6: 297-300

Serlin M J, Sibeon R G, Mossman S, Breckenridge A M, Williams J R B, Atwood J L, Willoughby J M T 1979 Cimetidine: interaction with oral anticoagulants in man. Lancet ii: 317-319

Shaw R G, Bury R W, Mashford M L, Breen K J, Desmond P V 1980 Effect of cimetidine on disposition of orally-administered chlormethiazole. 14th Annual Meeting Australasian Society of Clinical Experimental Pharmacology: Abstract 63

Warburton S, Opie L H, Kennelly B M, Muller F O 1979 Does cimetidine alter the cardiac response to exercise and propranolol? South African Medical Journal 55: 1125-1127
Wilkinson M L, O'Driscoll R, Kiernan T J 1981 Cimetidine and pancreatitis. Lancet i: 610-611
Wood L, Grice J, Petroff V, McGuffie C, Roberts R K 1980 Effect of cimetidine on the disposition of theophylline. Gastroenterological Society of Australia, Abstracts of the Annual Scientific Meeting, Melbourne: 8

31. Postmarketing surveillance

D. Colin-Jones*, M. J. S. Langman, D. H. Lawson, M. P. Vessey
*Queen Alexandra Hospital, Portsmouth

Current methods for detecting the pattern and frequency of adverse reactions following the marketing of a new drug are clearly inadequate. Various proposals have been advanced in attempts to improve matters, using schemes that, for instance, depend upon limited initial release and compulsory registration of adverse events.

We have used the opportunity provided by the marketing of cimetidine to test the feasibility of a scheme designed to detect serious adverse events occurring subsequently in a group of patients identified initially at the time of prescription of the drug in ordinary practice. In addition we have sought to collect a group of control individuals to determine if the frequency of adverse events can be related to the rate at which such events ordinarily occur in the population.

METHOD

The study was designed so that approximately 2500 recipients of cimetidine would be identified and enrolled at each of four centres in the UK: Glasgow, Nottingham, Oxford and Portsmouth. At each centre prescriptions for cimetidine were collected by physicians who agreed to cooperate in the study. In Glasgow, Oxford and Portsmouth local pharmacists helped, whilst in Nottingham prescriptions for the drug were collected as they passed through the responsible office of the Prescription Pricing Authority. On average over 90 per cent of physicians and general practitioners indicated their willingness to help, and the Department of Health and Social Security, after advice from the Committee on Safety of Medicines, agreed to the collaboration of the Prescription Pricing Authority.

Once prescriptions have been notified to the study centre a research worker visits the prescriber and records the patient's name, age, sex and NHS number and details of the reason for the prescription, and the number of tablets prescribed. Control patients are also identified at the same visit. These are matched for age and sex, with the patient receiving cimetidine and are drawn at random from the complete registration list of the co-operating practitioner.

Control individuals must have been in contact with the practice within the preceding year. This restriction is used to reduce the chances that individuals who have left the practice but failed to notify their move are followed by mistake.

Since a hundred or more practitioners may be participating in the study at any one centre, the first visit often takes place after a delay of about three months from notification. For the purposes of comparison, possible adverse effects of cimetidine are noted with effect from the date of the initial identified prescription. Control individuals are studied from the date of the initial visit of the research worker to the practitioner, so that the time period over which the findings in cimetidine takers are reviewed starts slightly earlier than, but substantially overlaps with, the time period considered in the controls. Cimetidine has now been marketed for several years so that the test cohort contains some individuals who have been previous takers of the drug. The inclusion of this group is of value because it increases the size of the group of heavier and more prolonged users, who might therefore be more prone to adverse effects of the drug.

At the initial visit a note is made of any possible adverse event already recorded in patients since the prescription of cimetidine. The main indicator of such an adverse event has been hospital referral or death, but general practitioners' records of such events are also noted if specifically recorded as causing withdrawal of cimetidine. Records of hospital referrals are scrutinised and the reasons noted. In general these can be divided into referrals directly concerned with cimetidine prescription such as diagnostic or follow-up visits because of digestive disease, and other events. For each category a division is made whether or not the condition was present before the initial prescription. The causes of any deaths are established from death certificates, and additional details sought from hospital or general practitioner case notes wherever possible.

Practitioners are visited again about 15 months after the initial visit and on this occasion details of hospital contact or death are noted for both patient and controls, and where possible details of patterns of cimetidine prescription are verified. In the controls, as in the patients, hospital referrals are divided according to whether or not the conditions present were already present at the time of the initial identification of that individual.

An initial time period of one year of follow-up has been chosen for the study both in patients and in controls. At the end of this period records are sent to a central computing facility, under code to maintain confidentiality. Death certificate, hospital discharge diagnosis and out-patient diagnosis are coded according to the I.C.D. classification (9th Revision) and the data are entered on the computer files for analysis.

FINDINGS

Patients and controls have now been identified and limited follow-up data are available on the first group of 2000 who have completed one year's surveillance.

Table 31.1 shows the mean ages of the patients and controls, and Table 31.2 shows the indications for treatment in the patients at each of the individual centres. In general patients and controls from each of the four centres have proved to be of equivalent age distribution, and the proportions diagnosed as digestive disorders have accounted for some two-thirds of the totals at each of the centres.

Table 31.1 Mean ages of patients and controls

Centre	Men		Women	
	Patients	Controls	Patients	Controls
A	51	51	56	56
B	53	53	58	58
C	46	47	52	52
D	50	50	54	54

Table 31.2 Indications for treatment (%)

	Centre			
	A	B	C	D
Gastric or duodenal ulcer	65	56	57	64
Oesophageal disease	7	15	6	2
Other	28	29	37	36

Patterns of hospital outpatient attendance are shown in Table 31.3; there have been very many more by cimetidine takers than by controls, but the difference is considerably reduced if attendances for digestive disorders are excluded from consideration.

Table 31.3 Outpatient attendance

(all patients)	Treated	Control
1	560	360
2	179	58
more than 2	78	8
Excluding digestive disease (all patients)		
1	398	344
2	79	51
more than 2	19	6

Detailed analyses of the reasons for hospital attendance are not yet available, but Tables 31.4 and 31.5 show figures for inpatients and outpatients separated into broad diagnostic categories. There has been a consistently greater tendency for cimetidine takers to attend clinics or to be admitted to hospital, and this has held true for all diagnostic categories outside digestive disorders except for neurological disorders.

The preliminary data allow a number of tentative conclusions to be drawn. The

Table 31.4 Diagnoses after hospital attendance — inpatients

	Treated	Control
Total	620	221
Digestive	256	18
Endocrine	20	7
Mental disorders	20	17
Musculo-skeletal	27	11
Respiratory	33	13
Cardiovascular	80	57
Neurological	15	11

Table 31.5 Diagnoses after hospital attendance — outpatients

	Treated	Control
Total	1725	695
Digestive	716	41
Endocrine	56	40
Mental disorders	77	32
Musculo-skeletal	167	89
Respiratory	78	53
Cardiovascular	146	105
Neurological	82	88

method of surveillance is plainly practicable, because most doctors and pharmacists agree to co-operate. We cannot be sure that all prescriptions are collected and returned, but it seems likely again that the great majority of cimetidine prescriptions are retrieved by co-operating pharmacists and by the Pricing Authority.

Comparison of the hospital outpatient and inpatient attendances of cimetidine takers and non-takers shows a generally increased frequency both for digestive and non-digestive disorders in cimetidine takers. It seems likely that this increased frequency is due in great part to a higher overall disease frequency in the cimetidine takers compared with the control group. In this context it should be noted that whereas the cimetidine takers must be current attenders of their general practitioners to obtain prescriptions, the controls are not necessarily current attenders, though they should have consulted within the previous twelve months.

The questionnaires used in the surveillance scheme will allow distinction between disorders known to have been present before cimetidine use and those which arise later. The excess of cimetidine takers over non-takers in certain specific non-digestive disease categories may reflect deliberate use of cimetidine but prescribed indirectly for associated disorders. Thus patients with musculo-skeletal disorders may receive cimetidine because of dyspepsia associated with the use of non-steroidal anti-inflammatory agents. Similarly, cimetidine may be preferred as a medical rather than a surgical treatment for an ulcer in individuals who by reason of associated cardiovascular or other disease are thought unfit for radical treatment.

CONCLUSIONS

Early findings in a postmarketing surveillance study are presented. The technique which depends upon the identification and retrieval of ordinary practice prescriptions and then comparison of outcome in treated patients and in controls is practical and seems likely to produce useful results.

ACKNOWLEDGMENTS

We are grateful to Mrs Margaret Edmond, Mr Tom Lucas, Mrs Maureen Rillie and Mrs Shirley Wood for their work in conducting the study, and to Mr John Beresford for help with the computing. Financial support from Smith Kline & French Laboratories Ltd. is gratefully acknowledged.

Discussion on Safety of Cimetidine in Treatment

Chairman: A. M. Breckenridge

Professor Breckenridge. How many of these adverse effects seen with cimetidine may be due to drug interactions? How many may be due to other drugs that the patients are taking, because of the effect that cimetidine has on the disposition of other agents? Professor Langman referred to the incidence of musculoskeletal disorders. Could that in any way be related to other drug therapy?

Professor Langman. We do not yet know the pattern of existing illness within our cimetidine takers. We will be able to sort this out because written into our protocol is a record of whether or not the diseases which turn up in the inpatients and outpatients had been previously diagnosed.

Professor Breckenridge. Is it possible that some of these cardiovascular findings may be due to other drugs that the patients are taking?

Professor Langman. Yes.

Dr Boyce. Looking back, as I did recently, at some of the individual case reports of bradycardia, there is no mention of the administration of other compounds, such as propranolol. We have to keep an open mind at this stage.

Dr Rowley-Jones. I feel that we would have become aware of the interaction with warfarin by spontaneous reporting alone. There has been no suggestion from the spontaneous reporting system, either in this country or elsewhere, over about the past four years that drug interactions are occurring with cimetidine in such frequency as to account for the adverse events that are reported to us.

Dr Spence. Dr Brimblecombe told us that with the doses of cimetidine normally used therapeutically it is very unlikely that any patients will become achlorhydric. I, and perhaps other clinicians in the audience, wonder whether the occasional patient may do so — there may perhaps be evidence to that end. Considering that the vast majority of patients treated with cimetidine do not have gastric function studies carried out, it would be reassuring to know whether in the animal studies, using very high doses as compared to the doses in humans, some of those animals are permanently achlorhydric, in spite of the fact that over the years there has been no report of the development of gastric carcinoma.

Dr Brimblecombe. Gastric acidity has not been measured in these particular animals because it would have upset the protocol of the study. However gastric function has been studied in other rats given cimetidine, about 1 g/kg/day. They were not completely achlorhydric, but were achlorhydric, at a guess, for about 22 of 24 hours. Again, these dogs have not been studied per se, but with parallel experiments using 144 mg/kg/day the animals were nearly achlorhydric for perhaps between 20 and 22 hours a day.

Professor Breckenridge. How good are the rat and the dog as models for what is being studied?

Dr Brimblecombe. Not much is known about dogs as models for carcinogens. The rat certainly responds well to nitrosamines in producing gastric carcinomas. With MNNG, the substance which has some structural resemblance to nitrosocimetidine, it is very easy to produce gastric tumours in rats. In that sense, I suppose it can be said that the rat is a good model.

Professor Breckenridge. I have never heard of dogs being used.

Dr Ruddel. I agree that the evidence for an association between cimetidine and gastric cancer is entirely anecdotal and quite unconvincing. However I do not accept the conclusions of Muscroft (*Lancet* 1981, i: 408) that bacterial overgrowth does not occur in the patient who is feeding and taking cimetidine (cf *Lancet* 1971 i: 784).

Another problem is the difficulty of interpreting the negative long-term data in Dr Brimblecombe's rats and dogs. Members and submembers of the group of carcinogens about which we are talking are both organ-specific and species-specific. In addition, one possible problem is that one of the groups of patients treated for a long time with cimetidine are those with gastric ulcer. These are a different population from those with duodenal ulcer and may possibly have an additional risk factor which differentiates them quite markedly from the animal model. This factor is their potentially unstable gastric epithelium. The rats and dogs have a normal gastric mucosa, whereas many patients who have a gastric ulcer have atrophic gastritis and intestinal metaplasia. Dr Brimblecombe will be aware that this epithelial abnormality has been suggested as being potentially premalignant, and it may therefore be particularly susceptible to carcinogens.

Dr Brimblecombe. Our experience is exactly the same as Muscroft's that bacterial colonisation does not occur very differently in control situations to cimetidine-treated situations in fed subjects. Much more work needs to be done.

In the animal models, known carcinogens, such as nitrosamine carcinogens, do produce tumours in rats. In studies with MNNG in which the gastric mucosa has been damaged, MNNG produces tumours more rapidly than if the gastric mucosa is undamaged. However, MNNG still produces tumours very rapidly even in animals with undamaged gastric mucosa. If cimetidine is a carcinogen, or is being converted into a carcinogen in these rats, it would be expected with these enormous doses over two years to produce tumours even when the gastric mucosa is undamaged. All that can be done is to relate this to experience with other compounds. It is very difficult to say whether or not the rat is the right or the wrong species.

I should add that there were no tumours anywhere else, except Leydig-cell tumours of the testes, which have been reported, and are benign.

Dr Muscroft. The problems of extrapolating from one species to another are problems throughout the whole of cancer work, and are not peculiar to cimetidine.

Dr Wormsley. It has recently been shown that cimetidine and gastric juice are mutagenic. The claim that they did not affect the Ames test must therefore be modified. We have to wait to find out whatever cimetidine does, or will turn out to do to the stomach and to other viscera, because nitrosamines will be absorbed. At present there is no evidence of its carcinogenicity.

Cimetidine is a good drug, but we have found that lymphocyte transformation is dramatically enhanced by cimetidine but not by ranitidine. Similarly, levels of luteinizing hormone and testosterone levels are altered quite markedly by cimetidine but not by ranitidine. I do not know whether these differences mean that they are not H_2 effects.

Dr Vickers. If cimetidine enhances lymphocyte proliferation, it may not be an H_2-mediated effect. We have compounds structurally similar to cimetidine which do not have H_2-antagonist activity, but do enhance lymphocyte proliferation. Other compounds structurally different from cimetidine will not enhance proliferation so that this particular effect is not H_2-receptor mediated.

Dr Crossley. Dr Wormsley's findings did not occur in our controlled studies — except for those on testosterone, which also occurred in the antacid group. It is curious, and I have no explanation for it.

Mr Elder. There are important methodological difficulties in the histological criteria for the diagnosis of early gastric cancer, both in animals and in man, and many pathologists may have to revise their diagnostic criteria. It is important that the terms 'epithelial dysplasia' and 'intra-epithelial dysplasia' should be looked at by Smith Kline and French in their rats. I understand from Dr Duncan, of ICI, that this was the crucial point upon which the fate of tiotidine depended.

The serious business, I think, of the Company and of others in the field is to measure and quantify both risk and benefit. What it comes down to is whether we can identify nitrosocimetidine in gastric juice. The answer is that we do not yet know.

Dr Brimblecombe. I take the point entirely. I was present at the FDA hearing when ICI presented their data. We have seen nothing in our rats remotely approaching what ICI observed in theirs. The critical point is whether or not nitrosocimetidine is formed, and the technological problems are horrendously difficult.

Dr Elder. Yes, I appreciate that. As a surgeon, I have no means of entering into this particular field.

Although Dr Brimblecombe stated that MNNG is much more active than nitrosocimetidine in doing whatever it does to generate alkylating species, nevertheless nitrosocimetidine was active. I suppose that someone is either pregnant or not pregnant, but not just a *little* pregnant. It is a very important distinction. Nitrosocimetidine has been shown to be active, but it is not known whether it is present.

Dr Brimblecombe. It depends on whether we agree with the threshold theory or the all-or-none theory and there is great debate about that too.

Dr Asquith. Dr Vickers mentioned that cimetidine may affect the size of the suppressor T cell pool. If it is accepted that certain autoimmune disease, in theory at least, can be dependent on the size of that pool, has anyone studied the incidence of tissue autoantibodies in people, particularly on long-term cimetidine? In theory, it could be picked up many years before any autoimmune disease might develop. A similar approach was made to practolol when tissue antibodies started to be picked up long before there was any tissue manifestation.

Dr Vickers. I do not think I said, and certainly did not mean to imply, that cimetidine could alter the size of the suppressor T cell pool. I meant to indicate that it might alter the function of that pool.

Yes, people have looked at autoantibody levels. After cimetidine had been given for a period of up to two years to immunologically-normal patients with Zollinger-Ellison syndrome, there was no alteration in autoantibody levels.

Professor Breckenridge. A large number of points have been raised in this session, some of which have been answered and others which will continue to be a matter of interest as time goes by.

Index